Current Topics in Microbiology and Immunology

224

Editors

Springer
Berlin
Heidelberg
New York
Barcelona
Budapest
Hong Kong
London
Milan
Paris
Santa Clara
Singapore
Tokyo

C-Myc in B-Cell Neoplasia

14th Workshop on Mechanisms in B-Cell Neoplasia

Edited by M. Potter and F. Melchers

With 94 Figures

Springer

MICHAEL POTTER, M.D.
Chief
Laboratory of Genetics
Building 37, Room 2B04
National Cancer Institute
National Institutes of Health
37 Convent Drive MSC4255
Bethesda, MD 20892-4255
USA

Professor Dr. FRITZ MELCHERS
Director
Basel Institute for Immunology
Grenzacherstr. 487
CH-4005 Basel
Switzerland

Cover Illustration: **DHFR gene amplification in fully developed plasmacytoma.** Arrows point to amplified *DHFR sequences as detected by FISH. Nuclei are counterstained with DAPI (4', 6'-diamidino-2-phenylindole) (from Taylor et al., this volume)*

Cover design: Design & Production GmbH, Heidelberg

ISSN 0070-217X
ISBN 3-540-62892-4 Springer-Verlag Berlin Heidelberg New York

Library of Congress Catalog Card Number 15-12910
Printed in Germany

Typesetting: Camera-ready by authors

SPIN: 10551875 27/3020 – 5 4 3 2 1 0 – Printed on acid-free paper

Preface

The papers in this book were presented at the 14th Mechanisms in B-cell Neoplasia meeting that was held in Bethesda, Maryland October 21–23, 1996. In 1995 the organizers decided that the format of the meeting would be changed and that specific topics relevant to B-cell neoplasia would be discussed. This year's topic is on the c-myc oncogene in B-cell neoplasia which has been discussed in virtually every previous meeting. Some of the presentations announced for the first time dramatic advances in our understanding of c-myc and because this subject has become highly complex it was thought that devoting the whole meeting to this theme would be appropriate. The book, therefore, represents a review of many aspects of the myc problem but by no means is truly comprehensive. In a recent Medline search there were 8,505 references to myc, fully illustrating the magnitude of the interest and depth of this field. The organizers of the meeting have each contributed review chapters that summarize different aspects of the meeting.

We thank the National Cancer Institute for sponsoring this workshop and the staff of Cygnus, Inc., for their outstanding organizational assistance. The organizers are most grateful to Vickie Rogers for assembling the book and dealing with the editorialization of the manuscripts.

MICHAEL POTTER
FRITZ MELCHERS

Table of Contents

List of Contributors

(Their addresses can be found at the beginning of their respective chapters.)

Alland, L. 159
Andersson, J. 67
Arora, T. 261
Arsura, M. 91
Austen, M. 123
Bahram, F. 191
Barlogie, B. 257
Bath, M.L. 221
Bellas, R.E. 91
Bergsagel, P.L. 277, 283
Bino, T. 149
Birshtein, B.K. 73
Brents, L. 283
Brents, L.A. 277
Calame, K. 57
Cerni, C. 123
Chen, C. 73
Chen, K. 159
Chesi, M. 277, 283
Chun, Y.S. 181
Clurman, B.E. 231
Collins, I. 33
Cory, S. 221
Cultraro, C.M. 149
Dang, C.V. 131, 181
Davis-Smyth, T. 33
Depinho, R.A. 159
Dolde, C. 181
Donjerković, D. 103
Duncan, R.C. 33
Echlin, D.R. 169
Eilers, M. 137
Eisenman, E.N. 115
Elefanty, A.G. 221
Epstein, J. 257
Ezhevsky, S. 103
Feinman, R. 257
Fitzgerald, M.J. 91
Francis, D.A. 83
Goltz, J. 159
Grdina, T. 103
Hänel, F. 137
Harris, A.W. 221
Hausner, P.F. 251
Henriksson, M. 123
Hilfenhaus, S. 123
Huppi, K. 67, 277
Hurlin, P.J. 115
Jalava, A. 201
Janz, S. 241, 251
Jelinek, D.F. 261
Jones, G.M. 251
Koury, J. 257
Kovalchuk, A.L. 241
Krylov, D. 169
Kuehl, W.M. 277, 283
Larsson, L.-G. 191
Lee, H. 91
Lee, L.A. 131
Levens, D. 33
Lewis, B.C. 181
Li, Q. 181
Lin, Y. 57
Little, R.D. 73
Lobanenkov, V.V. 231
Lüscher, B. 123, 191
Lüscher-Firzlaff, J.M. 123
Maddox, B. 103
Mai, S. 201
Marcu, K.B. 1, 47

The c-myc Story: Where we've been, Where we seem to be Going

M. Potter and K. B. Marcu[1]
National Cancer Institute, NIH, Bethesda, MD 20892, USA
[1] State University of New York at Stony Brook, Stony Brook, NY 11794, USA

History and Landmark Discoveries

The history of c-*myc* spans the panorama of discovery and technological development of our understanding of oncogenes. It begins indirectly in the early part of the century with the observations of Wilhelm Ellermann and Olaf Bang in 1908-9 who demonstrated that erythroleukemias in chickens could be transmitted with cell free filtrates. At the time there was prevailing doubt about the neoplastic nature of this leukemic process; even Ellermann and Bang thought it "represented an infection" (see [1]). The discovery was not heralded as a great conceptual breakthrough; but it nonetheless left a lasting impression. Two years later Peyton Rous, then a young investigator at the Rockefeller Institute in New York, successfully transmitted a fibrosarcoma arising in a Plymouth Rock chicken with cell free filtrates. Although there was greater acceptance of the neoplastic nature of this sarcoma, the result presented a perplexing problem because no one could explain how a tumor of the same histological type could be transmitted by a (cell free filtrate) virus. Within a year continued reports of other tumors in chickens that were transmissable by cell free extracts were described by Rous himself and Fujinami. Eventually, this enigma and the demands of WWI occasioned Rous himself to abandon this work. The first avian tumor that was found to contain what was to be later identified as v-*myc* was the Murray-Begg endothelioma known as MH-2 [2,3]. The virus ultimately isolated from this tumor contained both v-*myc* and v-*raf-1* [4]. In 1964-65 the prototypic *v-myc* producing MC29 strain was isolated in Bulgaria and was now thought to be a myelocytoma. Two additional myelocytomatosis viruses, the CMII virus in 1964 and OK10 in 1977, were isolated. The origin of these viruses was described by Thomas Graf and Hartmut Beug who grouped the four viruses, MH2, MC29, OK10 and CMII, based on their transformation of monocytes [3,5]. The MC29 virus induced a spectrum of different tumor types in chickens, including myelocytomas (from which the acronym myc was derived), endotheliomas, renal and hepatic tumors [6]. The myelocytomas appeared to develop in bone marrow cavities, and the predominant cell types were myelocytes that filled the intersinusoidal spaces in various bone marrow cavities. In vitro these viruses transformed cells of the monocyte macrophage lineage [3].

The viruses of MC29 and MH-2 were isolated by Peter Duesberg, Peter Vogt and Klaus Bister between 1977 and 1979 [5,7]. RNA fingerprints (made by using RNase T1 resistant oligonucleotides) revealed that the four transforming viruses, MH-2, MC29, OK10 and CMII, contained a common characteristic genetic element that was associated with transformation, i.e., the v-*myc* oncogene. Myc was not found in other transforming viruses, including the Rous Sarcoma Virus.

The first association of c-*myc* with B cell neoplasia came with the landmark discoveries of William Hayward, Benjamin Neel, Harriet Robinson, Joanna Fang and Susan Astrin in 1981 [8], who first found that ALV induced lymphomas in the chicken were consistently associated with retroviral insertions into the 5' end of the c-*myc* gene. Avian leukosis (lymphomas) as a disease was of great economic importance, as it was the most common neoplasm in this species and was often responsible for decimating flocks of chickens when they were still relatively young birds. These lymphomas were known to develop in the Bursa of Fabricius and were of B cell origin. This association was based upon histological evidence of preneoplastic lesions (transformed follicles) in the bursa [9] and the compelling experimental finding that lymphomagenesis in chickens was prevented by bursectomy [10]. The first paper by Hayward *et al.* was soon followed by the identification of the c-*myc* protooncogene as the consistent target of the retroviral insertion [11]. Retroviral promoter insertion became a new form of oncogenic mutagenesis and established a new direction in cancer research [12]. In the bursal lymphoma model this process had two important biological features. First, the mutations were consistent, that is, they were common to virtually all bursal lymphomas. Second, the cellular target of the insertional process was a B cell (see NEIMAN *et al.*, this book).

As crucial as this discovery was to the field of B cell neoplasia and oncogenesis, a second one in a non-virus associated mammalian system that followed within a year was equally sensational. Growing evidence indicated that the t(8;14) chromosomal translocation was a consistent translocation in both sporatic and endemic Burkitt lymphomas [13]. Then Ohno *et al.* studied a series of early transfer generation paraffin oil induced peritoneal plasmacytomas (PCTs) and found they all had either t(12;15) or t(6;15) [14]. Both of these had been previously seen in PCTs [15]. The location of the Ig heavy chain complex on chromosome (chr) 12 and the kappa light chain locus on chr 6 [16] suggested one of the partners in the translocation was an immunoglobulin (Ig) gene [14]. Several labs described rearranged Ig heavy chain switch DNA sequences that contained non-Ig DNA. These were known as NIARDs [17], LyRs [18] or NIRDs [19]. Harris *et al.* then demonstrated that the NIARD squence was on chr

15, not chr12, proving that the cloned rearranged DNA resided at the 12;15 chromosomal translocation breakpoint [20]. The identity of these non-Ig sequences was at first a mystery but then two almost simultaneous studies led to its identity. Dalla-Favera *et al.* [21] demonstrated that the human c-*myc* locus was on chr 8 at the 8;14 breakpoint. Grace Shen-Ong, Elizabeth Keath, Steven Piccoli and Michael Cole, strongly influenced by the findings of Hayward, Neel and Astrin, attacked this problem from a different direction by examining c-*myc* gene structure in plasmacytomas where they found it to be rearranged and recombined with an immunglobulin heavy chain switch region on chr 12 in the T(12;15) translocations [22]. The homologue T(8;14), which was known to be a consistent translocation in Burkitt's lymphomas [13,23], was also associated with myc/Ig recombinations [21]. Many papers bearing the 1982 date appeared almost simultaneously as a number of laboratories were actively pursuing this problem. The pace of modern biomedical science, the rapid communication both formal and informal and the number of active laboratories will make it difficult for historians to unravel the sequence of events in the 1981-2 period.

From studies on the cellular localization of v-*myc* it was a well established fact that the c-*myc* product was sequestered primarily in the nucleus. In cell transformation studies Hartmut Land, Luis Parada and Robert Weinberg had shown that oncogenes could be separated into two complementary groups, one located in the nucleus and the other in the cytoplasm [24]. The prototypic oncogene in the nuclear group was *myc* and in the cytoplasmic group was *Ha-ras*. Alone, these genes failed to transform rat embryo fibroblasts but did immortalize them.

Myc was long suspected of being a sequence specific DNA binding protein [25,26] and by structural comparison to other E box DNA binding proteins was assigned to be one of the founding members of the basic-helix-loop-helix family of dimerizing transcription factors [27]. However, the sequence specificity of Myc's DNA binding activity remained unknown until 1990 when Blackwell *et al.* identified CACGTG as the six base pair core of the Myc binding motif [28]. This was quickly followed by the ground-breaking work of Blackwood and Eisenman in 1991 [29] who demonstrated that the Myc DNA binding activity *in vivo* was a heterodimeric complex of Myc and Max, another though previously unknown basic-helix-loop-helix transcription factor. These findings established the primary generic function of c-*myc* as a transcripitional regulator.

Myc Trangenic and Knock-out Mice

c-*myc* transgenic mice were developed in 1984 using a normal mouse v-*myc* gene driven by MMTV promoters [30]. These mice developed a high incidence of mammary adenocarcinomas but also other tumors [31,32]. In 1985 a second type of transgene was constructed using c-*myc* driven by immunoglobulin enhancers thus ensuring c-*myc* would be expressed in B cells [33]. These mice developed a high incidence of early B cell lymphomas. A striking polyclonal expansion of the early B cell population was noted and many of these mice developed clonal B cell tumors. These occurred after several months and were thought to be due to additional stochastic oncogenic changes in the cells in the expanded populations.

c-*myc* plays a fundamental role in development. Mice carrying the null mutations for c-*myc* die in utero between 9.5-10.5 days [34]. The embryos are smaller, and there are organ defects. Cell lines derived from these embryos continued to proliferate *in vitro*, but the reasons why this is possible have not been elucidated. In studies of experimental cell lines that are haploid for c-*myc* it has been shown that the cells have prolonged intermitotic periods [35].

Regulation of c-*myc* Gene Transcription and Protein

c-*myc* function is regulated by at least five means based on present information: 1) transcription, 2) stability of the mRNA, 3) post-translational modifcations of the Myc proteins, 4) stability of the Myc protein, and 5) the rate of formation of the effector complexes with its partner Max. These are shown schematically in Figure 1.

Transcription

The transcriptional regulation of c-*myc* presents another complex problem in the understanding of this gene and its product. Figure 2 illustrates that up to 20 or so transcription factors have been documented to recognize control elements within the promoter regions of the murine and human c-*myc* genes. c-*myc* was the first cellular gene shown to be tightly regulated by transcriptional elongation [36-38]. This phenomenon has been extensively studied and molecularly defined to represent stalled RNA polymerase II initiation complexes which are proximally paused on the major c-*myc* P2 transcription start site [39-42]. Effective engagement of RNA polymerase complexes held back on P2 start are regulated in a positive fashion by growth factors and in a negative way by differentiation inducers (reviewed in [43]). Such a flexible mode of gene control would provide cells with a rapid means of accumulating Myc upon the initiation of cell cycle progression programs and a way to rapidly deplete Myc upon commitment to differentiation pathways [43]. Interestingly, loss of regulated polymerase pausing

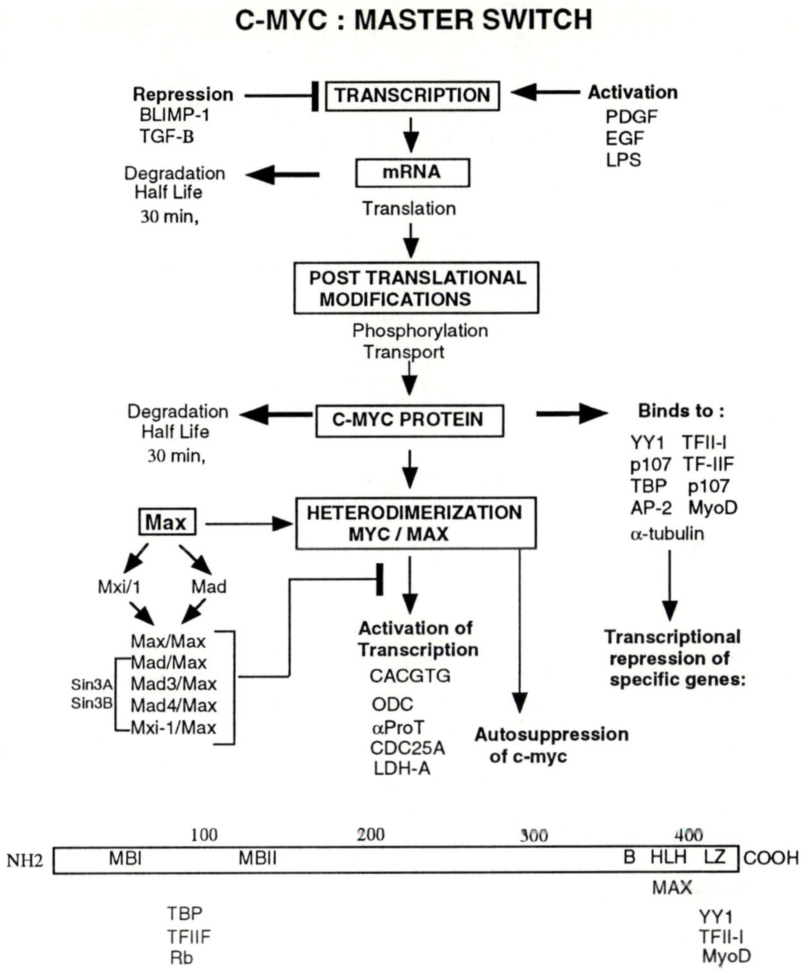

Fig. 1. Dynamics of the c-*myc* gene, mRNA, and protein and some of the known genes that are positively (activation) or negatively (suppression, repression) regulated by c-*myc*, recently reviewed in Henriksson and Luscher [44]. The Myc/Max heterodimer is required for transformation, apoptosis, and cellular proliferation. In the inset is a diagram of the c-Myc protein based on the one described by Prendergast and Ziff [45]. Specific binding sites on the c-Myc protein have been described for TBP [46,47], TFII-F [48], TFII-I [49],YY1 [50], MyoD [51], AP-2 [52], α-tubulin [53], BIN-1 (a tumor suppressor like factor [54] and MIZ-1 (see SCHNEIDER, this book). Myc also binds in vitro to the RB tumor suppressor [47] which can potentially stimulate its transactivation potential [55], while in contrast its binding to the p107 Rb-like tumor suppressor in vivo inhibited its transactivation function [56,57]. Mad3 and Mad4 [58]. Mad and Mxi interactions with Sin3A and 3B [59,60].

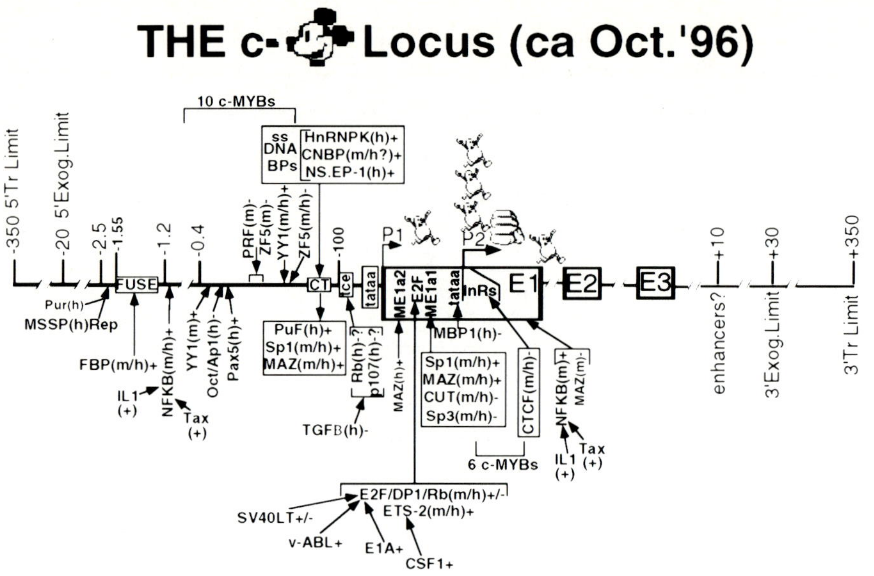

Fig. 2. Anatomy of the c-*myc* gene's environs and locations of binding sites of its putative, regulatory factors. Myc promoter paused RNA polymerase II initiation complexes are represented by a closed fist and freely engaged polymerase complexes by a jolly clown. The three Myc exons are boxed with the size of the first regulatory exon expanded to reveal the target sites of several transcription factors. The locations of binding sites of some twenty transcription factors are indicated with some of these factors themselves being encoded by proto-oncogenes or tumor suppressor genes [61-70]. Some Myc control elements have been shown to bind multiple factors which may have similar and/or opposing effects on Myc control in different cell types or physiological circumstances. Most of these factors recognize duplex DNA [61,71-78] but several uniquely bind to single stranded DNA [79-83]. Positive and negative acting factors are indicated by (+) and (-) and mouse and human by (m) and (h), respectively. The c-*myc* locus possesses no known stong transcriptional enhancers but several weak enhancer-like elements have been identified 3' of the third exon [84]. The physical limits of human c-*myc* genes transfected into tissue culture cells and the farthest known 5' and 3' translocation breakpoints are denoted by Exog. Limit [85] and Tr limit [86,87], respectively. In some instances, the response or target elements of growth factors and cytokines are also shown [63,88-90].

within the c-*myc* first exon is one of the consequences of chromosome translocations invading the c-*myc* locus (or chromatin domain). Dominant acting transcriptional enhancers and/or locus controlling regions of either the immunoglobulin heavy or light chain gene loci are likely responsible for the abrogation of the c-*myc* promoter proximal pause [85,91-93]. Furthermore, reconstructed c-*myc* genes containing all three exons and varying amounts of its 5' and 3' flanking sequences are not appropriately regulated in the tissues of transgenic mice [94] nor in cultured cells [85] implying that distant, dominant acting control elements are also likely to be important players in normal c-*myc* transcriptional control.

Myc is also subject to transcriptional autosuppression directly or indirectly *in vivo* by Myc/Max heterodimers, and this function structurally overlaps with Myc domains required in cellular transformation [95]. Myc family members reciprocally repress each other, strongly suggesting a conserved control mechanism [96]. Such a "Myc safety valve" may be critical to normal physiological growth control as many transformed cells have lost autocontrol of endogenous c-*myc* while other immortal cell lines (retaining contact inhibition of growth) maintain their Myc autoregulation loop [95,97]. Domains of human c-Myc protein required for autosuppression and cooperation with ras oncogenes are overlapping [97]. The Myc negative autoregulation mechanism requires Myc-Max association and involves the c-*myc* P2 minimal promoter [97]. Interestingly, it has long been known that the normal c-*myc* allele in plasma cell tumors and Burkitt lymphomas is transcriptionally silent, implying that the translocations activate a transcriptionally silent c-*myc* locus [43,98].

LEVENS *et al.* (this book) discuss the role of DNA conformation and topology in the regulation of c-*myc* transcription. They point out that at least 2 factors that bind to c-*myc* sequences recognize motifs in a 3 dimensional context, *i.e.*, with supercoiled DNA (hn RNP K) or single stranded DNA (FUSE binding protein). This raises intriguing questions about how the c-*myc* locus becomes accessible for transcription and possibly illegitimate recombination. Still not understood is how the *Pvt1* locus, positioned several hundred kilobases away from c-*myc*, can affect the transcription (see SIWARSKI, this book).

An important recent development has been the indentification of the Plasmacytoma Repressor Factor (PRF) as the product of the *Blimp1* gene (see ZOU *et al.*, this book). Expression of *Blimp1* is associated with terminal differentiation of B cells and repression of the *c-myc* promoter. This association may explain one facet of *Blimp1* action in terminal differentiation, mainly by shutting down c-*myc* transcription and cell cycling activity.

Stability of c-*myc* mRNA

The stability of c-*myc* mRNA has been extensively studied since Dani and colleagues originally reported myc mRNAs possess extremely short half lives [99]. Recently, in the literature Yeilding *et al.* [100] have used a PCR based strategy to compare the stability of normal c-*myc* and mutant c-*myc* genes that have been co-introduced into target cells. This obviates the use of inhibitors that potentially introduce artefacts. They have identified 2 regions in the c-*myc* gene that affect mRNA half life, one in the 3' UTR and the other in exon-3. Mutations in these regions extend the half life of the c-*myc* message from its normal limit of around 30 minutes to several hours. WILLIS *et al.* (this book) discuss a new aspect of mRNA physiology regulation at the level of the association of the c-*myc* message with polysomes.

Post Translational Modificiations of c-Myc Protein

Post translational modification of the Myc protein include phosphorylation and transport of the protein from cytoplasm to nucleus. These modifications have not figured strongly as regulatory mechanisms. However, SCHNEIDER *et al.* (this book) have identified a new gene, *Miz1* (Myc zinc finger protein), whose product complexes with Myc and whose function is not yet determined. Schneider *et al.* speculate that the interaction of Myc with Miz may stabilize and facilitate the transport of Myc protein into the nucleus.

Binding of Myc Protein to Other Proteins

There are a growing number of proteins to which Myc binds, not through its HLHLZ domains (as with Max), but through other domains, which includes TFII-I, YY1, possibly myoD, Rb, cyclin D1 and Miz1 as the major candidates. Several of these are transcriptional regulators, *i.e.*, TFII-I and YY1 (see LEE and DANG, this book). Several of the functions governed by these interactions are repressive rather than stimulatory. The molecular interactions of Myc with these elements are through other regions.

Stability of the Myc Protein

An important property of the Myc protein is its scarcity in the cell. It has been estimated a cycling fibroblast may contain only 3000 to 6000 molecules per cell [101]; further, the estimated half life of the Myc protein molecule is approximately 20 minutes. The disposition of the available molecules is then potentially critical as discussed by SCHNEIDER *et al.* The short half life of Myc protein of 20 to 30 minutes [102], coupled with the evidence that c-*myc* is expressed throughout the cell cycle, suggests that the activation of this gene must be sustained in cycling cells.

Heterodimerization with Max

The Myc/Max heterodimer plays an important role in cellular proliferation, apoptosis and transformation. The heterodimer binds to the CACGTG motif that is found now in a number of genes, including alpha prothymosin, ornithine decarboxylase, CDC25A phosphatase [103,104] and possibly LDH-A (see DANG *et al.* and personal communication). The role of Myc/Max heterodimers in transcriptional suppression is not yet clear; increasing evidence for suppression through alternate pathways involving binding to *Inr* motifs is gaining support ([105] and discussion herein by LEE). The Myc/Max heterodimer has also recently been shown to mediate autosuppression of endogenous c-*myc* genes and a minimal Myc promoter driven reporter gene [97].

Binding to Other Transcription Factors

In addition to the formation of heterodimers with Max, Myc protein interacts with a growing number of other factors implicated in transcription, e.g., TBP, TFII-F, TFII-I and YY1. Some of these interactions result in repression of transcription [49,105,106] or differentiation [51]. Myc has also been shown to repress transcription through motifs located in the 143aa amino terminal transactivating domain, specifically the two highly conserved regions myc BOX I [54] and myc BOX II [106]. Direct interaction of Myc with factors involved in transcription initiation, i.e., TBP and the RAP74 subunit of TFII-F, has also been described [48]. Many of these interactions are complex and involve participation of more than one motif on Myc. Much remains to be learned, and progress may depend upon a better understanding of the three dimensional structure of this protein and its allosteric variations.

Deregulation of c-*myc* Transcription in B Cell Neoplasms: Some Unanswered Questions

Highly consistent involvement of c-*myc* occurs in certain common models of B lineage derived tumors: bursal lymphomas by viral integration and mouse plasmacytomas, rat immunocytomas and Burkitt lymphomas by chromosomal translocations. This suggests that deregulation of c-*myc* in B cells is a pivotal and possibly the initial step in neoplastic transformation of some cells in the B lymphocyte lineage. Although there have been many studies on c-*myc* in multiple myeloma, it appears that the chromosomal translocation mechanism is only rarely found in this disease (see KUEHL *et al.*, BERGSAGEL *et al.,* WILLIS *et al.* and JELINEK *et al.*, this book, for further discussions of this interesting problem). Possibly, there is a commensurate disorder in c-*myc* expression that does not depend upon chromosomal translocation. This question is not resolved.

This raises a basic question: what constitutes deregulation? Is deregulation the loss of one or more controls over c-*myc* transcription? If so, there may be multiple kinds of deregulation that could be categorized as qualitative deregulations. Along this line it is interesting to note that there now appear to be at least two kinds of c-*myc* autosuppression (see ZOU, this book and [97]). The more familiar deregulations are extensive "take-overs" of c-*myc* transcription (as with certain chromosomal translocations or 5' retroviral insertions) that result in readily detectable quantitative increases in c-*myc* transcription. These are quantitative deregulations, including some associated with autosuppression. The apparent paucity in c-myc transcripts (3000-6000 per cell) suggests the amount of c-*myc* protein may be limited. Not all of the c-*myc* protein molecules at any given time may reach effective levels to form meaningful interactions with the many proteins (see Fig. 1) to which c-*myc* can bind. We need to establish some kind of hierarchy of the reactions based on rates of complex formation (and on binding constants?) to assess the importance of these reactions. These must be related to specific activations or repressions. We are still a long way from resolving these difficult questions, but we may be coming to the end of the concept that myc activity can be measured by just a few reactions.

In the mammalian systems chromosomal translocation is the principle mechanism for pathologically activating c-*myc*. This process is probably facilitated by immunoglobulin heavy chain switching which is associated with late B cell proliferative activity. Presumably, the Ig DNA in switch regions is nicked and spliced, making available numerous opportunities for illegitimate exchanges to nearby available open DNA sequences. c-*myc* seems to be preferentially caught up in this exchange for reasons that are not understood on a molecular basis. Is there an underlying physiological reason why the Igh and c-*myc* loci on the different chromosomes are brought into close enough proximity in the same sector of the nucleus to permit these illegitimate exchanges?

Another remarkable though poorly understood aspect of this phenomenon is that c-*myc* is universally involved in the genesis of virtually all known plasma cell tumors and Burkitt lymphomas, and despite the great redundancy built into mammalian transcriptional control networks and the existence of the highly related N-*myc* and L-*myc* genes (whose encoded proteins also heterodimerize uniquely with Max), only c-*myc* seems to do the trick. This strongly implies that inappropriate c-*myc* control may deregulate cellular physiology in a cell type specific fashion. Given that c-myc/max, L-myc/max and N-myc/max and homodimers of the very related USF basic-helix-loop-helix transcription factor all bind to the same CACGTG DNA sequence elements, these cell type specific c-*myc* functions are likely to reside in unique parts of c-*myc*'s structure, perhaps associated with its transcriptional activation domains (see review by Henriksson and Luscher [44]). Conceivably, B lymphocyte specific transcriptional co-activators or co-repressors may interface in unique ways with c-*myc*, thereby establishing regulatory pathways unique to mature B cells. Clearly, critically important questions like these still need to be addressed.

The full impact of c-*myc* deregulation is not attained at the B lymphocyte stage but does reveal itself when the B lymphocytes develop into plasma cells. As plasma cells are usually the end stage of B lymphocyte development and are associated with loss of cycling ability, the deregulated c-*myc* could facilitate sustained cycling. The detection of c-*myc*/Ig illegitimate recombinations by nested PCR amplifications (see JANZ and MULLER, this book) in the lymphoid tissues of normal mice suggests that the chromosomal translocation process can begin in B lymphocytes and supports a survival advantage hypothesis for cells carrying the translocation. More data to support this notion is needed.

We have no direct evidence that the deregulation of c-*myc* transcription *per se* drives B cells through successive cell cycles in a "Sorcerer's Apprentice"-like fashion, *i.e.*, myc is not turning on all the essential buttons to drive the cells through the cycle. This is not to say that myc is not an essential factor in cell cycling. c-*myc* appears to be much like a complex molecular switch that receives multiple inputs and channels them, either negatively or positively, to control other sets of genes. One property though that does seem to be safe to conclude is that c-*myc* does not govern a single function or even a single category of functions, e.g., solely cell cycling functions. Despite a wealth of information about c-*myc* we still do not have a clear picture about how it works *in vivo*.

Possibly, the sustained high transcription of c-*myc* operates in a different way in oncogenesis than by facilitating processes essential for proliferation. Galaktionov *et al.* [103] have evidence that c-*myc* increases the production of CDC25 phosphatases, and this could drive cells to override the G1 checkpoint. Such an action could lead to the accumulation of unwanted mutations and genomic instability. Further work is needed to evaluate this question.

References

1. Shimkin MB. (1980) Classics of experimental oncology. NIH Publication No. 80-2150. NIH Pub 80-2150:328-360
2. Begg AM. (1927) A filterable endothelioma of the fowl. Lancet :912-915
3. Graf T, Beug H. (1978) Avian leukemia viruses: interaction with their target cells in vivo and in vitro. Biochim Biophys Acta 516:269-299
4. Sutrave P, Bonner TI, Rapp UR, Jansen HW, Patschinsky T, Bister K. (1984) Nucleotide sequence of avian retroviral oncogene v-mil: homologue of murine retroviral oncogene v-raf. Nature 309:85-88

5. Bister K, Duesberg PH. (1979) Genetic structure of avian acute leukemia viruses. Cold Spring Harbor Symp Quant Biol 44:801-822
6. Mladenov Z, Heine U, Beard D, Beard JW. (1967) Strain MC29 avian leukosis virus. Myelocytoma, endothelioma, and renal growths: pathomorphological and ultrastructural aspects. J Natl Cancer Inst 38:251-285
7. Duesberg PH, Vogt PK. (1979) Avian acute leukemia viruses MC29 and MH2 share specific RNA sequences: evidence for a second class of transforming genes. Proc Natl Acad Sci U S A 76:1633-1637
8. Hayward WS, Neel BG, Astrin S. (1981) Activation of a cellular onc gene by promoter insertion in ALV-induced lymphoid leukosis. Nature 290:475-480
9. Cooper MD, Payne LN, Dent PB, Burmester BR, Good RA. (1968) Pathogenesis of avian lymphoid leukosis. I. Histogenesis. J Natl Cancer Inst 41:373-378
10. Peterson RDA, Burmester BR, Fredrickson TN, Purchase HG, Good RA. (1964) Effect of bursectomy and thymectomy on the development of visceral lymphomatosis in the chicken. J Natl Cancer Inst 32:1343-1354
11. Neel BG, Hayward WS, Robinson HL, Fang J, Astrin SM. (1981) Avian leukosis virus-induced tumors have common proviral integration sites and synthesize discrete new RNAs: oncogensis by promoter insertion. Cell 23:323-334
12. Payne GS, Bishop JM, Varmus HE. (1981) Multiple arrangements of viral DNA and an activated host oncogene (c-myc) in bursal lymphomas. Nature 295:209-214
13. Zech L, Haglund U, Nilsson K, Klein G. (1976) Characteristic chromosomal abnormalities in biopsies and lymphoid cell lines from patients with Burkitt and non-Burkitt lymphomas. Int.J.Cancer 17:47-56
14. Ohno S, Babonits M, Wiener F, Spira J, Klein G, Potter M. (1979) Nonrandom chromosome changes involving the Ig gene-carrying chromosomes 12 and 6 in pristane-induced mouse plasmacytomas. Cell 18:1001-1007
15. Yosida MC, Moriwaki K. (1975) Specific marker chromosomes involving a translocation (12;15) in a mouse myeloma. Proc Jpn Acad 51:588
16. Hengartner H, Meo T, Muller E. (1978) Assignment of genes for immunoglobulin kappa and heavy chains to chromosomes 6 and 12 in mouse. Proc Natl Acad Sci U S A 75:4494-4498
17. Harris LJ, Lang RB, Marcu KB. (1982) Non-immunoglobulin-associated DNA rearrangements in mouse plasmacytomas. Proc Natl Acad Sci U S A 79:4175-4179
18. Adams JM, Gerondakis S, Webb E, Mitchell J, Bernard O, Cory S. (1982) Transcriptionally active DNA region that rearranges frequently in murine lymphoid tumors. Proc Natl Acad Sci U S A 79:6966-6970
19. Calame K, Kim S, Lalley P, Hill R, Davis M, Hood L. (1982) Molecular cloning of translocations involving chromosome 15 and the immunobuliin C-alpha gene from chromosome 12 in two murine plasmacytomas. Proc Natl Acad Sci U S A 79:6994-6998
20. Harris LJ, D'Eustachio P, Ruddle FH, Marcu KB. (1982) DNA sequence associated with chromosome translocations in mouse plasmacytomas. Proc Natl Acad Sci USA 79:6622-6626
21. Dalla-Favera R, Bregni M, Erikson J, Patterson D, Gallo RC, Croce CM. (1982) Human c-myc oncogene is located on the region of chromosome 8 that is translocated in Burkitt lymphoma cells. Proc Natl Acad Sci USA 79:7824-7827
22. Shen-Ong GL, Keath EJ, Piccoli SP, Cole MD. (1982) Novel myc oncogene RNA from abortive immunoglobulin-gene recombination in mouse plasmacytomas. Cell 31:443-452
23. Lenoir GM, Taub R. (1987) Chromosomal translocations and oncogenes in Burkitt's lymphoma. In: Golman JM, Harnden DH (eds) Genetic rearrangements in leukaemia and lymphoma. Churchill-Livingstone, New York, pp 152-172
24. Land H, Parada LF, Weinberg RA. (1983) Tumorigenic conversion of primary embryo fibroblasts requires at least two cooperating oncogenes. Nature 304:596-602
25. Donner P, Greiser-Wilke X, Moelling K. (1982) Nuclear localization and DNA binding of the transforming gene product of avian myelocytomatosis virus. Nature 296:262-265

26. Persson H, Leder P. (1984) Nuclear localization and DNA binding properties expressed by the human c-myc oncogene. Science 225:718-721
27. Murre C, McCaw PS, Baltimore D. (1989) A new DNA binding and dimerization motif in immunoglobulin enhancer binding, daughterless, MyoD, and myc proteins. Cell 56:777-783
28. Blackwell TK, Kretzner L, Blackwood EM, Eisenman RN, Weintraub H. (1990) Sequence-specific DNA binding by the c-Myc protein. Science 250:1149-1151
29. Blackwood EM, Eisenman RN. (1991) Max: a helix-loop-helix zipper protein that forms a sequence-specific DNA-binding complex with Myc. Science 251:1211-1217
30. Stewart TA, Pattengale PK, Leder P. (1984) Spontaneous mammary adenocarcinomas in transgenic mice that carry and express MTV/myc fusion genes. Cell 38:627-637
31. Pattengale P, Leder A, Kuo A, Stewart T, Leder P. (1986) Lymphohematopoietic and other malignant neoplasms occurring spontaneously in transgenic mice carrying and expressing MTV/myc fusion genes. Curr Top Microbiol Immunol 132:9-16
32. Leder A, Pattengale PK, Kuo A, Stewart TA, Leder P. (1986) Consequences of widespread deregulation of the c-myc gene in transgenic mice: multiple neoplasms and normal development. Cell 45:485-495
33. Adams JM, Harris AW, Pinkert CA, Corcoran LM, Alexander WS, Cory S, Palmiter RD, Brinster RL. (1985) The c-myc oncogene driven by immunoglobulin enhancers induces lymphoid malignancy in transgenic mice. Nature 318:533-538
34. Davis AC, Wims M, Spotts GD, Hann SR, Bradley A. (1993) A null c-myc mutation causes lethality before 10.5 days of gestation in homozygotes and reduced fertility in heterozygous female mice. Genes Devel. 7:671-682
35. Shichiri M, Hanson KD, Sedivy JM. (1993) Effects of c-myc expression on proliferation, quiescence, and the G0 to G1 transition in nontransformed cells. Cell Growth Differen 4:93-104
36. Bentley DL, Groudine M. (1986) A block to elongation is largely responsible for decreased transcription of c-myc in differentiated HL60 cells. Nature 321:702-706
37. Eick D, Bornkamm GW. (1986) Transcriptional arrest within the first exon is a fast control mechanism in c-myc gene expression. Nucleic Acids Res 14:8331-8346
38. Nepveu A, Marcu KB. (1986) Intragenic pausing and anti-sense transcription within the murine c-myc locus. EMBO J. 5:2859-2865
39. Strobl LJ, Eick D. (1992) Hold back of RNA polymerase II at the transcription start site mediates down-regulation of c-myc in vivo. EMBO J. 11:3307-3314
40. Krumm A, Meulia T, Brunvand M, Groudine M. (1992) The block to transcriptional elongation within the human c-myc gene is determined in the promoter-proximal region. Genes Dev 6:2201-2213
41. Krumm A, Hickey LB, Groudine M. (1995) Promoter-proximal pausing of RNA polymerase II defines a general rate-limiting step after transcription initiation. Genes Dev 9:559-572
42. Wolf DA, Strobl LJ, Pullner A, Eick D. (1995) Variable pause positions of RNA polymerase II lie proximal to the c-myc promoter irrespective of transcriptional activity. Nucleic Acids Res 23:3373-3379
43. Marcu KB, Bossone SA, Patel AJ. (1992) myc function and regulation. Annu Rev Biochem 61:809-860
44. Henriksson M, Luscher B. (1996) Proteins of the Myc network: essential regulators of cell growth and differentiation. Adv Cancer Res 68:109-182
45. Pendergast GC, Ziff EB. (1992) A new bind for Myc. Trends Genet. 8:91-96
46. Matheswaran S, Lee H, Sonenshein GE. (1994) Intracellular association of the protein product of the c-myc oncogene with the TATA-binding protein. Mol.Cell.Biol. 14:1147-1152
47. Hateboer G, Timmers HTM, Rustgi AK, Billaud M, van 't Veer LJ, Bernards R. (1993) TATA-binding protein and the retinoblastoma gene product bind to overlapping epitopes on c-Myc and adenovirus E1A protein. Proc Natl Acad Sci USA 90:8489-8493

48. McEwan IJ, Dahlman-Wright K, Ford J, Wright APH. (1996) Functional interaction of the c-Myc transactivation domain with the TATA binding protein: evidence for an induced fit model of transactivation domain folding. Biochemistry 35:9584-9593
49. Roy AL, Carruthers C, Gutjahr T, Roeder RG. (1993) Direct role for Myc in transcription initiation mediated by interactions with TFII-I. Nature 365:359-361
50. Shrivastava A, Saleque S, Kalpana GV, Artandi S, Goff SP, Calame K. (1993) Inhibition of transcriptional regulator Yin-Yang-1 by association with c-Myc. Science 262:1889-1892
51. La Rocca SA, Crouch DH, Gillespie DA. (1994) c-Myc inhibits myogenic differentiation and myoD expression by a mechanism which can be dissociated from cell transformation. Oncogene 9:3499-3508
52. Gaubatz S, Imhof A, Dosch R, Werner O, Mitchell P, Buettner R, Eilers M. (1995) Transcriptional activation by Myc is under negative control by the transcription factor AP-2. EMBO J. 14:1508-1519
53. Alexandrova N, Niklinski J, Bliskovsky V, Otterson GA, Blake M, Kaye FJ, Zajac-Kaye M. (1995) The N-terminal domain of c-Myc associates with alpha-tubulin and microtubules in vivo and in vitro. Mol.Cell.Biol. 15:5188-5195
54. Sakamuro D, Elliott KJ, Wechsler-Reya R, Prendergast GC. (1996) BIN1 is a novel MYC-interacting protein with features of a tumour suppressor. Nature Genet 14:69-77
55. Adnane J, Robbins PD. (1995) The retinoblastoma susceptibility gene product regulates Myc-mediated transcription. Oncogene 10:381-387
56. Beijersbergen RL, Hijmans EM, Zhu L, Bernards R. (1994) Interaction of c-Myc with the pRb-related protein p107 results in inhibition of c-Myc-mediated transactivation. EMBO J. 13:4080-4086
57. Gu W, Bhatia K, Magrath IT, Dang CV, Dalla-Favera R. (1994) Binding and suppression of the Myc transcriptional activation domain by p107. Science 264:251-254
58. Hurlin PJ, Queva C, Koskinen PJ, Steingrimsson E, Ayer DE, Copeland NG, Jenkins NA, Eisenman RN. (1995) Mad3 and Mad4: novel Max-interacting transcriptional repressors that suppress c-myc dependent transformation and are expressed during neural and epidermal differentiation. EMBO J. 14:5646-5659
59. Ayer DE, Lawrence QA, Eisenman RN. (1995) Mad-Max transcriptional repression is mediated by ternary complex formation with mammalian homologs of yeast repressor Sin3. Cell 80:767-776
60. Schreiber-Agus N, Chin L, Chen K, Torres R, Rao G, Guida P, Skoulchi AI, DePinho RA. (1995) An amino-terminal domain of Mxi1 mediates anti-Myc oncogenic activity and interacts with a homolog of the yeast transcriptional repressor SIN3. Cell 80:777-786
61. Hay N, Takimoto M, Bishop JM. (1989) A FOS protein is present in a complex that binds a negative regulator of MYC. Genes Dev 3:293-303
62. Takimoto M, Quinn JP, Farina AR, Staudt LM, Levens D. (1989) fos/jun and octamer-binding protein interact with a common site in a negative element of the human c-myc gene. J Biol Chem 264:8992-8999
63. Kessler DJ, Duyao MP, Spicer DB, Sonenshein GE. (1992) NF-kappa B-like factors mediate interleukin 1 induction of c-myc gene transcription in fibroblasts. J Exp Med 176:787-792
64. Hamel PA, Gill RM, Phillips RA, Gallie BL. (1992) Transcriptional repression of the E2-containing promoters EIIaE, c-myc, and RB1 by the product of the RB1 gene. Mol Cell Biol 12:3431-3438
65. Cogswell JP, Cogswell PC, Kuehl WM, Cuddihy AM, Bender TM, Engelke U, Marcu KB, Ting JP. (1993) Mechanism of c-myc regulation by c-Myb in different cell lineages. Mol Cell Biol 13:2858-2869
66. Oswald F, Lovec H, Moroy T, Lipp M. (1994) E2F-dependent regulation of human MYC: trans-activation by cyclins D1 and A overrides tumour suppressor protein functions. Oncogene 9:2029-2036

67. Wolf DA, Hermeking H, Albert T, Herzinger T, Kind P, Eick D. (1995) A complex between E2F and the pRb-related protein p130 is specifically targeted by the simian virus 40 large T antigen during cell transformation. Oncogene 10:2067-2078

68. Wong KK, Zou X, Merrell KT, Patel AJ, Marcu KB, Chellappan S, Calame K. (1995) v-Abl activates c-myc transcription through the E2F site. Mol Cell Biol 15:6535-6544

69. Lee H, Arsura M, Wu M, Duyao M, Buckler AJ, Sonenshein GE. (1995) Role of Rel-related factors in control of c-myc gene transcription in receptor-mediated apoptosis of the murine B cell WEHI 231 line. J Exp Med 181:1169-1177

70. Herzinger T, Wolf DA, Eick D, Kind P. (1995) The pRb-related protein p130 is a possible effector of transforming growth factor beta 1 induced cell cycle arrest in keratinocytes. Oncogene 10:2079-2084

71. Hiebert SW, Lipp M, Nevins JR. (1989) E1A-dependent trans-activation of the human MYC promoter is mediated by the E2F factor. Proc Natl Acad Sci U S A 86:3594-3598

72. Bossone SA, Asselin C, Patel AJ, Marcu KB. (1992) MAZ, a zinc finger protein, binds to c-MYC and C2 gene sequences regulating transcriptional initiation and termination. Proc Natl Acad Sci U S A 89:7452-7456

73. DesJardins E, Hay N. (1993) Repeated CT elements bound by zinc finger proteins control the absolute and relative activities of the two principal human c-myc promoters. Mol Cell Biol 13:5710-5724

74. Riggs KJ, Saleque S, Wong KK, Merrell KT, Lee JS, Shi Y, Calame K. (1993) Yin-yang 1 activates the c-myc promoter. Mol Cell Biol 13:7487-7495

75. Numoto M, Niwa O, Kaplan J, Wong KK, Merrell K, Kamiya K, Yanagihara K, Calame K. (1993) Transcriptional repressor ZF5 identifies a new conserved domain in zinc finger proteins. Nucleic Acids Res 21:3767-3775

76. Roussel MF, Davis JN, Cleveland JL, Ghysdael J, Hiebert SW. (1994) Dual control of myc expression through a single DNA binding site targeted by ets family proteins and E2F-1. Oncogene 9:405-415

77. Dufort D, Nepveu A. (1994) The human cut homeodomain protein represses transcription from the c-myc promoter. Mol Cell Biol 14:4251-4257

78. Berberich SJ, Postel EH. (1995) PuF/NM23-H2/NDPK-B transactivates a human c-myc promoter-CAT gene via a functional nuclease hypersensitive element. Oncogene 10:2343-2347

79. Duncan R, Bazar L, Michelotti G, Tomonaga T, Krutzsch H, Avigan M, Levens D. (1994) A sequence-specific, single-strand binding protein activates the far upstream element of c-myc and defines a new DNA-binding motif. Genes Dev 8:465-480

80. Negishi Y, Nishita Y, Saegusa Y, Kakizaki I, Galli I, Kihara F, Tamai K, Miyajima N, Iguchi-Ariga SM, Ariga H. (1994) Identification and cDNA cloning of single-stranded DNA binding proteins that interact with the region upstream of the human c-myc gene. Oncogene 9:1133-1143

81. Michelotti EF, Tomonaga T, Krutzsch H, Levens D. (1995) Cellular nucleic acid binding protein regulates the CT element of the human c-myc protooncogene. J Biol Chem 270:9494-9499

82. Michelotti GA, Michelotti EF, Pullner A, Duncan RC, Eick D, Levens D. (1996) Multiple single-stranded cis elements are associated with activated chromatin of the human c-myc gene in vivo. Mol Cell Biol 16:2656-2669

83. Filippova GN, Fagerlie S, Klenova EM, Myers C, Dehner Y, Goodwin G, Neiman PE, Collins SJ, Lobanenkov VV. (1996) An exceptionally conserved transcriptional repressor, CTCF, employs different combinations of zinc fingers to bind diverged promoter sequences of avian and mammalian c-myc oncogenes. Mol Cell Biol 16:2802-2813

84. Mautner J, Joos S, Werner T, Eick D, Bornkamm GW, Polack A. (1995) Identification of two enhancer elements downstream of the human c-myc gene. Nucleic Acids Res 23:72-80

85. Mautner J, Behrends U, Hortnagel K, Brielmeier M, Hammerschmidt W, Strobl L, Bornkamm GW, Polack A. (1996) c-myc expression is activated by the immunoglobulin

kappa-enhancers from a distance of at least 30 kb but not by elements located within 50 kb of the unaltered c-myc locus in vivo. Oncogene 12:1299-1307

86. Joos S, Haluska FG, Falk MH, Henglein B, Hameister H, Croce CM, Bornkamm GW. (1992) Mapping chromosomal breakpoints of Burkitt's t(8;14) translocations far upstream of c-myc. Cancer Res 52:6547-6552

87. Zeidler R, Joos S, Delecluse HJ, Klobeck G, Vuillaume M, Lenoir GM, Bornkamm GW, Lipp M. (1994) Breakpoints of Burkitt's lymphoma t(8;22) translocations map within a distance of 300 kb downstream of MYC. Genes Chromosomes Cancer 9:282-287

88. Pietenpol JA, Stein RW, Moran E, Yaciuk P, Schlegel R, Lyons RM, Pittelkow MR, Munger K, Howley PM, Moses HL. (1990) TGF-beta 1 inhibition of c-myc transcription and growth in keratinocytes is abrogated by viral transforming proteins with pRB binding domains. Cell 61:777-785

89. Roussel MF, Cleveland JL, Shurtleff SA, Sherr CJ. (1991) Myc rescue of a mutant CSF-1 receptor impaired in mitogenic signalling. Nature 353:361-363

90. Duyao MP, Kessler DJ, Spicer DB, Bartholomew C, Cleveland JL, Siekevitz M, Sonenshein GE. (1992) Transactivation of the c-myc promoter by human T cell leukemia virus type 1 tax is mediated by NF kappa B. J Biol Chem 267:16288-16291

91. Strobl LJ, Kohlhuber F, Mautner J, Polack A, Eick D. (1993) Absence of a paused transcription complex from the c-myc P2 promoter of the translocation chromosome in Burkitt's lymphoma cells: implication for the c-myc P1/P2 promoter shift. Oncogene 8:1437-1447

92. Madisen L, Groudine M. (1994) Identification of a locus control region in the immunoglobulin heavy-chain locus that deregulates c-myc expression in plasmacytoma and Burkitt's lymphoma cells. Genes Dev 8:2212-2226

93. Hortnagel K, Mautner J, Strobl LJ, Wolf DA, Christoph B, Geltinger C, Polack A. (1995) The role of immunoglobulin kappa elements in c-myc activation. Oncogene 10:1393-1401

94. Lavenu A, Pournin S, Babinet C, Morello D. (1994) The cis-acting elements known to regulate c-myc expression ex vivo are not sufficient for correct transcription in vivo. Oncogene 9:527-536

95. Penn LJZ, Brooks MW, Laufer EM, Littlewood TD, Morgenstem JP, Evan GI, Lee WMF, Land H. (1990) Domains of human c-myc protein required for autosuppression and cooperation with ras oncogenes are overlapping. Mol.Cell.Biol. 10:961-966

96. DePinho RA, Schreiber-Agus N, Alt FW. (1991) myc family oncogenes in the development of normal and neoplastic cells. Adv Cancer Res 57:1-46

97. Facchini LM, Chen S, Marhin WW, Lear JN, Penn LZ. (1997) The Myc negative autoregulation mechanism requires Myc-Max association and involves the c-myc P2 minimal promoter. Mol.Cell.Biol. 17:100-114

98. Spencer CA, Groudine M. (1991) Control of c-myc regulation in normal and neoplastic cells. Adv Cancer Res 56:1-48

99. Dani C, Blanchard JM, Piechaczyk M, El Sabouty S, Marty L, Jeanteur P. (1984) Extreme instability of myc mRNA in normal and transformed human cells. Proc Natl Acad Sci U S A 81:7046-7050

100. Yeilding NM, Rehman MT, Lee WMF. (1996) Identification of sequences in c-myc mRNA that regulate its steady-state levels. Mol.Cell.Biol. 16:3511-3522

101. Waters CM, Littlewood TD, Hancock DC, Moore JP, Evan GI. (1991) c-myc protein expression in untransformed fibroblasts. Oncogene 6:797-805

102. Hann SR, Eisenman RN. (1984) Proteins encoded by the human c-myc oncogene: differential expression in neoplastic cells. Mol Cell Biol 4:2486-2497

103. Galaktionov K, Chen X, Beach D. (1996) Cdc25 cell-cycle phosphatase as a target of c-myc. Nature 382:511-517

104. Galaktionov K, Lee AK, Eckstein J, Draetta G, Meckler J, Loda M, Beach D. (1995) CDC25 phosphatases as potential human oncogenes. Science 269:1575-1577

105. Lee LA, Dolde C, Barrett J, Wu CS, Dang CV. (1996) A link between c-Myc-mediated transcriptional repression and neoplastic transformation. J.Clin.Invest. 97:1687-1695

106. Li LH, Nerlov C, Prendergast G, MacGregor D, Ziff EB. (1994) c-Myc represses transcription in vivo by a novel mechanism dependent on the initiator element and Myc box II. EMBO J. 13:4070-4079

B-lymphocyte-lineage Cells from Early Precursors to Ig-secreting Plasma Cells: Targets of Regulation by the myc/mad/max Families of Genes?

F. Melchers
Basel Institute for Immunology, Grenzacherstraße 487, CH-4005 Basel, Switzerland

Up- and down-regulation of the expression of c-myc, together or against its partners of the myc/mad/max gene families and the more recently discovered miz-1 (see papers in this volume, in particular Austen et al., Schneider et al., Schreiber-Agus et al.), is thought to control expression of genes involved in the proliferation and differentiation of cells. Very few lineages of cellular development have been studied *in vivo* and *in vitro* in comparable detail as B-lineage cells have at many different stages from an early precursor cell to the final stage of an Ig-secreting plasma cell (see [Chen and Alt 1993, Cumano et al 1992, Cumano et al 1994, Decker et al 1991, Era et al 1994, Hardy 1992, Hardy et al 1994, Hayashi et al 1990, Kincade et al 1994, Löffert et al 1994, Nossal 1994, Osmond 1991, Rajewsky 1992, Rolink et al 1994a] for a collection of relevant references). Deregulation of c-myc expression occurs as a consequence of chromosomal translocations to the IgH- and L-chain J segments which are frequently found in human Burkitt's lymphomas, or to the IgH switch regions which are detected in mineral oil-induced mouse plasmacytomas [Potter and Wiener 1992, Shen-Ong et al 1982]. This signifies the importance of the control of expression of the myc/mad/max-gene families in normal and neoplastic B-lymphocyte development. It is surprising how incomplete our knowledge is of the patterns of qualitative and quantitative expression of the myc/mad/max gene family members on mRNA as well as on protein level, as protein complexes either in the cytoplasm or in the nucleus, during B lymphocyte development and differentiation. This paper summarizes this development and, furthermore, defines the points in this development where the balance between proliferation, differentiation and apoptosis of B-lineage cells can be influenced by *in vitro* experimentation. It hopes to inspire a sophisticated analysis of myc/max/mad and miz and their family members in B cell development and differentiation.

Development from Early Precursors to Mature B Cells without Proliferation and without the Expression of Ig

Normal B lymphocyte development requires proliferation and differentiation of cells to fill the compartments of the primary and secondary lymphoid organs.

Also, the system selects for antigen-receptor-expressing cells, so that all other, receptor-negative cells which arise from non-productive V(D)J rearrangements during development in the primary organs do not appear in the secondary, peripheral sites of the system. However, B-lymphocyte cellular development can, nevertheless, be observed in cases where no functional Ig-molecules can be made, due to either naturally occurring or experimentally induced genetic defects with functions in the B-lineage. These developmental steps are difficult, if not impossible to observe in the deficient animals *in vivo* since the cells with differentiated properties but without Ig expression die rapidly. They can, however, be monitored *in vitro*. Expression of a transgenic form of bcl-2 under the control of the $E_{\mu H}$-enhancer greatly helps so that these Ig-negative forms of B-lineage cells survive without interfering with programs of (proliferation and) differentiation [Grawunder et al 1993].

First, precursor B cells (pre B-I) cells of H-chain-gene-deficient mice, or with H chain deficiencies can be induced *in vitro* to sterile κ transcription, followed by $V_{\kappa}J_{\kappa}$-rearrangement and κL chain expression by removing them in tissue culture from the stimulatory influence of interleukin-7 (IL-7) [Grawunder, et al. 1993].

Second, further differentiation of *ex vivo*-isolated or *in vitro*-proliferating B-lineage precursors leading to the expression of a mature B cell marker (CD23) and the induction of (sterile) transcription of the εH-chain gene locus can be achieved by the co-operative activating action of CD40-specific mAb and IL-4, without the necessity for expression of Ig and the RAG2 gene product. Furthermore, it is also independent of the SCID mutation [Rolink et al 1996b].

This *in vitro* differentiation occurs without proliferation. Nevertheless, Sμ-Sε-switch recombination can be induced, and seen *in vitro* in H chain gene loci that are in VDJ non-rearranged, germline configuration. This means that Sμ-Sε-switch recombination does not require the RAG-2 gene product. On the other hand, efficient Sμ-Sε-switch recombination does not occur in SCID B-lineage cells, hence requires the DNA-dependent protein kinase that is associated with the murine SCID defect.

Normal B Cell Development from Precursors to Mature Cells *in vivo*

B cells are generated in waves. In the mouse, a first wave in embryonic blood and the placenta is succeeded by a second wave in fetal liver [Melchers 1979, Rolink et al 1993b]. Throughout life, cells continue to be generated in bone marrow at a rate of 5 x 10^7 cells per day in the mouse (approximately 10^3-fold more in man), of which 2-5% become mature, surface-Ig (sIg)-positive cells of the periphery. Most newly generated B cells, therefore, die at the site where they have been generated. Some cells might die by apoptosis, but other mechanisms of cell destruction (such as phagocytosis) must be envisaged, since bcl-2-transgenic mice have normal, and not ever increasing levels of B cells in primary and secondary lymphoid organs [Strasser et al 1991].

From pluripotent stem cells which are the ancestors of the different lineages of blood cells, progenitors develop that are committed to the B lineage. A collection of intracellular and surface-bound marker molecules has allowed the separation of subpopulations of B-lineage cells from fetal liver and bone marrow, and single-cell PCR analyses of the status of the Ig gene loci have been useful to order these cell populations on their way from a pluripotent stem cell to mature, antigen-reactive B cells [Ehlich et al 1994, Rolink et al 1994b, ten Boekel et al 1995]. Many early cells of B lymphocyte development find themselves, and function, in close contact with an environment of stromal cells which provides specific contacts and cytokines that regulate the proliferation and differentiation of B lineage cells [Era, et al. 1994, Kincade, et al. 1994]. IL-3 and IL-7 have been identified as such cytokines in the mouse, and c-kit and flk-2 are membrane-bound tyrosine kinases on B lineage precursors which interact with their corresponding membrane-bound ligands on stromal cells [Era, et al. 1994, Ogawa et al 1991, Rolink et al 1991a, Rolink et al 1991b, Winkler et al 1994].

The earliest signs of a cell to be committed to the B lineage of development is the transcription of the non-rearranged, germline μ heavy (H) chain gene locus, the transcription of the V_{preB} and λ_5 genes encoding the surrogate light (SL) chain [Melchers et al 1993] and the activation of the machinery involved in rearrangements of segments of the Ig gene loci, i.e. the activation of terminal desoxyribonucleotidyl transferase (TdT) and the rearrangement-active genes RAG1 and RAG2 [Mombaerts et al 1992, Oettinger et al 1990, Schatz et al 1989, Shinkai et al 1992]. This occurs in cells which express B220 (CD45R), but do not yet express CD19 the two markers most commonly used in the characterization of B-lineage [Hardy, et al. 1994, Rolink et al 1996a]. The first Ig gene rearrangements, D_H segments to J_H segments, are already detectable in these cells. TdT is responsible for N sequence insertions at the joints of the rearrangements. TdT is active in the bone marrow but not in the fetal liver. Therefore, antibodies derived from bone marrow-generated B cells are N region diverse (in their H chains) those derived from the fetal liver are not. Single cell PCR analyses of the conformation of the Ig gene loci in the different B-lineage precursors in mouse and human bone marrow has allowed to order these cells in their maturity of differentiation (Ehlich et al 1994, Ghia et al 1996, ten Boekel et al 1995).

This ordered rearrangement process continues in the next distinguishable B lineage cell population, which is B220 $(CD45)^+$, $CD19^+$, that also expresses c-kit and SL chain on the surface, and now has practically all H chain alleles D_HJ_H rearranged [Melchers 1995]

The next rearrangement in line is V_H to D_HJ_H on one of the two H chain alleles. Whenever this rearrangement occurs in-frame, a μH chain can be made. The μH chain combines with the SL chain and thus forms a pre B receptor. This development has several consequences which lead to a new cell population *in vivo*. In the proper environment of bone marrow or other B-lineage generating organs pre B-receptor-expressing cells are induced into cycle, hence these so called pre B-II cells are large. Since non-productively rearranged cells cannot form a pre B receptor, they do not expand by proliferation. Thus, productively rearranged, μH chain-expressing, pre B-receptor-positive cells outgrow this compartment, i.e. are positively selected. They no longer express c-kit and have completely down-regulated the rearrangement machinery, i.e. TdT, RAG1 and RAG2. As a new surface marker, they now express CD25 (TAC), the α-chain of the IL-2 receptor [Grawunder et al 1995]. Down-regulation of the rearrangement machinery is likely to be part of the mechanisms by which the second H chain allele is inhibited from a second, potentially productive V_H to D_HJ_H-rearrangement. Hence, it secures allelic exclusion, so that one B cell makes only one H chain.

Once a VDJ-rearranged H chain locus has been generated, the V_H expression in this locus might still be altered by gene replacements or gene conversions [Kleinfeld et al 1986, Reth et al 1986]. These secondary changes in V_H-expression, also termed V_H editing, are likely to occur at the stage of transition of a pre B-I to a pre B-II cell, after a first VDJ-rearrangement, and before the rearrangement machinery has been turned off. Large pre B-II cells proliferate *in vivo* for an estimated three to five cell cycles, lose pre B receptor expression, begin to re-express RAG1 and RAG2, and begin to transcribe the non-rearranged L chain gene loci κ and λ. While doing so, they fall into a resting state, become small, and are thus called small pre B–II cells. The rearrangement–active genes RAG1 and 2, but not TdT, are active; all cells now contain V_L-J_L-rearranged L chain gene loci, but no N-region insertions can be made. Half of them are productively rearranged and express the L chains in their cytoplasm, but not (yet) on their surface. The other half contain non-rearranged, or out-of-frame-rearranged L chain loci. Since the pre B-II cells have an active rearrangement machinery, they can engage in secondary V_L to J_L rearrangements, which in some cells might change non-productive to productive L chain gene loci, and which in other cells might change a productive L chain locus encoding an autoantigen-reactive Ig receptor (termed receptor L chain editing). Secondary L chain gene rearrangements might allow a B cell to express two L chains, whenever the rearrangement process allows both L chain alleles to be used. It has been seen that no more than 1-3% of all peripheral mature B cells express two L chains. Since less than 1% of all B cells have been seen to express two H chains, it remains true that for most B cells the rule that one B cell makes one antibody is valid. This is the basis for clonal selection in the immune system in which a given antigen selects from all the lymphocytes those which have a fitting receptor on their surface.

The up- and down-regulation of the activities of RAG1 and RAG2, and the opening and closing of the IgH, then IgL-loci, are events during early B cell development which are likely to make translocations of c-myc into the J-segment regions of the Ig loci more or less probable.

The rearrangement machinery continues to be active in the next cell population in-line, the immature, surface-IgM (sIgM)-expressing B cells [Ghia et al 1995, Rolink et al 1993a]. This, most likely, is useful in editing autoreactive B cells, and might even be induced by this autoreactivity [Nemazee et al 1991].

Development of Precursors to Immature B Cells *in vitro*

D_H-J_H-rearranged pre B-I cells can be induced *in vitro* to differentiate to $sIgM^+$ and $sIgM^-$ immature B cells when IL-7 is omitted from the tissue cultures of the cells grown previously on stromal cells in the presence of IL-7 [Rolink, et al. 1991a]. This differentiation occurs without proliferation, and is as effective with normal as with λ_5T pre B cells. This suggests that the pre B receptor does not control Ig L chain gene rearrangements, but promotes pre B cell proliferation *in vivo*, but not *in vitro*. The ratio of the numbers of $sIgM^+/sIgM^-$ cells developing in these differentiating culture indicate that Ig gene rearrangements occur randomly in- and out-of-frame.

Negative and Positive Selection

In vivo, in the proper environment of the primary lymphoid organ (i.e. bone marrow), the expression of an autoreactive Ig-receptor on immature B cells leads to the arrest of differentiation of this cell [Chen et al 1995b, Chen et al 1995a, Goodnow et al 1995, Nemazee, et al. 1991, Prak and Weigert 1995]. Since the autoreactive cells remain short-lived, they will die at this site of development in the primary lymphoid organ unless they can change their receptor specificity through secondary L-chain rearrangements [Young et al 1994]. In this way of arrest of differentiation, the emerging B cell repertoire is purged of all B cells which are autoreactive to antigens present and presented in the bone marrow. A classical case for such an autoantigen is double-stranded DNA, present in large quantities due to extensive cell death at this site of development [Andersson et al 1995, Chen, et al. 1995a].

Of the sIgM-expressing immature B cells which do not recognize an auto-antigen at this point of development, a small part (2-3%) are chosen each day to become mature, resting antigen-sensitive, sIgM/sIgD-double-expressing B cells which are allowed to migrate to the periphery and to eventually become longer-lived. Whether sIg is involved in this positive selection, i.e. whether self-antigens or foreign antigens are mandatory to make all immature B cells mature remains to be seen. However, B lineage cells which are defective in T-independent as well as T-dependent B cell activation through mutations in their btk and CD40 genes are unable to establish longer-lived peripheral, mature B cell compartments, although the precursor and immature B cell compartments in bone marrow are normally filled, indicating that during the transition from immature to mature B cells such stimulatory pathways are involved in the establishment of the peripheral, mature B cell compartments [Oka et al 1996].

Negative, and potential positive selecting steps of B cell development can, so far, not be executed under *in vitro* culture conditions.

Stimulation of Resting, Mature B Cells

Helper T cell-independent and dependent stimulation of mature, peripheral, antigen-reactive B cells leads to proliferation and maturation to Ig secretion. T cell-independent antigens stimulate, usually in extra-follicular regions of the secondary lymphoid organs, a burst of cell divisions and the maturation to IgM secretion within a week. Very little switching to other classes and no hypermutation of V-regions of Ig genes are usually observed in these T cell-independent B cell responses. By contrast, helper-T cell-dependent antigens stimulate in follicles and germinal centers in the secondary lymphoid organs an extended proliferation and maturation of B cells, which includes switching to downstream Ig classes (IgG, IgE, IgA) and hypermutation of Ig V-regions (reviewed by [Lane 1996, Stavnezer 1996, Storb 1996]). Once stimulated, the same B cells can respond to T cell-independent as well as T cell-dependent stimulatory signals (reviewed in [Armitage and Alderson 1995, Hathcock and Hodes 1996, Law and Clark 1994, Mond et al 1995], and papers in Immunological Reviews 99, 1987).

B cells can be stimulated polyclonally by polyclonal activators which appear to use T-independent or T-dependent pathways of antigenic stimulation. Thus, lipopolysaccharides (LPS) resemble T-independent antigenic stimulation of type I, IgM-specific antibodies plus IL-2 T-independent antigenic stimulation of type II, and CD40-specific antibodies (or CD40 ligand) and IL-2 or IL-4 T-dependent antigenic stimulation. At least one in 3 to 10 peripheral B cells can be stimulated in each of these three polyclonal ways of activation. Analysis of the growth kinetics of single clones of LPS-reactive, normal B cells has shown that these cells divide every 18 hours for at least 4 to 5 divisions. Within the first 125 hours of proliferation, every B cell in the clone divides, and every dividing B cell in this clone secretes sufficient amounts of Ig to form a hemolytic plaque [Andersson et al 1977]. The intensity of secretion, measured by the number of molecules of Ig secreted during the cell cycle, and the extent of morphological maturation, measured by the gradual loss of sIg and the gradual development of an endoplasmic reticulum containing large stores of intracellular Ig, increases with every cell division that the maturing B cell clone undergoes. Activated B cell blasts stimulated by T-independent polyclonal activators can be restimulated in T-dependent ways, indicating that the peripheral B cell repertoire is not divided into different compartments, but is largely crossreactive to T-dependent and T-independent stimulations.

Similarly, polyclonal stimulation by CD40-specific antibodies and IL-4, resembling T cell-dependent stimulation, leads to balanced proliferation and Ig-secretion within single activated B cells. After 2 to 3 days, switching to IgG_1 and IgE becomes measurable.

Proliferation Versus Maturation in Mature B Cells

Proliferation and maturation of mature B cells can be dissociated from each other. Inhibition of LPS-stimulated proliferation by hydroxyurea still allows the maturation to IgM secretion [Andersson and Melchers 1974]. On the other hand, stimulation of B cells by IgM-specific antibodies in cross-linking form induces proliferation without maturation to IgM secretion [Andersson et al 1974]. Resting small B cells exposed to cytokines secreted by helper T cells [Melchers et al 1980], later identified as IL-2 or IL-5 [Lernhardt et al 1987], mature to Ig-secreting cells in the absence of proliferation. In all these experimental conditions, a large part of all B cells participate in the reaction, making them reasonable targets for biochemical analyses.

Ever since the interactions of CD40 on B cells with CD40 ligand on activated helper T cells were identified as a central interaction that controls proliferation, differentiation (to Ig class switching and hypermutations) and apoptosis, a large body of information, which also attempts to define the roles of costimulatory molecules (e.g. B7-1, B7-2, CD19, CD21, CD23, CD35, CD38, cytokine and chemokine receptors, intracellular signalling pathways, etc.) in these processes, has been collected. They help to define different states of B cells in their reactions to become either plasma cells, memory cells, anergic cells or apoptotic cells.

As one more recent example, p50/nFκB-T and relB-T deletion mutant mice have been shown to be defective in B cell proliferation, but mature normally to Ig secretion and Ig class switching [Snapper et al 1996].

c-myc Expression During Normal B Cell Development

During the development of B lymphocytes from early progenitors in bone marrow to Ig-secreting plasma cells, up-regulating of c-myc expression is seen twice. It is first up-regulated to high levels in pro-, pre B-I and large pre B-II cells, and a second time again to high levels, when resting, mature, antigen-sensitive $sIgM^+/sIgD^+$ B cells are stimulated by antigen or by polyclonal activation. At the first precursor B cell stage of B cell development, up-regulation of c-myc is maintained at high levels during continued proliferation of cells through several cell cycles. At the second stage, up-regulation of c-myc precedes the entry of G_0-resting B cells into the cell cycle (see Francis *et al.,* this volume). At this mature stage of B cell proliferation, however, up-regulation of c-myc to high levels is not maintained but falls to low, if not undetectable levels in proliferating, mature B cells. At the first stage, the proliferating pre B cells maintain their state of differentiation as long as they are in contact with the stimulating environment of stromal cells and the cytokine IL-7 provided by the stromal cells, at the second stage they progressively mature to memory B cells and Ig-secreting plasma cells.

Expression of c-myc is down-regulated for the first time in development as large, cycling pre B-II cells become small, resting pre B-II and $sIgM^+$ immature B cells [Winkler, et al. 1994]. This transition coincides with the rearrangements of V_L to J_L segments in the Ig L chain gene loci. While the expression of TdT is turned off already in large pre B-II cells and, hence, might not be down-regulated by the loss of expression of c-myc, the re-expression of the rearrangement active genes (RAG1 and 2) at this point development might well be influenced by this loss of expression of c-myc. Similarly, the expression of surrogate L chain is down-regulated at this transition and loss of expression of c-myc might again be implied in this down-regulation (see literature in Taylor et al., this volume).

Mice that express c-myc under the control of the H chain enhancer $E_{\mu H}$ as a transgene, i.e. early in pre B cell development when the μ H chain gene locus is first expressed, have an expanded, continuously proliferating pre B-II-compartment in bone marrow [Adams et al 1985]. Hence, their lack of down-regulation of c-myc at the transition from large pre B-II to immature B apparently disturbs this transition.

Up- and down-regulation of c-myc at the second stage, i.e. in resting mature B cells activated from the G_0 state into the G_1 phase of the cell cycle, occurs synchronously, up within the first hours and down after 5-10 hours of stimulation in <u>all</u> cells [Kelly et al 1984]. However, these synchronously c-myc-activated cells enter the first cell cycle in an asynchronous fashion, so that a constant part of all cells enter the G-phase and the first mitosis from 12 to 24 hours after stimulation, to continue several cell cycles of 18 hours at low or undetectable levels of c-myc expression. Hence, the role of c-myc in the entry of B cells into cell cycle, and in the progression of these B cells in their balance of proliferation, differentiation and apoptosis though succeeding cycles remains unclear. It remains remarkable that a transgenic mouse strain which expresses c-myc under the control of a late, mature B cell- or plasma cell-specific promotor has not yet been generated. Such a transgenic construct might prevent the early, deregulated expression of c-myc observed in Eμ-myc-transgenic mice [Adams, et al. 1985] and should more appropriately simulate the deregulated expression achieved by the t12, 15 translocation of c-myc into the switch regions of the IgH locus [Potter and Wiener 1992].

Studies of c-myc Expression Control in Model Cell Systems

Since c-myc plays such general, important roles in the controls of cell proliferation, differentiation and apoptosis, its control of expression has been studied in many cell lineages, mostly in transformed and malignant cells representing such lineages. In the B-lymphocyte lineage, lymphomas and plasmacytomas have been studied (see papers by Zou et al., Scott et al. and Wu et al., this volume). Inappropriate over-expression of c-myc has been seen to promote apoptosis in some cells, although decreased levels may do the same in others. In the surface IgM-expressing WEHI 231 cells, signals mediated via surface IgM occupied by antibodies induce first up-, then down-regulation of c-myc expression. The cells are induced to die by apoptosis. Anti-sense S-oligonucleotides specific for c-myc inhibit apoptosis (Scott et al., this volume). During the up- and down-regulation of c-myc expression, it appears to be the second phase, i.e. the down-regulation which leads to apoptosis (Wu et al., this volume). The WEHI 231 cells have been taken as a model for tolerance induction in immature B cells (Scott et al., this volume, and 1986; [Benhamou et al 1990, Hasbold and Klaus 1990]). In this context, it is interesting to note that in normal, early B cell development, c-myc expression is down-regulated at the transition of large, pre B-receptor expressing pre B-II cells to small, resting pre B-II and immature B cells, i.e. <u>before</u> the expression of surface IgM and at the time when precursor B cells acquire the capacity to enter apoptosis.

However, while it is difficult to detect c-myc up- and down-regulation in normal immature, surface IgM-expressing B-lymphocytes of bone marrow, recent experiments by Scott et al [1996] indicate that in a mouse expressing the Sp6 anti-TNP monoclonal antibody as a transgenic receptor, TNP-dextran-induced apoptosis of transgenic, IgM-expressing B-lymphocytes of spleen can be inhibited by antisense c-myc. In the pathway of differentiation, these cells appear to be beyond the stage of an immature B cell in bone marrow and might be the example for peripheral, but not for central tolerance induction. Hence, while the molecular genetics and the signaling reactions involving c-myc in B lineage cells can be studied in detail in transformed cells (Scott et al., this volume, [Fukuda et al 1995]), the meaning of these reactions for normal cell physiology remains an enigma. Possible scenarios in normal B-lineage cells are discussed by Snow in this volume.

It is also clear from studies with transformed B lineage cells representing different stages of development (Zou et al., this volume) and with cells of different lineages (as one recent example, see [Fukada et al 1996]) that regulation of c-myc expression can target different genes in different cells, with the result that either proliferation, or terminal differentiation, or apoptosis may be affected.

While the efforts to dissect the different signaling pathways in the different cells and to identify target genes of the deregulated c-myc expression have already led to impressive results, it remains surprising how little has been done to study the changes in expression of c-myc together with its family members and partners on either RNA or protein levels.

Concluding Remarks

B cell development *in vivo* and *in vitro* has been studied so extensively that well over a dozen stages of cellular differentiation can be distinguished and ordered in mouse development. A similarly high number of cells begins to be discernible in humans. Furthermore, proliferation, differentiation and programmed cell death of cells can be dissected at more than one stage of this development. A wealth of B-lineage tumors, both of mouse and man, further add to the diversity of cells which can be located within B cell development. A multitude of transgenic and deletion mutation mice affects various stages in B cell development. Deregulation of c-myc is clearly implicated in the control of normal cellular development, and in deregulatory events leading to neoplasia. It seems very timely to combine the ever growing knowledge of the diversity of B-lineage cells of normal and mutant mice and man with the ever growing diversity of myc/mad/max gene family members in efforts to understand how the latter control the former.

Acknowledgment

The Basel Institute for Immunology was founded and is supported by F. Hoffmann-La Roche Ltd., Basel, Switzerland.

References

Adams JM, Harris AW, Pinkert CA, Corcoran LM, Alexander WS, Cory S, Palmiter RD, Brinster RL (1985) The c-myc oncogene driven by immunoglobulin enhancers induces lymphoid malignancy in transgenic mice. Nature 318: 533-538

Andersson J, Bullock WW, Melchers F (1974) Inhibition of mitogen stimulation of mouse lymphocytes by anti-mouse immunoglobulin antibodies. I. Mode of action. Eur J Immunol 4: 715-722

Andersson J, Coutinho A, Lernhardt W, Melchers F (1977) Clonal growth and maturation to immunoglobulin secretion in vitro of every growth-inducible B lymphocyte. Cell 10: 27-34

Andersson J, Melchers F (1974) Maturation of mitogen-activated bone marrow-derived lymphocytes in the absence of proliferation. Eur J Immunol 4: 533-539

Andersson J, Melchers F, Rolink A (1995) Stimulation by T cell independent antigens can relieve the arrest of differentiation of immature auto-reactive B cells in the bone marrow. Scand J Immunol 42: 21-33

Armitage RJ, Alderson MR (1995) B-cell stimulation. Curr Opin Immunol 7: 243-247

Benhamou LE, Cazenave PA, Sarthou P (1990) Anti-immunoglobulins induce death by apoptosis in WEHI-231 B-lymphoma cells. Eur J Immunol 20

Chen C, Nagy Z, Prak EL, Weigert M (1995b) Immunoglobulin heavy chain gene replacement: A mechanism of receptor editing. Immunity 3: 747-755

Chen C, Nagy Z, Radic MZ, Hardy RR, Huszar D, Camper SA, Weigert M (1995a) The site and stage of anti-DNA B-cell deletion. Nature 373: 252-255

Chen J, Alt F (1993) Gene rearrangement and B-cell development. Curr Op Immunol 5: 194-200

Cumano A, Kee BL, Ramsden dA, Marshall A, Paige CJ, Wu GE (1994) Development of B lymphocytes from lymphoid committed and uncommitted progenitors. In Immunol. Rev., G Möller, ed. Munksgaard (Copenhagen), pp. 5-33

Cumano A, Paige CJ, Iscove NN, Brady G (1992) Bipotential precursors of B cells and macrophages in murine fetal liver. Nature 356: 612-615

Decker DJ, Boyle NE, Koziol JA, Klinman NR (1991) The expression of the Ig H chain repertoire in developing bone marrow B lineage cells. J Immunol 146: 350-361

Ehlich A, Matin V, Müller W, Rajewsky K (1994) Analysis of the B-cell progenitor compartment at the level of single cells. Curr Biol 4: 573-583

Era T, Nishikawa S, Sudo T, Fu-Ho W, Ogawa M, Kunisada T, Hayashi S-I, Nishikawa S-I (1994) How B-precursor cells are driven to cycle. In Immunol. Rev., G Möller, ed. Munksgaard (Copenhagen), pp. 35-51

Fukada T, Hibi M, Yamanaka Y, Takahashi-Tezuka M, Fujitani Y, Yamaguchi T, Nakajima K, Hirano T (1996) Two signals are necessary for cell proliferation induced by a cytokine receptor gp130: involvement of STST3 in anti-apoptosis. Immunity 5: 449-460

Fukuda T, Kitamura D, Taniuchi I, Maekawa Y, Benhamou LE, Sarthou P, Watanabe T (1995) Restoration of surface IgM-mediated apoptosis in an anti-IgM-resistant variant of WEHI-231 lymphoma cells by HSI, a protein-tyrosine kinase substrate. Proc Natl Acad Sci 92: 7302-7306

Ghia P, Gratwohl A, Signer E, Winkler TH, Melchers F, Rolink AG (1995) Immature B cells from human and mouse bone marrow can change their surface light chain expression. Eur J Immunol 25: 3108-3114

Ghia P, ten Boekel E, Sanz E, de la Hera A, Rolink A, Melchers F (1996) Ordering of human bone marrow B lymphocyte precursors by single-cell polymerase chain reaction analyses of the rearrangement status of the immunoglobulin H and L chain gene loci. J Exp Med 184: 2217-2229

Goodnow CC, Cyster JG, Hartley SZ, Bell SE, Cooke MP, Healy JL, Akkaraju S, Rathmell JC, Pogue SL, Shokat KP (1995) Self-tolerance checkpoints in B lymphocyte development. In Advances in Immunology, FJ Dixon, ed. Academic Press (London), pp. 279-368

Grawunder U, Haasner D, Melchers F, Rolink A (1993) Rearrangement and expression of κ light chain genes can occur without μ heavy chain expression during differentiation of pre-B cells. Int Immunol 5: 1609-1618

Grawunder U, Leu TMJ, Schatz DG, WErner A, Rolink AG, Melchers F, Winkler TH (1995) Down-regulation of *RAG1* and *RAG2* gene expression in preB cells after functional immunoglobulin heavy chain rearrangement. Immunity 3: 601-608

Hardy RR (1992) Variable gene usage, physiology and development of Ly1+ (CD5+) B cells. Curr Op In Immunol 4: 181-185
Hardy RR, Carmack CE, Li YS, Hayakawa K (1994) Distinctive developmental origins and specificities of murine CD5$^+$ B cells. In Immunol. Rev., G Möller, ed. Munksgaard (Copenhagen), pp. 91-118
Hasbold J, Klaus GGB (1990) Anti-immunoglobulin antibodies induce apoptosis in immature B-cell lymphomas. Eur J Immunol 20: 1685-1690
Hathcock KS, Hodes RJ (1996) Role of the CD28-B7 costimulatory pathways in T cell-dependent B cell responses. In Advances in Immunology, FJ Dixon, ed. Academic Press (London), pp. 131-166
Hayashi S, Kunisada T, Ogawa M, Sudo T, Kodama H, Suda T, Nishikawa S, Nishikawa S (1990) Stepwise progression of B lineage differentiation supported by interleukin 7 and other stromal cell molecules. J Exp Med 171: 1683-1695
Kelly K, Cochran B, Stiles C, Leder P (1984) The regulation of c-myc by growth signals. Curr Top Microbiol Immunol 113: 117-126
Kincade PW, Medina KL, Smithson G (1994) Sex hormones as negative regulators of lymphopoiesis. In Immunol. Rev., G Möller, ed. Munksgaard (Copenhagen), pp. 119-134
Kleinfeld R, Hardy RR, Tarlington D, Dangl J, Herzenberg LA, Weigert M (1986) Recombination between an expressed immunoglobulin heavy chain gene and a germ-line variable gene segment in Ly1$^+$ Be cell lymphoma. Nature 322: 843-846
Lane P (1996) Development of B-cell memory and effector function. Curr Opin Immunol 8: 331-335
Law C-L, Clark EA (1994) Cell-cell interactions that regulate the development of B-lineage cells. Curr Opin Immunol 6: 238-247
Lernhardt W, Karasuyama H, Rolink A, Melchers F (1987) Control of the cell cycle of murine B lymphocytes: The nature of α- and β-B-cell growth factors and of B-cell maturation factors. Immunol Rev 99: 241-262
Löffert D, Schaal S, Ehlich A, Hardy RR, Zou Y-R, Müller W, Rajewsky K (1994) Early B-cell development in the mouse: Insights from mutations introduced by gene targeting. In Immunol. Rev., G Möller, ed. Munksgaard (Copenhagen), pp. 135-153
Melchers F (1979) Three waves of B lymphocyte development during embryonic development in the mouse. In Cell lineage, stem cells and cell determination. INSERM Symposium 10, N le Douarin, ed. Elsevier Science Publishers (Amsterdam), pp. 281-289
Melchers F (1995) The role of B cell and pre-B-cell receptors in development and growth control of the B-lymphocyte cell lineage. In Immunglobulin genes, T Honjo and FW Alt, eds. Academic Press (London)
Melchers F, Andersson J, Lernhardt W, Schreier MH (1980) H-2-unrestricted polyclonal maturation without replication of small B cells induced by antigen-activated T cell help factors. Eur J Immunol 10: 679-685
Melchers F, Karasuyama H, Haasner D, Bauer S, Kudo A, Sakaguchi N, Jameson B, Rolink A (1993) The surrogate light chain in B-cell development. Immunol Today 14: 60-68
Mombaerts P, Iacomini J, Johnson RS, Herrup K, Tonegawa S, Papaioannou VE (1992) RAG-1-deficient mice have no mature B and T lymphocytes. Cell 68: 869-877
Mond JJ, Vos Q, Lees A, Snapper CM (1995) T cell independent antigens. Curr Opin Immunol 7: 349-354
Nemazee D, Russell D, Arnold B, Haemmerling G, Allison J, Miller JF, Morahan G, Buerki K (1991) Clonal deletion of autospecific B lymphocytes. Immunol Rev 122: 117-132
Nossal GJV (1994) Differentiation of the secondary B-lymphocyte repertoire: The germinal center reaction. In Immunol. Rev., G Möller, ed. Munksgaard (Copenhagen), pp. 173-183
Oettinger MA, Schatz DG, Gorka C, Baltimore D (1990) RAG-1 and RAG-2, adjacent genes that synergistically activate V(D)J recombination. Science 248: 1517-1523
Ogawa M, Matzusaki Y, Nishikawa S, Hayashi SI, Kunisada T, Sudo T, Kina T, Nakauchi H, Nishikawa SI (1991) Expression and function of c-kit in hemopoietic progenitor cells. J Exp Med 174: 63-70
Oka Y, Rolink AG, Andersson J, Kamanaka M, Uchida J, Yasui T, Kishimoto T, Kikutani H, Melchers F (1996) Profound reduction of mature B cell numbers, reactivities and serum immunoglobulin levels in mice which simultaneously carry the XID and CD40-deficiency genes. Int Immunol 8: 1675-1685
Osmond DG (1991) Proliferation kinetics and the lifespan of B cells in central and peripheral lymphoid organs. Curr Opin Immunol 3: 179-185

Potter M, Wiener F (1992) Plasmactyomagenesis in mice: model of neoplastic development dependent upon chromosomal translocations. Carcinogenesis 13: 1681-1697

Prak EL, Weigert M (1995) Light chain replacement: A new model for antibody gene rearrangement. J Exp Med 182: 541-548

Rajewsky K (1992) Early and late B-cell development in the mouse. Curr Opin Immunol 4: 171-176

Reth M, Gehrmann P, Petrac E, Wiese P (1986) A novel V_H to V_HDJ_H joining mechanism in heavy-chain-negative (null) preB cells results in heavy-chain production. Nature 322: 840-842

Rolink A, Grawunder U, Haasner D, Strasser A, Melchers F (1993a) Immature surface Ig^+ B cells can continue to rearrange κ and λ L chain gene loci. J Exp Med 178: 1263-1270

Rolink A, Grawunder U, Winkler TH, Karasuyama H, Melchers F (1994b) IL-2 receptor a chain (CD25, TAC) expression defines a crucial stage in preB cell development. Int Immunol 6: 1257-1264

Rolink A, Haasner D, Nishikawa SI, Melchers F (1993b) Changes in frequencies of clonable preB cells during life in different lymphoid organs of mice. Blood 81: 2290-2300

Rolink A, Karasuyama H, Haasner D, Grawunder U, Martensson IL, Kudo A, Melchers F (1994a) Two pathways of B lymphocyte development in mouse bone marrow and the roles of surrogate L chain in this development. In Immunological Reviews, G Möller, ed. Munksgaard (Copenhagen), pp. 185-201

Rolink A, Kudo A, Karasuyama H, Kikuchi Y, Melchers F (1991a) Long-term proliferating early pre B cell lines and clones with the potential to develop to surface-Ig positive mitogen-reactive B cells *in vitro* and *in vivo*. EMBO J 10: 327-336

Rolink A, Streb M, Nishikawa SI, Melchers F (1991b) The *c-kit* encoded tyrosine kinase regulates the proliferation of early pre-B cells. Eur J Immunol 21: 2609-2612

Rolink A, ten Boekel E, Melchers F, Fearon DT, Krop I, Andersson J (1996a) A subpopulation of $B220^+$ cells in murine bone marrow does not express CD19 and contains NK cell-progenitors. J Exp Med 183: 187-194

Rolink AG, Melchers F, Andersson J (1996b) The SCID but not the RAG2 gene product is required for Sμ-Sε-heavy chain class switching. Immunity 5: 319-330

Schatz DG, Oettinger MA, Baltimore D (1989) The V(D)J recombination activating gene, RAG-1. Cell 59: 1035-1048

Scott DW, Livnat D, Pennell CA, Keng P (1996) Lymphoma models for B-cell activation and tolerance III. Cell cycle dependence for negative signalling of WEHI-231 B lymphoma cells by anti-μ. J Exp Med 164: 156-164

Shen-Ong GLC, Keath E, Picolli SP, Cole MD (1982) Novel myc oncogene RNA from abortive immunoglobulin gene recombination in mouse plasmacytomas. Cell 31: 443-452

Shinkai Y, Rathbun G, Lam KP, Oltz EM, Stewart V, Mendelsohn M, Charron J, Datta M, Young F, Stall AM, Alt FW (1992) RAG-2-deficient mice lack mature lymphocytes owing to inability to initiate V(D)J rearrangement. Cell 68: 855-867

Snapper CM, Rosas FR, Zelazowski P, Moorman MA, Kehry MR, Bravo R, Weih F (1996) B cells lacking Re1B are defective in proliferative responses, but undergo normal B cell maturation to Ig secretaion and Ig class switching. J Exp Med 184: 1537-1541

Stavnezer J (1996) Immunoglobulin class switching. Curr Opin Immunol 8: 199-205

Storb U (1996) The molecular basis of somatic hypermutation of immunoglobulin genes. Curr Opin Immunol 8: 206-213

Strasser A, Wittingham S, Vaux DL, Bath ML, Adams JM, Cory S, Harris AW (1991) Enforced BCL2 expression in B-lymphoid cells prolongs antibody responses and elicits autoimmune disease. Proc Natl Acad Sci USA 88: 8661-8665

ten Boekel E, Melchers F, Rolink A (1995) The status of Ig loci rearrangements in single cells from different stages of B cell development. Int Immunol 7: 1013-1019

Winkler TH, Melchers F, Rolink AG (1994) Interleukin-3 and interleukin-7 are alternative growth factors for the same B-cell precursors in the mouse. Blood 85: 2045-2051

Young F, Ardman B, Shinkai Y, Lansford R, Blackwell TK, Mendelsohn M, Rolink A, Melchers F, Alt FW (1994) Influence of immunoglobulin heavy- and light-chain expression on B-cell differentiation. Genes Dev 8: 1043-1057

Regulation of the C-Myc Gene

DNA Conformation, Topology, and the Regulation of *c-myc* Expression

D. Levens, R. C. Duncan, T. Tomonaga, G. A. Michelotti, I. Collins, T. Davis-Smyth, T. Zheng and E. F. Michelotti
The Laboratory of Pathology, National Cancer Institute, Bethesda, MD 20892, USA

The Problem of *c-myc* Expression

The *c-myc* protein, a basic leucine zipper helix-loop-helix transcription factor is a key regulator of life and death [1-4}. *c-myc* expression is coupled to a multitude of physiological processes and has been reported to be regulated by a long list of hormones, cytokines, lymphokines, nutritional status, development and differentiation. Myc levels can be pharmacologically perturbed, at least transiently, by a host of agents. Consistent with the notion that *c-myc* expression is tightly regulated, both the mRNA and protein products of this gene are extraordinairily short-lived, 30 minutes and 20 minutes, respectively [1-4]. In growing cells wide-ranging excursions in *c-myc* expression are generally not seen, attesting either to tight homeostatic regulation or constitutive expression of *c-myc*.

Numerous constitutive and inducible gene regulatory proteins have been reported to govern *c-myc* expression. Included among these proteins, are factors widely-recognized to be potent regulators of transcription in other settings such as the duplex DNA binding proteins NFκB, E2F, Sp1, BLIMP-1/PRF, and YY1 [5-9]. Sites for binding in vitro to the *c-myc* gene for other well-studied factors such as NF-I, octamer binding proteins, AP1 and RFX have been identified [10-12]. Some duplex DNA binding proteins such as MAZ and CTCF have been studied primairily as regulators of *c-myc* [13, 14]. In addition to the proteins enumerated above, binding or regulation of *c-myc* transcription by several non-standard transcription factors has been described. Among these are the single strand DNA binding proteins hnRNP K, FBP, CNBP, PUR, THZif-1, MSSP1 and MSSP2, as well as the candidate tumor suppressor protein/enzyme nm23/nucleotide disphosphate kinase [15-28]. A replication initiation zone has been mapped upstream of *c-myc* which binds the sequence specific single strand protein PUR which has been suggested to participate in both replication and transcription [29].

The *c-myc* locus suffers various forms of genetic damage in a variety of neoplasms. Translocations, amplification and viral insertions disrupt the arrangement of regulatory elements within and flanking the gene [1-4]. It appears that maintenance of the integrity of the chromsomal domain enveloping the *c-myc* gene is necessary to achieve proper transcriptional control in vivo. In addition mutations occur both within coding segments and in candidate cis-elements which may contribute to malignant transformation or tumor progression. Further evidence indicating that the correct long range chromosomal context is necessary for the physiological regulation, is the inability to recapitulate many, if not most, features of c-myc expression in transfection experiments; in transient, stable and transgenic assays including the c-myc structural gene as well as tens of thousands of 5' and 3' flanking sequence have all failed to recapitulate normal expression [30, 31]]. Despite more than a decade of investigation, the principles and even the patterns describing the transcriptional regulation of the human *c-myc* protooncogene remain enigmatic. No simple model explains how the myriad of signal transduction pathways, transcription factors and cis elements act to set the level of myc expression.

If the physiological function of *c-myc* expression is to facilitate cell division or to drive apoptosis, then the achievement of either of these goals lies many hours future to signal inciting increased expression. If only a pulse of enhanced *c-myc* expression were to trigger *c-myc* function, then tight moment to moment regulation of myc levels must exist . How might the final level of *c-myc* expression be determined? Several modes of feedback regulation as well as cross-regulatory circuits are likely to govern *c-myc* levels. Accummulating evidence suggests that *c-myc* acting either as a transcriptional activator or repressor contributes to the fine regulation of many genes, but thus far myc has not been proven to be an all or none switch for any downstream target. If *c-myc* were to govern the general readiness of a cell to divide through the adjustment of many different metabolic, anabolic and catabolic pathways, then the diversity of its candidate targets would be explained; yet this same diversity would dictate that no single end product feedback mechanism would dominate myc regulation. So the problem reduces to what features of the myc gene, RNA and protein might allow a rapid monitoring mechanism to constrain myc expression, yet permit an integrated response to the diverse inputs upon the gene.

Multiple Upstream Segments of the *c-myc* Gene are Single Stranded when *c-myc* is Expressed.

Several lines of evidence indicate that some upstream segments of the *c-myc* gene are not B-DNA, in vivo. Numerous studies have mapped and measured the intensity of DNase I hypersensitive sites within the chromatin of the *c-myc* locus [10, 32-34]. Although reactivity of these sites with DNase I is presumed to result from perturbation of normal chromatin architecture, the source of this disturbance is not known and conceivably might reflect alteration of factor binding, nucleosome positioning or DNA conformation. The presence or absence of individual sites correlates with the activity of the gene. Comparison of DNase I and S1 nuclease hypersensitive sites in activated or repressed *c-myc* genes reveals a striking concordance in the locations and intensity of the cleavage sites for each enzyme [35]. (**Fig. 1**)

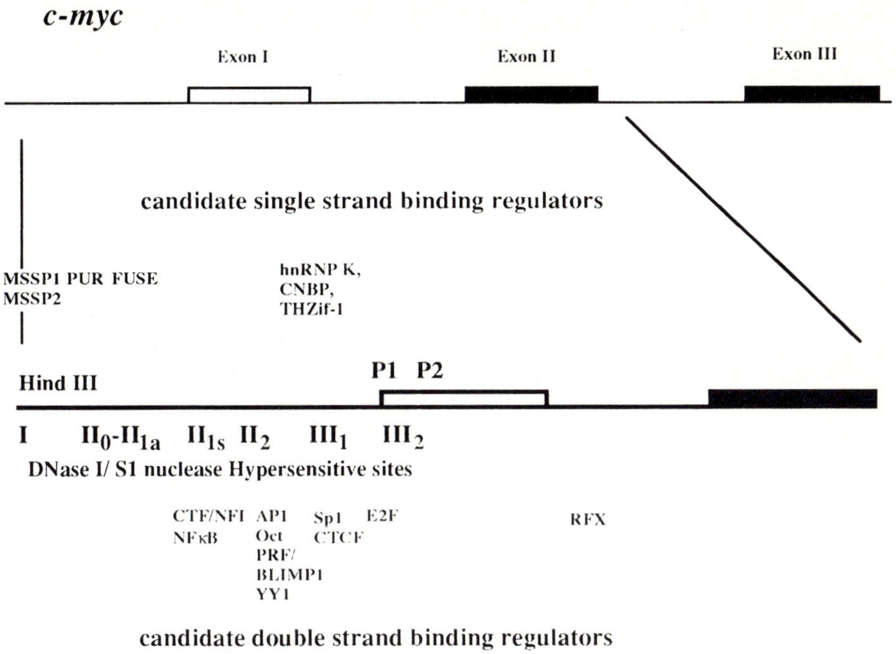

Fig. 1. Summary of sites of double strand or single strand recognizing sequence specific factors, relative to the promoters as well as DNase I or S1 nuclease hypersensitive sites of the *c-myc* gene.

Strong S1 sensitivity occurred as expected at P1 and P2, presumably reflecting the presence of open or engaged RNA polymerase complexes at the promoters. However S1 sensitivity was also noted in neuroblastoma cells (which do not express *c-myc)* at P1 and P2. Another site of strong S1 nuclease sensitivity was the CT-region, 100 - 150 nt upstream of P1. This region, comprised of five repeats of a nonanucleotide element, binds hnRNP K and CNBP; these proteins interact respectively with the C-rich and G-rich strands of this segment. Both highly sensitive and weaker zones of S1 sensitivity were noted. Among the latter was a sequence termed the far upstream element (FUSE) which interacts with a sequence specific, single strand nucleic acid binding protein. Binding sites for other single strand binding proteins including MSSP1 & 2 and PUR may be associated with S1 sensitivity. Another possible zone of non-B DNA in the general vicinity of FUSE and the PUR region has been reported to assume Z-DNA [36]. Although the simplest interpretation of S1 sensitivity is that segments of DNA are not duplex, other explanations including biochemical artefacts relating to the digestion conditions and DNA damage during preparation of nuclei might be entertained.

An independent, entirely in vivo method for modifying and mapping single stranded DNA, relies on the conformation sensitive reaction of KMnO4, with pyrimidines (especially thymine) coupled with ligation mediated PCR. This approach allows the identification of unpaired bases with single nucleotide resolution. This method confirmed the opening of P2 [37] and demonstrated opening at P1 in cells which make *c-myc*. Surprisingly, another pattern of $KMnO_4$

reactivity, distinct both from naked duplex DNA or active *c-myc* DNA, was seen in cells which express no *c-myc*, suggesting that repressed promoters are held in an alternate, non-B DNA conformation which is still sensitive to both permanganate and S1 nuclease [35].

FBP Binds to FUSE in a Bipartite Manner.

Prominent reactivity at FUSE, extending over an 80 nucleotide region was noted.(**Fig. 2**) On the non-template strand, only enhanced base modifications and no protections were noted. On the template strand both enhancements and protections from permanganate reactions were seen; protection from chemical modification would be expected at sites covered with protein. The pattern of reactivity produced by permanganate treatment of mixtures of purified recombinant FBP with supercoiled, but not linear DNA molecules bearing the FUSE region, closely mirrored the in vivo profile. Coupled with gel shift analysis revealing sequence specific recognition of the template strand FUSE by FBP, these results suggest that FBP may gain access to its cognate site, in vivo, in repsonse to processes that generate superhelical strain [35].

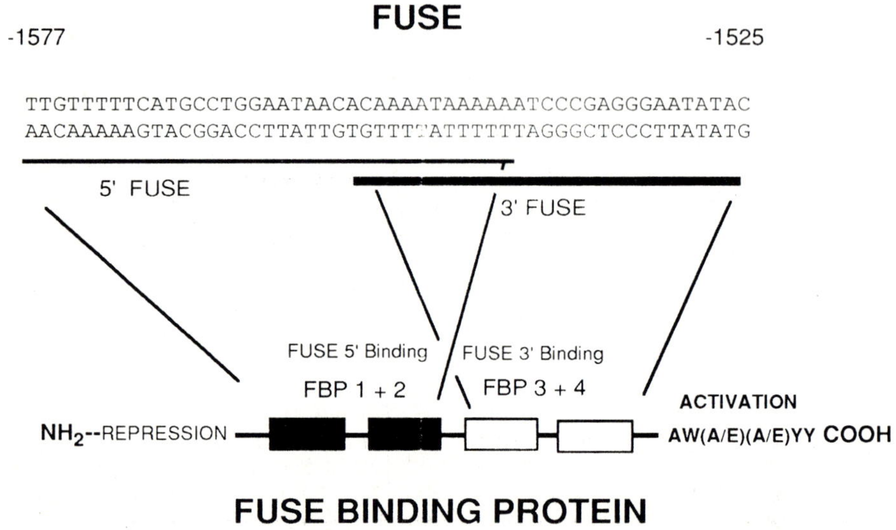

Fig. 2. Both the FUSE and FBP are bipartite with respect to recognition of the lower strand. The sequence of FUSE is shown collinear with the domains of FBP for schematic purposes only.

The central domain of FBP is composed of four tandemly repeated K-homology (KH) motifs [19]. Although the KH motif is often referred to as an RNA binding motif [38], in every instance where proteins possessing this structural element have been examined for DNA or RNA binding, the proteins bound to both [16, 39,40,41]. In the case of hnRNP K, the prototype for this family (hence the "K") the protein prefers DNA to RNA. Perhaps a better moniker would label the KH motif as a nucleic acid binding element. The third and fourth repeats of FBP's central domain interact strongly with the 3' segment of the FUSE in single stranded or supercoiled DNA. In contrast, repeats one and two, when separated from the remainder of FBP, interact only weakly with the 5' half of FUSE when single stranded and show no evidence of interaction with supercoiled DNA [35]. Thus melting of the full extent of FUSE by full-length FBP is likely to be anchored by the interaction of repeats three and four with 3' FUSE.

hnRNP K Binds Supercoiled DNA.

The region comprising the CT-element is sensitive to S1 nuclease and has single stranded character as assayed with $KMnO_4$. This region has been suggested to bind with a number of factors including Sp1, CTCF, nm23/Puf, CNBP, THZif-1 and hnRNP K [7, 14-18, 22,28]. Some of these have been reported to bind single stranded segments of the CT-element in electrophoretic mobility shift assays (EMSA). Incubation of recombinant hnRNP K with supercoiled DNA embracing the CT-region mimicked many of the features of permanganate sensitivity detected in vivo, whereas alone other factors did not perturb the reaction pattern of naked, supercoiled DNA. At the two most upstream repeats of the CT-element, CNBP enhanced and Sp1 repressed melting in conjunction with binding by hnRNP K. Thus combinations of single and double strand DNA binding proteins might expand the physiological repertoire of a given segment of DNA. Once again the binding of hnRNP K only to single stranded or supercoiled DNA would appear to couple the action of this molecule on DNA with processes either melting or torsionally straining the DNA.

FBP Possesses Potent Effector Domains to Modify Gene Expression.

If FBP and hnRNP K interact with cis-elements, in vivo and modify gene expression, then these proteins should either possess direct effector domains or should help to recruit other proteins which can modify transcription. In fact, each of these molecules has properties implicating them as transcription factors. The carboxyl terminus of FBP has a thrice repeated sequence motif, rich in tyrosine [19-21]. When fused to the Gal4 DNA binding domain, each of these repeats, singly or in combination, drives high levels of Gal4 UAS dependent activation 20]. The aromaticity of the tyrosines appears to be essential for activation as substitution of these residues with phenylalanine does not eliminate reporter expression, in contrast to replacement with other amino acids. The amino terminus of FBP supplied in cis- or in trans- is an efficient transcriptional repressor of activation by FBP or E1a activation domains [20]. Surprisingly, activation driven by the highly homologous carboxyl terminal domains of FBP2 and FBP3, which respectively share four or two copies of the tyrosine-rich activating segment, are relatively refractory to FBP N-terminal mediated repression, as is the actvation driven by the Herpes virus protein VP16 The molecular basis for this fine specificity is not yet known..

Although the pathways through which the FBP activates or represses gene expression remain to be elucidated, it appears that FBP has appropriate and potent molecular tools to modify gene expression.

hnRNP K has Many of the Properties Expected for a Transcription Factor.

hnRNP K binds to the CT-element in single stranded or supercoiled form, in vitro. In transfection studies, hnRNP K stimulates CT-element mediated activation only 3 -5 fold. Several problems interfer with the in vivo analysis of hnRNP K mediated transcriptional activation. First the protein is an abundant intranuclear molecule, and hence K-mediatedbasal activation is likely to preexist in most cells. Second, alone hnRNP K lacks either overwhelmingly potent activation or repression domains when assayed as Gal4-fusion proteins, thus potentially limiting the achievable magnitude of transactivationin transfections; and third other factors such as Sp1 may bind to some CT-elements confounding straightforward analysis. No matter how it acts or to what degree, if hnRNP K activates CT-elements in vivo, then it must first recognize those elements. Therefore, an approach was developed to demonstrate the capacity of hnRNP K to interact with CT-elements in vivo [18]. To circumvent the problems noted above, the potent VP16 activation domain was engrafted onto the carboxyl terminus of hnRNP K; in addition the gal4 DNA binding domain was fused with the amino terminus of hnRNP K-VP16 fusion, finally yielding yielding a triple chimera. The VP16 activation moiety was predicted to amplify either the response of a CT-element driven reporter gene to hnRNP K binding at CT-elements or of a Gal4 UAS driven reporter when bound to the Gal4 DNA binding domain of the triple fusion. Indeed, the predicted stimulation through CT-elements was observed, but only from transfected supercoiled reporter plasmids. Linearized reporters cwere not activated. In contrast this same triple chimera activated a Gal4 UAS reporter irrespective of the topology of the transfected DNA. Of course Gal4-VP16 supplied in trans- without fusion to hnRNP K, had no effect on CT-element driven activation and strongly activated Gal4 UAS reporters whether supercoiled or linear. Thus, hnRNP K can find and bind to CT-elements in vivo, however it seems to require the energetic assistance of negatively supercoiled (or underwound) DNA in order to gain access to its target sites [18].

In vitro transcription reactions programed with supercoiled templates could not be directly analyzed for their ability to support hnRNP K mediated activation, due to the overwhelming abundance of topoisomerase activity in Hela cell nuclear extracts. To test if hnRNP K could activate transcription in vitro, templates were generated bearing single stranded tails of either wild-type or mutant CT-elements [17]. These tailed templates were assayed for their ability to direct nuclear extracts to transcribe properly in presence or absence of hnRNP K. Stimulation of CT-element specific transcription was specifically activated by recombinant hnRNP K and was most prominent when hnRNP K was allowed synergize with AP1. (Although not specifically examined, it is presumabed synergy with some other transactivating factors would also occur).

Even if hnRNP K binds to CT-elements in DNA in vivo and in vitro, and stimulates transcription in vitro, it might not directly alter gene expression. If acting indirectly, hnRNP K might serve as an architectural transcription factor, governing DNA conformation and thereby determining which conventional factors have access to the TATA-promoter bound basal machinery. Alternatively, hnRNP K might serve directly as an activator or co-activator of transcription, itself binding with the transcription apparatus. Several experiments which were designed to distinguish between these alternatives, yielded evidence that hnRNP K forms complexes with transcriptional components in the absence of DNA. First, columns covalently coupled with hnRNP K efficiently removed factors required for activating transcription through the CT- and other cis-elements. Addition of a crude preparation enriched for TFIID (phospocellulose 1M fraction) restored the depeleted activating factors [17]. Second reciprocal "gst pull-down" experiments demonstrated the ability of in vitro translated hnRNP K to bind with a TATA binding protein (TBP)-glutathione-S-transferase fusion protein and of TBP to bind with an hnRNP K--gst fusion protein [17]. Extensive nuclease treatment did not alter these results indicating that nucleic acid bridges were not mediating the interactions observed. Third, hnRNP K was shown to co-immunoprecipitate specifically with epitope tagged TBP from cells stably transfected with DNA encoding the latter [17]. All of these results attest to the capacity of hnRNP K to bind with the transcription machinery in vivo and in vitro and suggest that hnRNP K may be capable of directly modifying transcription.

While the considerable evidence supports the notion that FBP and hnRNP K are at least part-time transcription factors, the extent of their involvement in the regulation of *c-myc* or other genes is unlargely unexplored.

Why Single Strand and Supercoil Binding Factors?

At least hypothetically there are functions which may be subsumed by proteins with the features of FBP and hnRNP K which might not be as easily filled by conventional factors. Both FBP and hnRNP K bind with supercoiled or single stranded DNA, but not with relaxed duplex. If the in vitro properties of these proteins mirror their in vivo function, then it is necessary to ask when is DNA supercoiled or single stranded in cells? What properties might be intrinsic to single stranded or supercoiled DNA which are not shared by conventional duplex? Because DNA melting within a topological domain changes the amount of supercoiling within that domain melting and supercoiling most often do not occur independent of each other. (A topological domain is formed any time one end of a segment of DNA is restrained from twisting about the helical axis relative to the other end. End-fixation can occur by anchoring ends to immobile nuclear structures and components. Segment ends can be also be fixed relative to each other through ligation into covalent circles or through the formation of protein bridges connecting proteins bound to fixed points along the DNA.) Nevertheless, for this discussion processes inevitably requiring strand separation will first be considered. In addition to transcription, DNA is singled stranded, at least transiently during replication, recombination, repair. These latter processes might therefore open CT-elements and FUSE for binding with hnRNP K or FBP, respectively, which then might stabilize the melted DNA at these sites. Hence the action of structure/sequence sensitive factors like FBP and hnRNP K on the *c-myc* gene, might serve to coordinate *c-myc* levels with key molecular processes governing cell growth. It is also possible that FBP and hnRNP K could play direct or accessory roles in replication, recombination or repair. However, because both CT-elements and FUSE retain single-stranded character throughout the cell cycle as assessed with permanganate, it seems unlikely that melting of these segments is temporally related to DNA synthesis or any other S-phase specific events.

Some Physical Properties are Very Different between Single Stranded and Duplex DNA.

Single stranded DNA has less flexural (bending) and torsional (twisting) rigidity than duplex DNA [42]. Hence the arrangement of chromatin loops and of the inter-protein loops formed between DNA bound factors--including the basal machinery-- is likely to be profoundly influenced by segements of melted DNA. Loops of single stranded DNA occurring at discrete, strategic sites may play a key role in determining the relative influence of individual, conventional duplex binding transcription factors on the *c-myc* promoter. In order for two DNA bound proteins to interact, their respective associating surfaces must lie along a common face of the double helix. Obviously, DNA must bend in order to bring together widely separated factors. The intervening DNA may also be forced to twist. Due to the periodicity of B-DNA (10.4 bp/turn), only a restricted set of positions allow any given protein-protein interaction to occur without necessitating winding or unwinding a fraction of a helical turn in order to force the interacting proteins together. The formation of the first protein-protein bridgeimposes constraints on the formation of additional complexes or upon the recruitment of additional DNA bound proteins into the complex. Clearly the formation of large supramolecular complexes involving the holo-enzyme, TFIIH, TBP-TAFs and upstream activators must be subjected to even more stringent topological and stereochemical constraints. DNA is not sufficiently flexible that passive deformation of its structure can simply be assumed. Studies on naked DNA indicate that DNA is actually quite rigid and resists twist (hence the difficulty typically encountered in attempting to cyclize short DNA fragments except in those instances when the 5' and 3' ends are in phase). The formation of the first protein-protein loop fixes the phases required by additional DNA bound factors over hundreds of base pairs, if this DNA is duplex. Yet in most studies the influence of upstream cis-elements is examined in vivo and in vitro with little consideration of the optimal positioning of these elements relative to each other or to the promoter, and still these studies generate useful results. Apparently DNA in vivo is somehow more torsinally flexible than predicted from its intrinsic B-form polymeric properties. One way to acquire this additional flexibility would be the creation of single stranded loops. Single strand loops are several hundred-fold more flexible to twist than is duplex DNA. Single stranded DNA loops as small as 3 bp [42]. virtually eliminate the requirement for correct phasing and facilitate the proper stereochemistry to allow the association of separated DNA segments. These small single stranded loops also exhibit increased flexibility to DNA bending. On a complex gene, such as *c-myc* the presence or absence of single stranded cis-elements in principle could determine which factors, and hence which signal transduction pathways, exert dominant influence on the promoter at any given moment.

DNA, in Most Cells, Most of the Time, is Negatively Supercoiled.

In prokaryotes torsional stress is tightly regulated and is coupled with the regulation of many genes. The degree of negative supercoiling is coupled with the metabolic state of the cell. Nutritional or genetic alterations of the ATP stores of E. coli alter the topological state of its DNA. Alteration of the superhelicity, in turn modulates the expression of many and efficacy of various transcriptional regulators. Thus alterations in DNA topology and the organismal reponse to these alterations constitute an important homeostatic device in prokaryotes [43]. Torsional stress is generated in prokaryotes by transcription and by DNA gyrase which intrinsically is capable of directly introducing negative (left-handed) supercoils into DNA in an ATP consuming reaction. Other type I and type II topoisomerases encoded by the bacterial genome or by invading bacteriophage modify the steady state levels of torsional stress [44].

In eukaryotes also, DNA is negatively supercoiled [44, 45]. However, most of the torsional stress in eukaryotic DNA has been restrained upon the surface of the nucleosomes compacting the genome; unless liberated, at least transiently, these supercoils are unlikely to influence the conformation of DNA or the binding of topology and single strand selective factors. The amount and distribution of free superhelical torsion--unrestrained supercoils-- in the mammalian genome is not known [45]. The energy stored in unrestrained supercoils is more apt to be exploited by proteins and processes preferring or requiring unwound DNA. Melting of negatively supercoiled DNA is energetically favored relative to relaxed B-DNA; thus in principle the action of molecules such as FBP and hnRNP K may be coupled with processes which generate supercoils. In eukaryotes most torsional stress is generated by RNA synthesis [44, 45]. The transcriptionally generated torsional stress has several possible fates: 1) It is depleted by the action of toposiomerases. 2) It is dissipated following strand scission. 3) It is constrained by fixation on nucleosomes (each nucleosome absorbs 1.7 negative supercoils). 4) It accummulates within a topologically closed domain bounded by protein-protein interactions, matrix attachment, etc. 5) It is dynamically transmitted off an unrestrained end. Under physiological conditions breaks and ends are too infrequent to provide a useful strategy for dissipating torsion. Most studies on the elastic and torsional properties of DNA have focused on the net accummulation of torsional stress within topologically closed boundaries. Clearly torsional forces are of sufficient magnitude that they must be included in any reckoning of the physical state of chromatin. Accummulation of positive supercoils ahead of RNA polymerase, in principle, could stall the forward progress of transcription [46]. Little consideration has been given to the potential involvement of torsional strain in the genesis of the promoter proximal pausing seen on many genes In these analyses, the energy associated with accummulated torsional stress is treated as a thermodynamic function of state directly related to the linking number of the domain. Due to the abundance of topoisomerase I and II with in the nuclei of most cells, there is no agreement as to the or extent to which supercoils accrue either at equilibrium or at steady state. Yet it seems unlikely that topoisomerases can instantaneously cancel the dynamic pulses of torsional stress transmitted by an elongating RNA polymerase. Although at one time it seemed that RNA polymerase simply revolved around the double helix thereby transducing no energy into the DNA structure, but rather dissipating it as friction directly into the nucleopasm, as the transcription complex is discovered to be more and more complex andbecomes more and more encumbered by macromolecular attachments with the nuclear matrix, upstream factors or splicing machinery, thereby creating intrachromosomal loops, etc., it seems that the energetics of rotating this molecular leviathan will become comparable to the potential energy of supercoiling DNA. Dynamic perturbation of upstream segments by an applied force has not been considered theoretically or experimentally. But since RNA polymerase generates more force than any molecular motor (including myosin) studied to date [47], it seems likely that the act of transcription might be inextricably associated with conformational perturbations of upstream DNA. Factors such as hnRNP K and FBP may be capable of sensing these perturbations through interactions with deformed DNA; if as appers likely, these factors also possess transcription effector domains, then they would be well-suited to feedback adjust ongoing transcription in real time. These same factors would be ill-suited for induction of silent genes, unless single stranded DNA were specifically propped open in repressed chromatin or unless unrestrained negative supercoils could be liberated prior to or during induction of the repressed genes.

A coupling between the DNA conformation of the *c-myc* gene, promoter activity, and elongation rates would further implicate chromatin structure, matrix/scaffold attachment and the relative position and distances of a multitude of elements as determinants of myc expression. Within this greater context, subtle deregulation of myc in response to translocations and viral insertions, even at great distances might result from disruption of the physiological balance of subtle inputs from many pathways. Similarly except on rare occassions, transfected myc genes would be unlikely to insert into a chromosomal domain equivalently topologically constrained and situated appropiately relative promoters, origins of replication, protein-protein loopsby attachments to nuclear matrix and equivalently situated relative to other promoters, replication zones, protein-protein loops, matrix attachment sites, etc. in order to correctly tune *c-myc* trancription. Well studied genes responding to one or few well characterised signals or biological processes might not be expected to utilize the same fine tuning devices operating on *c-myc*. If *c-myc* expression is coupled with the overall metabolic condition of the cell then, as in bacteria DNA supercoiling might provide one mechanism for the integration of many pathways. It is provocative that processes and treatments which are known to modify DNA topology such as topoismerase inhibitors, strand breakage due to irradiation, etc. decrease *c-myc* transcription [48]. This decrease does not reflect global inhibition of mRNA transcription as other genes such as vimentin and jun are up-regulated by these same treatments, in the same cells. A complete description of gene regulation may well require an accurrate depiction of the generation, transmission and dissipation of the mechanical as well as chemical forces operating on the genome.

References

1. Cole MD (1986) The myc oncogene: its role in transformation and differentiation. Annu Rev Genet 20: 361-84 (1986)

2. Spencer CA, Groudine M (1991) Control of c-myc regulation in normal and neoplastic cells. Adv Cancer Res 56:1-48

3. Marcu KB, Bossone SA, Patal AJ (1992) myc function and regulation: Ann Rev Biochem 61:809-860

4. Evan, GI, Littlewood, TD (1993) The role of c-myc in cell growth Curr Opin Genet Dev 3:44-49

5. Duyao MP, Buckler AJ., Sonnenshein, GE (1990) Interaction of an NF-kappa B-like factor with a site upstream of the c-myc promoter. Proc Natl Acad Sci USA 87:4727-473

6. Hiebert, SW, Lipp, M, Nevins, JR (1989) E1A-dependent trans-activation of the human c-myc promoter is mediated by the E2F factor. Proc Natl Acad Sci USA 86:3594-3598

7. DesJardins, E, Hay, N (1993) Repeated CT-elements bound by zinc finger proteins control the absolute and relative activities of the two principal human c-myc promoters Mol Cell Biol 13:5710-5724

8. Kakkis, E, Riggs KJ, Gillespie W, Calame K (1989) A transcriptional repressor of c-myc. Nature 339:718-721

9. Riggs KJ, Saleque S, Wong KK, Merrell KT, Lee JS, Shi Y, Calame K (1993) Yin-yang 1 activates the c-myc promoter. Mol Cell Biol 13:7487-7495

10. Siebenlist U, Hennighausen L, Battey J, Leder P (198) Chromatin structure and protien binding in the prtative regulatory region of the c-myc gene in Burkitt lymphoma Cell 37: 381-391

11. Takimoto M, Quinn JP, Farina AR, Staudt LM, Levens D (1989) Fos/jun and octamer-binding protein interact with a common site in a negative element of the human c-myc gene. J Biol Chem 264:8922-8999

12. Alesse E, Krutzsch H, Michelotti G, Levens D (1996) Mol Cell Diff 4:127-148

13. Bossone SA, Asselin C, Patel AJ, Marcu, KB (1992) MAZ, a zinc finger protein, binds to c-myc and C2 gene sequences regulating transcriptional initiation and termination. Proc Natl Acad Sci USA 89:7452-7456

14. Filippova GN, Fagerlie S, Klenova EM, Myers C, Dehner Y, Goodwin G, Neiman PE, Collins SJ Lobanenkov VV (1996) An exceptionally conserved transcriptional repressor, CTCF, employs different combinations of zinc fingers to bind diverged promoter sequences of avian and mammalian c-myc oncogenes. Mol Cell Biol 16: 2802-2813

15. Takimoto, M, Tomonaga, T, Matunis, M, Avigan, M, Krutzsch, H, Dreyfuss, G, and Levens, D (1993)Specific binding of heterogeneous ribonucleoprotein particle protein K to the human c-myc promoter, in vitro. J Biol Chem 268:18249-18258

16. Tomonaga T, Levens D (1995) Heterogeneous nuclear ribonucleoprotein K is a DNA binding transactivator. J Biol Chem 270: 4875-4881

17. Michelotti EF, Michelotti GA, Aronsohn AI, Levens D (1996) Heterogenous Nuclear Ribonuclearprotein K Is a Transcription Factor Mol Cell Biol 16:2350- 2360

18. Tomonaga T, Levens D (1996) Activating transcription from single stranded DNA Proc Natl Acad Sci USA 93:5830-5835

19. Duncan RD, Bazar L, Michelotti G, Tomonaga T, Krutzsch H, Avigan M, Levens D (199). A sequence-specific, single strand binding protein activates the far upstream of c-myc and defines a new DNA binding motif. Genes Dev. 8: 465-480.

20. Duncan R, Collins I, Tomonaga T, Zheng T, Levens D (1996) A Unique Sequence Motif is Found in the Carboxyl-Terminal Domain of the Single-Strand-Binding Protein FBP. Mol Cell Biol 16:2274-2282

21. Davis-Smyth T, Duncan RC, Zheng T, Michelotti G, Levens D (1996) The Far Upstream Element-binding Proteins Comprise an Ancient Family of Single-strand DNA -binding Transactivators. J Biol Chem 271:31679-31687

22. Michelotti E, Tomonaga T, Krutzsch H, Levens D (1995) Cellular nucleic acid binding protein regulates the CT-element of the human c-myc protooncogene. J Biol Chem 270: 9494-9499

23. Bergemann AD, Johnson EM (1992) The HeLa Pur factor binds single-stranded DNA at a specific element conserved in gene flanking regions and origins of DNA replication. Mol Cell Biol 12: 1257-1265

24. Bergemann AD, Ma Z-W, Johnson EM (1992) Sequence of cDNA comprising the human pur gene and properties of the encoded protein. Mol Cell Biol 12: 5673-5682

25. Sakatsume O, Tsuti H, Wang Y, Gao H, Tang X, Yamauchi T, Murata T, Itakura K, Yokoyama KK (1996) Binding of THZif-1, a MAZ-like Zinc Finger Protein to Nuclease-hypersensitive Element in the Promoter Region of c-Myc Protooncogene. J Biol Chem 271:31322-31333.

26. Negishi Y, Nishita Y, Saegusa Y, Kakizaki I, Galli I, Kihara F, Tamai K, Miyajama N, Iguchi-Ariga S, Ariga H (1994) Identification and cDNA cloning of single stranded DNA binding proteins that interact with the region upstream of the human c-myc gene. Oncogene 9:1133-1143

27. Takai T, Nishita Y, Iguchi-Ariga S, Ariga, H (1994) Molecular cloning of MSSP-2, a c-myc gene single-strand binding protein: characterization of binding specificity and DNA replication activity. Nucleic Acids Res 22:5576-5581

28. Postel EH, Berberich SJ, Flint SJ, Ferrone CA (1993) Human c-myc Transcription Factor PuF Identified as nm23H2 Nucleoside Diphosphate Kinase, a Candidate Suppressor of Tumor Metastasis. Science:478-480

29. Vassilev L, Johnson EM (1990). An initiation zone of chromosomal DNA replication located upstream of the c-myc gene in proliferating HeLa cells. Mol Cell Biol 10: 4899-4904

30. Mautner, J, Behrends, U, Hortnagel, K, Brielmeier, M, Hammerschmidt, W, Strobl, L, Bornkamm, GW, Polack, A (1996) c-myc expression is activated by the immunoglobulin kappa-enhancers from a distance of at least 30 kb but not by elements located within 50 kb of the unaltered c-myc locus in vivo. Oncogene 12: 1299-1307

31. Lavenu, A, Pourin, S, Babinet, C, Morello, D (1994) The cis-acting elements known to regulate c-myc expression ex vivo are not sufficient for correct transcription in vivo. Oncogene 9: 527-536

32. Dyson P, Littlewood T, Forster A, Rabbitts TH (1985) Chromatin structure of transcriptionally active and inactive human c-myc alleles. EMBO J 4:2885-2891

33. Grosso LE, Pitot HC (1985) Chromatin structure of the c-myc gene in HL-60 cells during alterations of transcriptional activity .Cancer Res 45: 5035-41

34. Bentley D L, Groudine M (1986) A block to elongation is largely responsible for decreased transcription of c-myc in differentiated HL60 cells. Nature 321: 702-706

35. Michelotti GA, Michelotti EF, Pullner A, Duncan RC, Eick D, Levens D (1996) Multiple Single-Stranded cis Elements Are Associated with Activated Chromatin of the Human c-myc Gene In Vivo. Mol Cell Biol 16:2656-2669

36. Wittig B, Wolfl S, Dorbic T, Vahrson W, Rich A (1992) Transcription of human c-myc in permeabilized nuclei is associated with formation of Z-DNA in three discrete regions of the gene. EMBO J 11: 4653-466.

37. Krumm A., Meulia T, BrunvandM, Groudine M (1992) The block to transcriptional elongation within the human c-myc gene is determined in the promoter-proximal region. Genes Dev 6: 2201-2213

38. Siomi H, Matunis MJ, Michael WM, Dreyfuss G (1993) The pre-mRNA binding K protein contains a novel evolutionarily conserved motif.Nucleic Acids Res 21: 1193-1198

39. Siomi H, Choi M, Siomi MC, Nussbaum RL, Dreyfuss G (1994) Essential role for KH domains in RNA binding: impaired RNA binding by a mutation in the KH domain of FMR1 that causes fragile X syndrome. Cell 77: 33-39

40. Ashley CT, Wilkinson KD, Reines D, Warren ST (1993FMR1 protein: conserved RNP family domains and selective RNA binding. Science 262: 563-566

41. Wong G, Muller O, Clark R, Conroy L, Moran MF, Polakis P, McCormick F (1992) Molecular cloning and nucleic acid binding properties of the GAP-associated tyrosine phosphoprotein p62. Cell 69: 551-558

42. Kahn J, Yun E, Crothers D (1994) Detection of localized DNA flexibility. Nature 368: 163-166

43. Jensen PR, Loman L, Petra B, Van derWeijden C, Westerhoff HV (1995) Energy Buffering of DNA Structure Fails when Escerichia colia Runs Out of Substrate. J Bact 177:3430-3426

44. Cozzarelli NR, Wang JC (1990) DNA topology and its biological effects. Cold Spring Harbor Laboratory, Cold Spring Habor Press, NY

45. Freeman LA, Garrard WT (1992) DNA Supercoiling in Chromatin Structure and Gene Expression. Crit Rev Eukaryotic Gene Expr. 2:165-209

46. Liu LF, Wang JC (1987) Supercoiling of the DNA template during transcription. Proc Natl Acad Sc. USA 84: 7024-7027.

47. Yin H, Wang MD, Svoboda K, Landick R, Block SM, Gelles J (1995) Transcription Against an Applied Force. Science 270:1653-1657

48. Aller P, Rius C, Mata F, Zorilla A, Cabanas C, Bellon T, Bernabeu C (1992) Camptothecin induces differentiation and stimulates the expression of differentiation-related genes in U937 human promonocytic leukemia cells. Cancer Res 52: 1245-1251

Differential Regulation of the c-MYC P1 and P2 Promoters in the Absence of Functional Tumor Suppressors: Implications for Mechanisms of Deregulated MYC Transcription

K. B. Marcu, A. J. Patel and Y. Yang
Department of Biochemistry and Cell Biology, Institute for Cell and Developmental Biology, State University of New York at Stony Brook, Stony Brook, NY 11794, USA

Introduction

The c-MYC polypeptide plays critical roles in cellular proliferation and differentiation and its dysregulation can lead to abnormal growth, neoplasia and death [1,2]. MYC normally initiates a cell cycle progression program culminating in S phase whilst enforced MYC expression can inhibit cellular differentiation programs and excessive levels of MYC lead to the induction of apoptosis (programmed cell death) [1-3]. The MYC polypeptide functions as a transcriptional activator (a member of the basic-helix-loop-helix family of heterodimerizing proteins) and as such is very likely the master regulator of many genes in diverse cellular contexts [1,2,4]. The pivotal contributions of the MYC polypeptide to cellular gene control and physiology are accomplished by its own tight regulation [1,2,5]. The c-MYC polypeptide and its mRNA are extremely short lived in vivo and are generally expressed at low levels in normal proliferating cells [2,5]. Minor fluctuations in MYC protein and/or mRNA levels can have dramatic outcomes on cellular physiology. Consequently, mammalian MYC gene expression is subject to tight control at multiple levels.

MYC transcription is principally controlled by two promoters regulating both the initiation and effective elongation of MYC mRNAs [2,5]. P2 is the predominant start site, giving rise to 75-90% of cytoplasmic MYC RNAs, whereas P1 generates 10-25% of them. Differential MYC promoter usage has been observed in a variety of cell types with ratios of P1:P2 varying from 0.1 to 1.0 in normal proliferating cells. Circumstances under which the promoter ratio approaches 1.0 or higher have generally been associated with abnormal MYC control. The P2 promoter possesses a TATAA box and two functional initiator (InR) motifs thereby providing multiple pathways for the activation and repression of MYC transcription [2,6]. The murine and human c-MYC promoter regions have been well characterized with about 20 transcription factors having been shown to bind and/or modulate the P1 and P2 promoters [2,7-22]. Most of these factors have positive effects on either P1 or P2 activity or both and some have negative effects. The majority recognize sequences within 400 bp 5' of the P1 start site or in between P1 and P2. Some factor binding sites are unique to the murine and human MYC genes and others are evolutionarilly conserved.

MYC was one of the first cellular genes shown to be subject to transcriptional blockage [23-25]. Nuclear run-on transcription assays performed with proliferating or differentiating human and murine cells revealed a strong block to MYC transcriptional elongation within the gene's first non-coding exon [2,5]. For constitutively active or recently silenced c-MYC genes (visa vi inducible differentiation programs), most RNA polymerase II initiation complexes reside in a paused configuration on the P2 start site, except for long term repressed Myc alleles which do not retain stalled intiation complexes [2,5,26-30]. Processive engagement of such "promoter proximally paused" polymerase II complexes can be enhanced or inhibited by diverse cellular stimuli thereby providing a rapid, differential mode of gene control. [2,5,23-25,31-33]. Loss of transcriptional blockage has been shown to contribute to abnormal MYC regulation [2,5]. The physical invasion of the c-MYC locus by the enhancers and/or locus controlling regions (LCRs) of other chromosomal loci results in dysregulated c-MYC control as evidenced by a shift in promoter usage in favor of P1 and a dramatic, complete loss of transcriptional blockage [2,5,34-36]. The phenomenon of MYC transcriptional blockage has been defined as RNA polymerase holdback or promoter proximal pausing [28,29]. A combination of refined nuclear run-on assays and in vivo mapping of single stranded DNA with potassium permanganate (a single strand selective reagent) on MYC chromosomal loci in mammalian cells have revealed that the majority of RNA polymerase II complexes are actually tethered to the P2 promoter start site [28,29]. Induction of cellular differentiation programs then result in the rapid loss of processive polymerase complexes with all P2 initiation complexes being fixed at the P2 start site. The mechanism of promoter proximal pausing may involve the modulation of recruitment of TFIIH (a general transcription factor complex) required for the effective initiation, clearance and establishment of an elongation competent RNA polymerase holoenzyme [37-39]. Conversion of RNA polymerase II into an elongation mode is believed to in part require the phophorylation of CTD amino acid repeats at its carboxy-terminus mediated by a cell cycle regulated TFIIH associated kinase activity [38,39]. TFIIH recruitment and its mechansim of action are believed to be modulated by the combinatorial effects of DNA bound activators, their interacting co-activators and a "mediator complex" associated with the CTD tail of RNA pol II in vivo which integrates signals for the initiation complex [6,38-41].

Extensive promoter reconstruction experiments have revealed two aspects of the normal MYC promoter as being necessary and sufficient to mediate P2 promoter proximal polymerase pausing: (a) a wild type ME1a1 site positioned about 44 to 58 bp 5' of the P2 start site [26,42], (b) a combination of TATAAA and initiator (InR) elements and (c) a variety of other upstream activator binding sites required for full promoter activity [6]. The ME1a1 element (a 14 bp $GAAG_3AG_4AG_3$ motif 3' of the E2F site in mouse and human) has multiple potentially positive and negative effector functions for the P1 and P2 start sites. The Sp1 and MAZ zinc finger proteins both bind ME1a1 and the former has been shown to transactivate the c-MYC promoter [7,8,43]. MAZ has been shown to have differential effects on the properties of the ME1a1 element that are highly dependent on its regulatory context [44,45]. The CUT homeodomain protein binds to the ME1a1 site and repressed the activity of a MYC promoter driven reporter gene [18]. The same ME1a1 mutations affect Sp1 and MAZ binding [8,44 and other unpublished results] but do not appear to affect CUT binding [18] indicating that it interacts with different though overplapping parts of ME1a1. Interestingly, deletion of the ME1a1 site abrogated the P2 promoter proximal pausing of RNA polymerase [26]. Mutation of the G4 core of the murine ME1a1 site, which abrogates both Sp1 and MAZ binding, has differential negative effects on P2 activity dependent on the cellular context [7,8,43]. The ME1a1 element may represent a molecular switch in c-MYC transcriptional control targeting factors that promote initiation complex assembly and modulating the processivity of the assembled initiation complex and MAZ may participate in both of these processes [7,44-46]. Substitution of the ME1a1 motif by heterologous control elements in combination with downstream TATAAA and InR motifs reconstituted the promoter proximal pause effect implying that this phenomenon could be more general for other cellular genes [6]. However, these experiments were performed with an exogenous MYC gene bearing a portion of the regulatory elements of the endogenous c-MYC locus and these exogenous MYC genes were not serum growth factor responsive like the endogenous c-MYC locus (Mark Groudine, personal communication). More importantly, a key aspect of in vivo c-MYC control was not reconstituted in these latter experiments. Specifically, the presence or absence of the observed promoter proximal pause was not correlated with effective MYC readthrough transcription but it rather behaved like a constitutive, characteristic of the wild type promoter [6]. This is fundamentally different to strong negative effects on MYC mRNA accumulation manifested by the differentiation induced, "promoter proximal pause" at chromosomal MYC loci.

In spite of this extensive knowledge of MYC gene control, we have yet to decipher the mechanistic basis for deregulated MYC transcription. Which cellular controls over MYC have been altered in transformed contexts such that promoter usage shifts from P2 to P1 concomitant with a loss in P2 proximal pausing? What trans-acting factors are largely responsible for these changes? Here, we examined elements regulating P2 promoter activity in cells lacking the RB and P53 tumor supressors as a consequence of enforced expression of the Adenovirus E1A and SV40 LT genes. We show that the P1 and P2 transcripts are differentially controlled by elements residing in between them. No one element was particularly critical for P2 activity (including the well characterized E2F site) while multiple elements acted in concert. Interestingly, the P1 promoter appears to be intrinsically stronger than P2 in this transformed cellular context but its strength is masked not by P2 interference but by negative elements residing within the P2 promoter.

Results and Discussion

Multiple P2 promoter elements act in concert to mediate the output of the P1 and P2 start sites

To determine the individual and combined role(s) of P2 promoter elements for MYC transcriptional control, a group of single and double site directed mutations between the P1 and P2 start sites were generated within a 1.7 Kb murine MYC promoter fragment (WTMBg) [2,7,47]. Six site single and four double site directed mutants between the ME1a2 and ME1a1 P2 promoter elements are displayed in Fig. 1. Mutations were designed by PCR techniques or by more standard in vitro mutagenesis methods [7,48]. Some single mutations inactivated nuclear factor binding to the cores of the ME1a2, E2F and ME1a1 sites (mutants m6, m7 and m23) [7,47,48] while others had less significant effects on factor binding (mutants m8 and m1) and one mutant converted the 3' portion of the Me1a1 GA box into a high affinity Sp1 GC motif. Four double mutants in the ME1a1 (m3), ME1a1/ME1a2 (m2 and m5) and ME1a1/E2F (m6) sites were prepared by combining the PCR generated single mutants. All mutations were confirmed by restriction mapping and DNA sequencing. Mutant MYC promoters were fused to either CAT or human β−globin reporter genes and introduced by a modified calcium phosphate technique into the highly transfectable BING human epithelial line [49,50]. BING cells are a derivative of 293T/17 cells which stably express Adenovirus E1A and SV40 LT genes making them phenotypically negative for the P53 and retinblastoma (RB) tumor suppressors [50,51]. Transfections were monitored by introduction of a CMV promoter driven β-gal reporter gene and in situ β-gal staining revealed up to 95% transfection efficiency. A representative set of RNAse protections are displayed in Fig. 1 and analyzed in Fig. 2. None of the site directed mutations altered the size of the wild type P2 transcript whilst each P1 product was severed into two bands (denoted P1*) which also provided confirmation of each mutation in the exogenously expressed MYC RNAs. Surprisingly, the E2F site 5' of P2 is not essential for its activity even in the presence of free E2F/DP-1 complexes which are not associated with functional

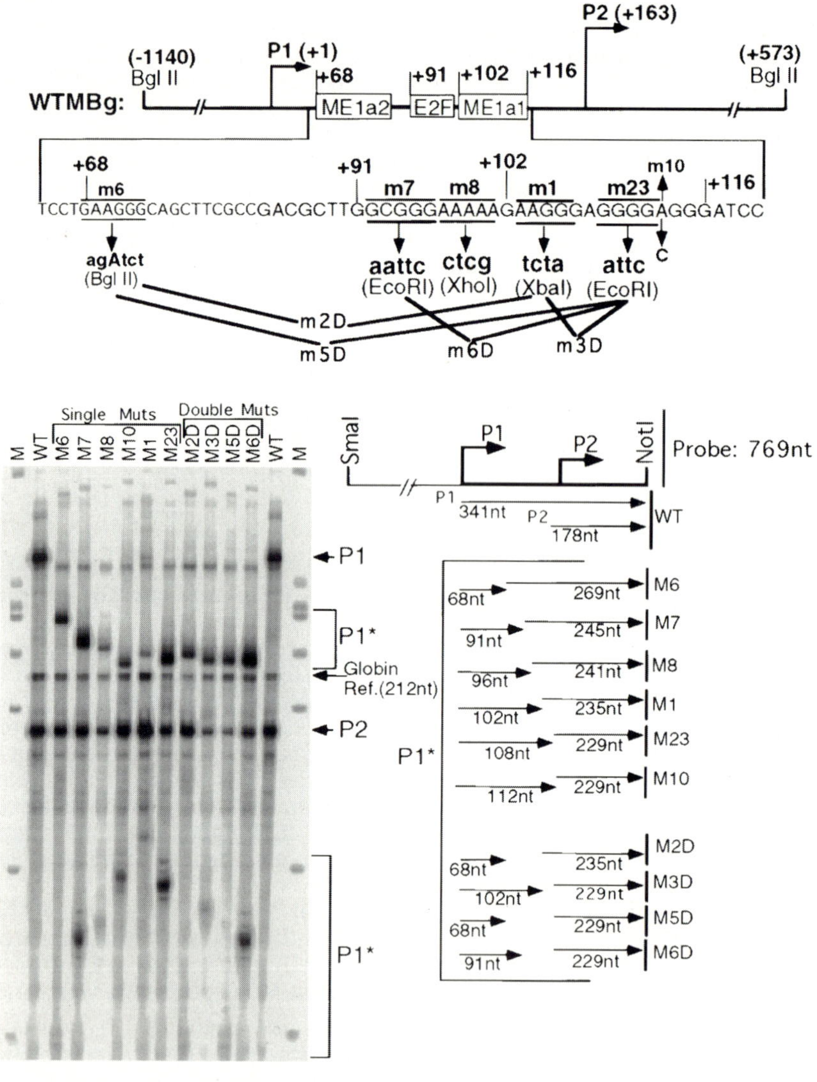

Fig. 1. Top: Locations of the P1 and P2 start sites, nuclear factor binding sites, single and double site sirected mutations. Each mutation generated aunique restriction enzyme site. Bottom: RNAse protections of MYC-reporter chimeras transiently expressed in BINGcells. 10 μg of each MYC construct was co-transfected with 1.0μg of a mouse β-globin gene reference control. MYC and globin probes were mixed and hybridizations performed overnightat 55°C in 50% formamide. Wild type MYC P1 and P2, mutant P1* and mouse β-globin transcripts are indicated.

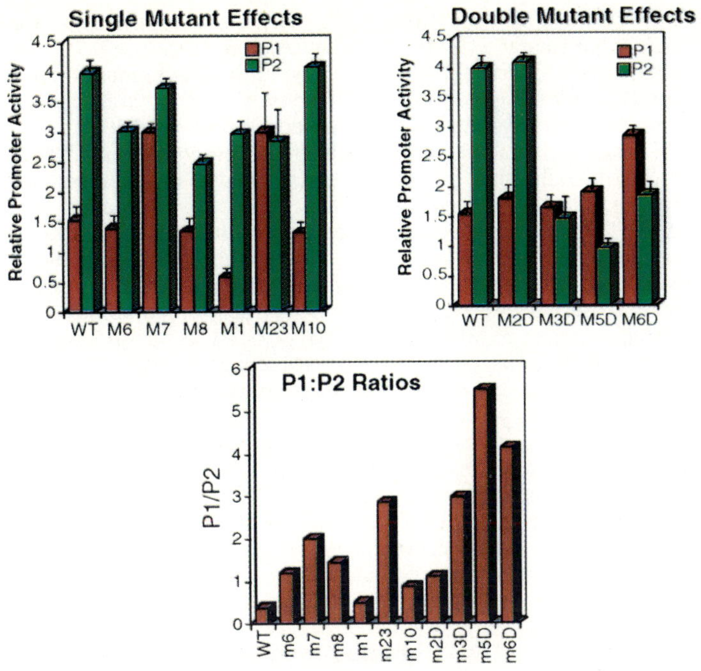

Fig. 2. Quantitative comparisons of single and double P2 promoter mutations on P1 and P2 activites. The relative effects of each mutation are shown in comparison to the wild type promoter (after correcting for transfection variations with the β-globin control) and the same findings are also expressed as P1:P2 ratios. Each experiment was performed three times in duplicate.

pRB, p107 or p130 proteins. Adenovirus E1A and SV40 LT protein dependent transactivation of P2 transcription has been previously reported but each of these former studies either employed 5' P2 deletion mutations (removing considerably more 5' sequence than the P2 E2F site) [11,52,53] or site directed E2F mutations in the context of a -70 minimal P2(ΔP1) promoter [11]. More recently, we demonstrated that this same E2F site was dispensable for v-ABL reponsiveness in the context of a full MYC promoter, though akin to these former E1A and LT studies it was required in a minimal P2 promoter (5' end at -70 relative to P2 at +1) [48]. Use of a such a minimal P2 promoter in the BING line also revealed complete dependence of a wild type E2F site for P2 activity (data not shown). We conclude that additional, uncharacterized E2F sites (most likely located 5' of P1 start) are functionally redundant with the 5' P2 E2F site. In addition, loss of either the ME1a1 or ME1a2 elements have modest inhibitory effects on P2. However, double site directed mutations in ME1a1, ME1a1/ME1a2 or ME1a1/E2F all had severe inhibitory effects for P2 function indicating that they act in concert with each other. A MYC P2 promoter with a high affinity Sp1 site has comparable P1 and P2 activities to the wild type. Surprisingly, mutation of an A run in between the E2F and ME1a1 sites (mutant M8) was the most negative of the single mutants for P2 (60% of wild type function) either indicating that other unknown DNA binding factors are required for P2 activity or that these sequences are in some way required for optimum interactions between the ME1a1, ME1a2 and E2F sites.

Finally, sequences spanning the E2F and MElal sites have unprecendented, significant effects on the accumulation of P1 transcripts independent of their effects on P2 activity. This is most evident for the E2F site directed mutant M7 which has doubled its P1 activity with no significant effect on P2 and a similar magnitude effect for P1 is observed with the MElal site directed mutant M23. These results clearly show for the first time that P1 and P2 transcripts do not interfere with each other but akin to earlier studies also support the notion that P2 promoter elements have dual functions for P1 and P2 activity [7,42,47,54,55]. These observations are specific in that all other single mutants either had no effect on P1 except for M1 which was inhibitory. Double mutations appear to have compensitory effects on P1. Interestingly, the M1 and M23 mutants both reside within the MElal site but their P1 effects are dramatically opposite while their double mutant exhibits near wild type P1 function. These findings suggest that different portions of the MElal sequence differentially modulate P1 transcript processivity. Nuclear run-on assays are in progress to determine if these diverse effects on P1 activity occur at the level of polymerase processivity as we strongly suspect. Earlier studies of the human c-MYC promoter in X. laevis oocytes revealed that sequences overlapping the MElal site contributed to the termination of P1 transcripts upstream of P2 [54,56] and two other studies revealed that a wild type MElal sequence can specifically contribute to the pausing and/or premature termination of upstream transcription units in mammalian cells [42,44]. However, the results presented here indicate for the first time that different portions of the MElal site have strong negative and positive effects on P1 activity.

Effects of MAZ and its DNA binding domain on exogenous P1 and P2 activities

We next determined the effects of the MAZ zinc finger protein on the wild type and MElal mutant c-MYC promoters. Earlier circumstantial evidence implicated MAZ as a transcriptional activator of MElal and related GA box sequences [7,45,57]. More recently over-expressed MAZ was directly shown to be more potent than Sp1 for activating multiple MElal-like sequences in the serotonin 1α receptor gene's promoter [46]. The results of co-transfections of wild type MAZ or M5ZF (a truncated version containing the protein's carboxy-proximal five zinc fingers) and wild type or M23 mutant MYC promoter/reporter constructs into BING cells are shown in Fig. 3. MAZ modestly stimulated the wild type P2 promoter and had a less significant effect on P1. However, its albeit modest effect on P2 was abolished with the M23 site directed MElal mutant. In addition, M5ZF strongly inhibited the activities of P1 and P2 but was weakly stimulating for the M23 mutant version. Exogenous MAZ and M5ZF proteins were revealed by western blotting with the HA epitope specific 12CA5 monoclonal antibody [58] and their sequence specific DNA binding was also confirmed by gel mobility shifts with an MElal probe (data not shown). The steady state levels of MAZ and M5ZF proteins were several fold higher than endogenous MAZ. Taken together these results suggest that MAZ has the potential to activate P2 via the MElal element. The stronger inhibitory effects of M5ZF either suggests that: (1) endogenous MAZ is not limiting in BING cells but can be competed out by its DNA binding domain which may function as a trans-dominant negative version of the protein on exogenous constructs in this cellular context or (2) M5ZF over-expression is interfering with other in vivo positive effector proteins also operating via the MElal site. It is conceiveable that MAZ may be incapable of stimulating the accumulation of P2 transcripts not because of an inability to stimulate transcription initiation but due to limitations imposed by insufficient polymerase processivity. Consequently, nuclear run-on assays are in progress to determine if the direct effects of MAZ on transcriptional activities are comparable. The latter experiments will also reveal if the inhibitory effects of M5ZF on P1 and P2 are at the levels of transcriptional initiation or elongation.

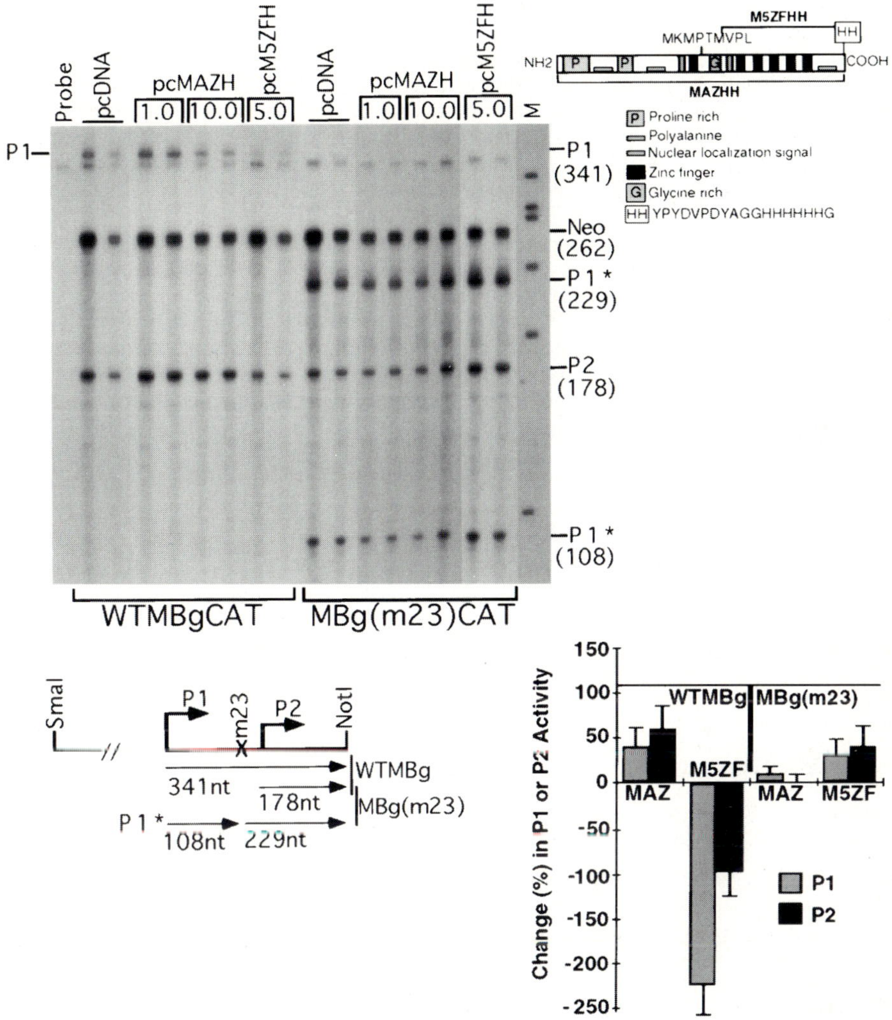

Fig. 3. Effects of MAZ on wild type and ME1a1 mutant MYC promoters. WT and m23 mutant MYC promoter CAT reporters were co-transfected with different amounts of MAZ or M5ZF(MAZ) driven by the CMV promoter in pcDNA(Neo). RNAse protections were performed for MYC P1 and P2 with Neo as a reference control. Negative controls were transfected with comparable amounts of the empty pcDNA(Neo) vector. MAZ, M5ZF and the MYC RNAse mapping probe are shown. MAZ and M5ZF proteins were carboxy-tagged with a hemaglutinin epitope (HA) [58] and histidines to facilitate their detection by westerm blotting and gel mobility shifts. Multiple similar experiments were averaged and analyzed as a function of the wild type or m23 mutant MYC promoter activities. Effects of 1-10 μg of MAZ and M5ZF were comparable.

Conclusions

The results presented herein reveal, that control of the murine c-MYC P1 and P2 promoters in transformed cells lacking the RB and P53 tumor supressors, requires the concerted interaction of multiple elements residing in between the P1 and P2 start sites. Surprisingly, the well characterized E2F element of the P2 promoter was found to be redundant in this context. Positive and negative elements affecting P1 activity were identified and their modes of action were independent of occlusion by the P2 start site. Furtheremore, the MAZ zinc finger protein was found to be a modest, ME1a1-dependent activator while its DNA binding domain was a strong ME1a1 dependent inhibitor of P1 and P2 activities.

We propose that initiation at the P1 start site is intrinsically stronger than P2 in cells lacking tumor suppressors but its effective output is impeded by negative effectors interacting at the P2 promoter, most likely influencing the processivity of P1 transcripts. Exogenous MYC-reporter constructs bearing 1.7 Kb of promoter sequences are sensitive to this negative phenomenon. Subsequent comparisons of the control of chromosomal and exogenous MYC genes in this cellular context will reveal if the former have escaped such P1 repression or if other genetic events are required to achieve full deregulated MYC transcription in neoplasia.

Acknowledgements

This research was supported by American Cancer Society grant VM-120.

References

1. Luscher B, Eisenman RN (1990) New light on MYC and MYB: Part 1. Myc. Genes & Dev. 4: 2025-2035.
2. Marcu KB, Bossone SA and Patel AJ (1992) Myc function and regulation. Annu Rev Biochem 61: 809-860.
3. Evan GI et al (1992) Induction of apoptosis in fibroblasts by c-myc protein. Cell 69: 119-128.
4. Murre C, McCaw PS and Baltimore D (1989) A new DNA binding and dimerization motif in immunoglobulin enhancer binding, daughterless, MyoD, and myc proteins. Cell 56: 777-783.
5. Spencer CA and Groudine M (1991) Control of c-myc regulation in normal and neoplastic cells. Adv Cancer Res 56: 1-48.
6. Krumm A, Hickey LB and Groudine M (1995) Promoter-proximal pausing of RNA polymerase II defines a general rate- limiting step after transcription initiation. Genes Dev 9: 559-572.
7. Bossone SA, Asselin C, Patel AJ and Marcu KB (1992) MAZ, a zinc finger protein, binds to c-MYC and C2 gene sequences regulating transcriptional initiation and termination. Proc Natl Acad Sci U S A 89: 7452-7456.
8. DesJardins E and Hay N (1993) Repeated CT elements bound by zinc finger proteins control the absolute and relative activities of the two principal human c-myc promoters. Mol Cell Biol 13: 5710-5724.
9. Riggs KJ, Saleque S, Wong KK, Merrell KT, Lee JS, Shi Y and Calame K (1993) Yin-yang 1 activates the c-myc promoter. Mol Cell Biol 13: 7487-7495.
10. Hay N, Takimoto M and Bishop JM (1989) A FOS protein is present in a complex that binds a negative regulator of MYC. Genes Dev 3: 293-303.

11. Hiebert SW, Lipp M and Nevins JR (1989) E1A-dependent trans-activation of the human MYC promoter is mediated by the E2F factor. Proc Natl Acad Sci U S A 86: 3594-3598.
12. La RF, Pierce JW and Sonenshein GE (1994) Differential regulation of the c-myc oncogene promoter by the NF-kappa B rel family of transcription factors. Mol Cell Biol 14: 1039-1044.
13. Lipp M, Schilling R and Bernhardt G (1989) Trans-activation of human MYC: the second promoter is target for the stimulation by adenovirus E1a proteins. Oncogene 4: 535-541.
14. Negishi Y, et al (1994) Identification and cDNA cloning of single-stranded DNA binding \ proteins that interact with the region upstream of the human c-myc gene. Oncogene 9: 1133-1143.
15. Numoto M, et al (1993) Transcriptional repressor ZF5 identifies a new conserved domain in zinc finger proteins. Nucleic Acids Res 21: 3767-3775.
16. Roussel MF, Davis JN, Cleveland JL, Ghysdael J and Hiebert SW (1994) Dual control of myc expression through a single DNA binding site targeted by ets family proteins and E2F-1. Oncogene 9: 405-415.
17. Duncan R, Bazar L, Michelotti G, Tomonaga T, Krutzsch H, Avigan M and Levens D (1994) A sequence-specific, single-strand binding protein activates the far upstream element of c-myc and defines a new DNA-binding motif. Genes Dev 8: 465-480.
18. Dufort D and Nepveu A (1994) The human cut homeodomain protein represses transcription from the c- myc promoter. Mol Cell Biol 14: 4251-4257.
19. Berberich SJ and Postel EH (1995) PuF/NM23-H2/NDPK-B transactivates a human c-myc promoter-CAT gene via a functional nuclease hypersensitive element. Oncogene 10: 2343-2347.
20. Filippova GN, et al (1996) An exceptionally conserved transcriptional repressor, CTCF, employs different combinations of zinc fingers to bind diverged promoter sequences of avian and mammalian c-myc oncogenes. Mol. Cell. Biol. 16: 2802-2813.
21. Michelotti EF, Tomonaga T, Krutzsch H and Levens D (1995) Cellular nucleic acid binding protein regulates the CT element of the human c-myc protooncogene. J Biol Chem 270: 9494-9499.
22. Michelotti EF, Michelotti GA, Aronsohn AI and Levens D (1996) Heterogeneous nuclear ribonucleoprotein K is a transcription factor. Mol. Cell. Biol. 16: 2350-2360.
23. Bentley DL and Groudine M (1986) A block to elongation is largely responsible for decreased transcription of c-myc in differentiated HL60 cells. Nature 321: 702-706.
24. Nepveu A and Marcu KB (1986) Intragenic pausing and anti-sense transcription within the murine c-MYC locus. EMBO J. 5: 2859-2865.
25. Eick D and Bornkamm GW (1986) Transcriptional arrest within the first exon is a fast control mechanism in c-myc gene expression. Nucleic Acids Res 14: 8331-8346.
26. Miller H et al (1989) A cis-acting element in the promoter region of the murine c-myc gene is necessary for transcriptional block. Mol Cell Biol 9: 5340-5349.
27. Spencer CA, LeStrange RC, Novak U, Hayward WS and Groudine M (1990) The block to transcription elongation is promoter dependent in normal and Burkitt's lymphoma c-myc alleles. Genes Dev 4: 75-88.
28. Strobl LJ and Eick D (1992) Hold back of RNA polymerase II at the transcription start site mediates down-regulation of c-myc in vivo. Embo J 11: 3307-3314.
29. Krumm A, Meulia T, Brunvand M and Groudine M (1992) The block to transcriptional elongation within the human c-myc gene is determined in the promoter-proximal region. Genes Dev 6: 2201-2213.
30. Wolf DA, Strobl LJ, Pullner A and Eick D (1995) Variable pause positions of RNA polymerase II lie proximal to the c-myc promoter irrespective of transcriptional activity. Nucleic Acids Res 23: 3373-3379.
31. Nepveu A, Marcu KB, Skoultchi AI and Lachman HM (1987) Contributions of transcriptional and post-transcriptional mechansims to the regulation of c-MYC expression in mouse erythroleukemia cells. Genes & Dev. 1: 938-945.
32. Nepveu A et al (1987) Alternative modes of c-MYC regulation in growht factor-stimulated and differentiating cells. Oncogene 1: 243-250.
33. Lindsten T, June CH and Thompson CB (1988) Multiple mechanisms regulate c-myc gene expression during normal T cell activation. Embo J 7: 2787-2794.
34. Strobl LJ, Kohlhuber F, Mautner J, Polack A and Eick D (1993) Absence of a paused transcription complex from the c-myc P2 promoter of the translocation chromosome in Burkitt's lymphoma cells: implication for the c-myc P1/P2 promoter shift. Oncogene 8: 1437-1447.

35. Madisen L and Groudine M (1994) Identification of a locus control region in the immunoglobulin heavy- chain locus that deregulates c-myc expression in plasmacytoma and Burkitt's lymphoma cells. Genes Dev 8: 2212-2226.
36. Polack A, Feederle R, Klobeck G and Hortnagel K (1993) Regulatory elements in the immunoglobulin kappa locus induce c-myc activation and the promoter shift in Burkitt's lymphoma cells. Embo J 12: 3913-3920.
37. Goodrich JA and Tijan R (1994) Transcription factors IIE and IIH and ATP hydrolysis direct promoter clearance by RNA polymerase II. Cell 77: 145-156.
38. Svejstrup JQ, Vichi, P. and Egly, J-P. (1996) The multiple roles of transcription/ repair factor TFIIH. TIBS 21: 346-350.
39. Reines D, Conaway JW and Conaway RC (1996) The RNA polymerase II general elongation factors. TIBS 21: 351-355.
40. Roeder RG (1996) The role of general initiation factors in transcription by RNA polymerase II. TIBS 21: 327-335.
41. Bjorklund S and Kim Y-J (1996) Mediator of transcriptional regulation. TIBS 27: 335-337.
42. Dufort D, Drolet M and Nepveu A (1993) A protein binding site from the murine c-myc promoter contributes to transcriptional block. Oncogene 8: 165-171.
43. Majello B, De LP, Suske G and Lania L (1995) Differential transcriptional regulation of c-myc promoter through the same DNA binding sites targeted by Sp1-like proteins. Oncogene 10: 1841-1848.
44. Ashfield R, Patel AJ, Bossone SA, Brown H, Campbell RD, Marcu KB and Proudfoot NJ (1994) MAZ-dependent termination between closely spaced human complement genes. Embo J 13: 5656-5667.
45. Duncan DD, Stupakoff A, Hedrick SM, Marcu KB and Siu G (1995) A Myc-associated zinc finger protein binding site is one of four important functional regions in the CD4 promoter. Mol Cell Biol 1555: 3179-3186.
46. Parks CL and Shenk T (1996) The serotonin 1a receptor gene contains a TATA-less promoter that responds to MAZ and Sp1. J. Biol. Chem. 271: 4417-4430.
47. Asselin C, Nepveu A and Marcu KB (1989) Molecular requirements for transcriptional initiation of the murine c-MYC gene. Oncogene 4: 549-558.
48. Wong KK, Zou X, Merrell KT, Patel AJ, Marcu KB, Chellappan S and Calame K (1995) v-Abl activates c-myc transcription through the E2F site. Mol Cell Biol 15: 6535-6544.
49. Pear WS, Nolan GP, Scott ML and Baltimore D (1993) Production of high-titer helper-free retroviruses by transient transfection. Proc Natl Acad Sci U S A 90: 8392-8396.
50. Pear WS, Scott, M.L. and Nolan, G.P. (1994). Generation of high titer, helper-free retroviruses by transient transfection. *In* "Methods in Molecular Biology: Methods in Gene Therapy", pp. 1-8.
51. Dubridge RB et al (1987) Analysis of mutation in human cells by using an Epstein-Barr virus shuttle system. Mol. Cell. Biol. 7: 379-387.
52. Thalmeier K, Synovzik H, Mertz R, Winnacker EL and Lipp M (1989) Nuclear factor E2F mediates basic transcription and trans-activation by E1a of the human MYC promoter. Genes Dev 3: 527-536.
53. Batsche E, Lipp M and Cremisi C (1994) Transcriptional repression and activation in the same cell type of the human c-MYC promoter by the retinoblastoma gene protein: antagonisation of both effects by SV40 T antigen. Oncogene 9: 2235-2243.
54. Meulia T, Krumm A, Spencer C and Groudine M (1992) Sequences in the human c-myc P2 promoter affect the elongation and premature termination of transcripts initiated from the upstream P1 promoter. Mol Cell Biol 12: 4590-4600.
55. Roberts S, Purton T and Bentley DL (1992) A protein-binding site in the c-myc promoter functions as a terminator of RNA polymerase II transcription. Genes Dev 6: 1562-1574.
56. Wright S, Mirels LF, Calayag MC and Bishop JM (1991) Premature termination of transcription from the P1 promoter of the mouse c-myc gene. Proc Natl Acad Sci U S A 88: 11383-11387.
57. Kennedy GC and Rutter WJ (1992) Pur-1, a zinc-finger protein that binds to purine-rich sequences, transactivates an insulin promoter in heterologous cells. Proc Natl Acad Sci U S A 89: 11498-11502.
58. Field J, Nikawa J, Broek D, MacDonald B, Rodgers L, Wilson IA, Lerner RA and Wigler M (1988) Purification of a RAS-responsive adenylyl cyclase complex from Saccharomyces cerevisiae by use of an epitope addition method. Mol Cell Biol 8: 2159-2165.

Positive and Negative Regulation of c-*Myc* Transcription

X. ZOU*, Y. LIN*, S. RUDCHENKO and K. CALAME
Departments of Biochemistry and Molecular Biophysics and Microbiology, Columbia University College of Physicians and Surgeons, New York, NY 10032, USA

INTRODUCTION

The c-Myc proto-oncoprotein is well-known to play important roles in determining the growth and development of normal cells [1,2]. c-Myc is required for cells to exit G0 and to enter cycle and is induced as an immediate early gene in response to most mitogenic stimuli. In contrast to the requirement for c-*myc* expression in proliferating cells, c-*myc* expression is shut down in differentiating cells. In fact, addition of exogenous c-Myc blocks terminal differentiation of several hematopoietic cell lines [3-11] and of myogenic cells [12,13] while inhibitors of c-Myc expression accelerate terminal differentiation of promonocytic HL60 cells [14-16], M1 leukemic myeloid cells [17], F9 teratocarcinoma cells [18] and human esophagael cancer cells [19]. Finally, c-Myc plays a role in programmed cell death. Elevated levels of c-Myc can cause apoptosis in certain cells when other factors necessary for their proliferation are absent [20,21]. However, decreased levels of c-Myc can also cause apoptosis in Ramos and WEHI 231 B cell lines upon treatment with anti-immunoglobulin [22,23].

Given the importance of c-Myc in determining growth and differentiation decisions in normal cells, it is not surprising that deregulated expression of c-Myc plays a causal role in many tumors. Molecular mechanisms responsible for deregulated c-Myc expression include gene amplification, chromosomal translocation and retroviral insertion. However, there are also tumors where the mechanism(s) responsible for deregulated c-Myc expression are not well-understood.

We report here results from two studies focused on transcriptional regulation of c-*myc*. In the first, we have identified the mechanism which appears to be responsible for shutting down c-Myc expression in B lymphocytes upon their terminal differentiation to non-dividing plasma cells. This represents a case where c-*myc* is the target of a protein which drives terminal differentiation. In the second, we have studied how the v-Abl non-receptor tyrosine kinase activates transcription of the c-*myc* gene. This represents a case where the c-*myc* gene is a critical target of a transforming oncoprotein.

RESULTS

Plasmacytoma Repressor Factor Is Encoded by the *Blimp-1* Gene.

We have previously described a plasmacytoma-specific repressor of c-*myc* transcription termed Plasmacytoma Repressor Factor (PRF), which binds a site located 290 bp upstream of the P1 transcriptional start site in the c-*myc* gene [24,25]. The PRF site sequence is nearly identical to an interferon stimulated response element (ISRE) and to the positive regulatory domain 1 (PRD1) in the β–IFN promoter. Electrophoretic mobility shift assays were used to investigate the possible relationship between PRF and various proteins which are known to bind ISRE and PRD1 sites. First we found that oligonucleotide competitors containing either ISRE or PRD1 sequences competed for PRF binding, but that PRD1 sequences competed significantly better. IRF-1 and IRF-2 bind the PRF site, but antiserum to them does not affect the PRF complex. However, antiserum to Blimp-1, the murine homologue of PRF1-BF1 which binds to the PRD1

* The first two authors contributed equally to this work.

site, ablated formation of the PRF complex (not shown). Thus, PRF is immunologically related to PRD1-BF1/Blimp-1

Blimp-1 is induced upon stimulation of the BCL_1 B-cell lymphoma line with IL-2 + IL-5 [26]. Ectopic expression of Blimp-1 can drive B-cell terminal differentiation and Blimp-1 is expressed only in plasmacytomas and mature B cells; however its mechanism of action is not well-understood [26].

To investigate the functional relationship between PRF and Blimp-1, we tested the effect of ectopically expressed Blimp-1 on the activity of the c-*myc* promoter. Reporters dependent upon a c-*myc* promoter with either wild type or mutated PRF sites were cotransfected with a Blimp-1 expression plasmid into the 1881 pre-B cell line. Wild type and mutant promoters had similar activity in the absence of Blimp-1 (Fig. 1). However, expression of Blimp-1 repressed the wild type promoter 3-4 fold while the promoter harboring a mutation in the PRF site was not repressed (Fig. 1). Thus we

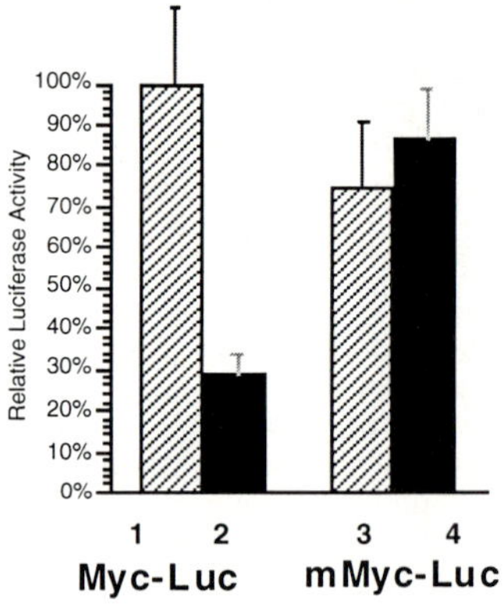

Fig. 1 Blimp-1 represses the *c-myc* promoter in a PRF site-dependent manner in pre-B cells. 2 μg of a luciferase reporter fused with either a wild type (BBluc) or PRF-deleted (mPRF BBluc) c-*myc* promoter [24] with 10 μg of blimp-1 expression vector (pBDP1-F) or expression vector control (pBDP1-B) [26] were transfected into 1881 pre-B cells by electroporation; cells were harvested 18 hr post-transfection and luciferase activities were measured. Results show the average of at least 3 independent transfections and the bars show standard deviations.

conclude that ectopic Blimp-1 represses c-*myc* transcription in pre-B cells and the repression depends upon the presence of the PRF site at -290 bp. Since the function of Blimp-1 is the same as that of PRF, these data, in conjunction with the *in vitro* binding studies, lead us to conclude that PRF is encoded by the *blimp-1* gene.

Blimp-1 induction during differentiation of BCL_1 cells is followed by a reduction in c-Myc.

BCL_1 is a mature B-cell line which terminally differentiates upon stimulation with IL2 + IL5 [27,28]. Blimp-1 is induced early in BCL_1 differentiaion [26]. Based on the ability of transfected Blimp-1 to repress the c-*myc* promoter, we predicted that differentiation-dependent induction of Blimp-1 in BCL_1 cells would cause a decrease in endogenous c-Myc. 72 hr after BCL_1 cells were treated with IL2 + IL5, differentiation was verified by increased immunoglobulin secretion and changes in cell size as indicated by changes in forward vs. orthogonal scatter (not shown). c-Myc levels during this period were assessed by immunoblot (Fig. 2A). Following a transient increase, c-Myc levels decreased approximately four fold between 1 and 2 hrs of IL2 + IL5 stimulation and remained low for 24 hr. Northern analyses showed that 1 hr after stimulation, *Blimp-1* mRNA increased approximately 5 fold, as previously reported [26] (Fig. 2B). These data are consistent with the notion that Blimp-1 represses endogenous c-*myc* transcription, leading to decreased c-Myc protein levels.

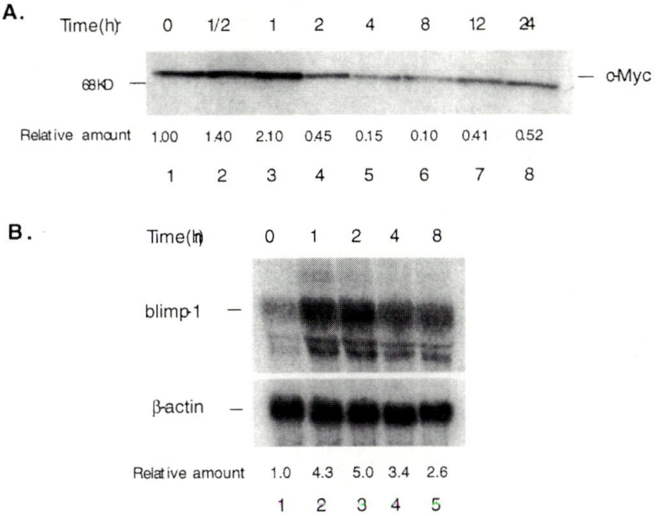

Fig. 2 Blimp-1 induction and c-Myc reduction during BCL_1 cell differentiation. (A) BCL_1 cells were treated with IL2 + IL5 and whole cell extracts were prepared at various time. 10 μg of each sample was electrophoresed on SDS-polyacrylamide gels (8%), transferred to a nitrocellulose membrane and immunoblotted with polyclonal antiserum raised against the C-terminus of murine c-Myc. The bands were quantitated and the amounts relative to that prior to treatment (0 hr) are shown below the lanes. (B) RNA was also prepared and analyzed by Northern blotting using a *blimp-1* cDNA probe (26) and a control *β–actin* probe. The relative amounts of *blimp-1* mRNA are given below the lanes.

Ectopic expression of Blimp-1 in 18-81 pre-B cells leads to a dramatic reduction of c-Myc and to apoptosis.

To obtain more direct evidence for the notion that Blimp-1 represses c-*myc* transcription in B cells, we stably transfected pre-B cells with a Blimp-1 expression plasmid containing the neo^R gene. However, few G418-resistant clones were obtained, demonstrating that over-expression of Blimp-1 suppressed cell growth as measured by neo^R colony formation (not shown). We speculated that Blimp-1-dependent suppression of growth might be caused directly by the decreased abundance of c-Myc. Therefore, we tested whether ectopic expression of c-Myc could reverse Blimp-1-dependent growth suppression. As before, few colonies were obtained with the Blimp-1 expression plasmid. However, co-expression of c-Myc partially reversed Blimp-1 suppression of growth. Compared to control antisense Blimp-1 and c-*myc* plasmids, transfections with Blimp-1 sense and c-*myc* plasmids gave 17-65% the number of control colonies, depending on the ratio of c-*myc* to Blimp-1 plasmid transfected. This demostrates that ectopic c-Myc blocks the growth suppressing effect of high Blimp-1 expression. The simplest interpretation of these results is that repression of *c-myc* transcription by over-expressed Blimp-1 is directly responsible for the failure of Blimp-1 over-expressing cells to grow.

To obtain additional support for this suggestion, we introduced an expression plasmid in which Blimp-1 was under the control of an inducible metallothionein promoter into 18-81 cells. Upon induction of Blimp-1 by cadmium, c-Myc levels decreased dramatically (Fig. 3A). Cadimum treatment also caused cell death and this death appeared to result from apoptosis, as indicated by the observed fragmentation of genomic DNA (Fig. 3B). Thus we conclude that Blimp-1 is a potent repressor of c-*myc* transcription in B cells and that in the context of Abelson-transformed pre-B cells, decreased c-Myc leads to programmed cell death.

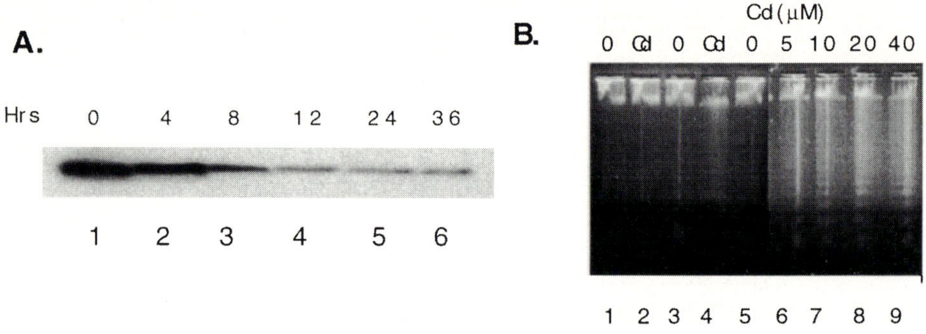

Fig. 3 Induction of Blimp-1 in 18-81 cells causes repression of c-Myc levels and apoptosis. 18-81 cells were transfected with sheep metallothionine promoter controlled Blimp-1 expression vector (MT-Blimp-1) and stable transfectants were generated. (A) The stably transfected 18-81 cells were treated with 20μM $CdCl_2$ and whole cell extracts were prepared at various time. 10μg of each sample was used for immunoblot with polyclonal anti-c-Myc antiserum. (B) The 18-81 cells were treated with or without 20μM $CdCl_2$(Lane 1 to 4) or various amount of $CdCl_2$. 36 hours later, the genomic DNA from each sample(~$1X10^6$ cells) was prepared and subjected to 1.5% agarose electrophoresis. Lane 1 and 2, 18-81 vector control cell line. Lane 3 to 9, MT-Blimp-1 transfected cell line.

Ras GTPase and Raf Ser/Thr Kinase Are Required for the Induction of c-*Myc* Transcription by v-Abl

Our previous work suggested that induction of c-*myc* transcription by v-Abl depended on initiation of a phosphorylation cascasde [29]. We wondered if this pathway involved activation of the Ras GTPase which, like induction of c-*myc* [30] is required for Abl-dependent transformation [31,32]. To test this hypothesis, we utilized our previously developed co-transfection assay [29]. v-Abl activated a c-*myc* promoter reporter approximately 6 fold compared with the appropriate control lacking v-Abl cDNA. However, in the presence of dominant negative Ras N17, v-Abl-dependent activation was completely ablated (Fig. 4A); similar results were obtained using a more truncated promoter from the c-*myc* gene (Fig. 4B). We then tested the effect of cotransfecting a plasmid encoding a constitutively active Ras mutant, Ras V12 [33]. Ras V12 activated c-*myc* transcription and v-Abl was unable to activate it further in the presence of Ras V12 (Fig. 4A). These results show that Ras GTPase activity is required downstream of v-Abl for v-Abl to activate c-*myc* transcription.

The serine/threonine kinase Raf1 is an immediate downstream effector for many Ras-dependent events [34] The same approach was used to ask if Raf1 was required for v-Abl-dependent activation of c-*myc* transcription. Expression of RafC4, a dominant negative form of Raf1 [35], efficiently inhibited activation of both c-*myc* promoters by v-Abl (Figs. 4B and 5A). In addition, a constitutively active mutant of Raf1, RafBXB [35] activates the c-*myc* promoter alone and there is no further activation with v-Abl (Fig. 5A). To be sure that expression of dominant negative forms of Ras and Raf did not inhibit activation of c-*myc* transcription non-specifically, we tested the ability of the p65 subuint of NF-κB to activate the c-*myc* promoter in the absence or presence of dominant negative Ras or Raf since NF-κB activation does not involve Ras or Raf. We cotransfected a p65 expression plasmid with -1100/+580Luc, a larger c-*myc* promoter reporter construct which contains the two NF-κB responsive sites [36,37], into 4A2 cells. p65 activated this reporter approximately 5 fold (Fig. 5B). In the presence of dominant negative Ras N17 or dominant negative RafC4, p65 still fully activated c-*myc* transcription. Thus we conclude that inhibition of v-Abl-dependent activation of c-*myc* transcription by Ras N17 and RafC4 is specific. Taken together these data demonstrate that activation of the Ras GTPase and Raf serine/threonine kinase are required

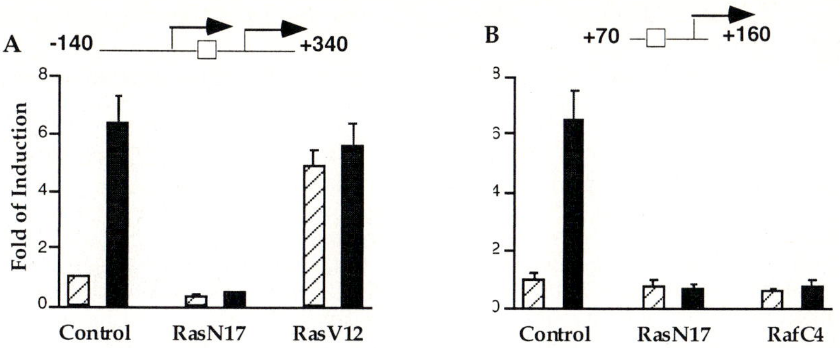

Fig. 4 Ras is required for v-Abl-Dependent Induction of c-Myc Transcription. 4A2 cells were transfected with 5μg of a luciferase reporter dependent upon regions of the murine c-*myc* promoter diagrammed above the data and expression plasmids for v-Abl and dominant negative (N17) or constitutive active (V12) Ras, indicated below. The striped bars were transfected with 5μg pLTR, the control expression plasmid. The filled bars were transfected with 5μg pAB160-19wt, expression plasmid encoding wild type v-Abl. The average luciferase activity of unstimulated cells transfected with vector plasmid was set as 1. The fold-induction shown is the mean and standard deviation determined from three independent transfections of one representative experiment.

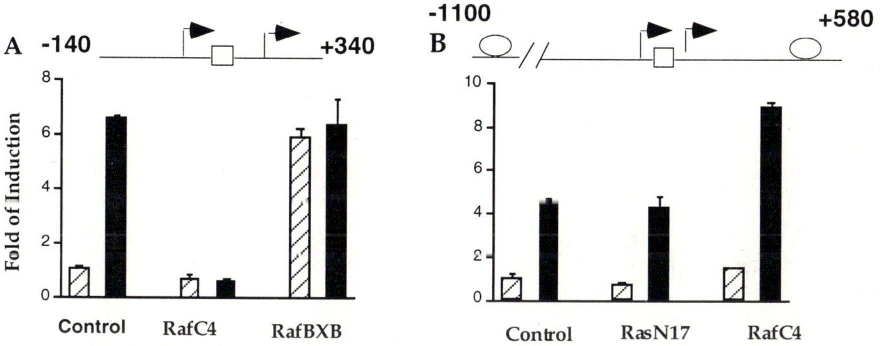

Fig. 5 Raf1 is Required for v-Abl-Dependent Activation of c-*Myc* Transcription. A. 4A2 cells were cotransfected as in Fig. 4 with a luciferase reporter dependent upon the c-*myc* promoter and expression vectors for DN Raf (C4) or constitutively active Raf (BXB). Hashed bars are control and filled bars are with a v-Abl expression plasmid. B. A reporter dependent upon a larger fragement of the c-*myc* promoter was cotransfected with expression plasmids for DN Ras or Raf without (hashed) or with (filled) an expression plasmid for p65.

downstream effectors for v-Abl-dependent transactivation of c-*myc* transcription. In a parallel set of experiments, using a dominant negative form of the Rac GTPase, we found that Rac was not required for v-Abl to induce c-*myc* transcription in this system (data not shown).

v-Abl Activates Cyclin-dependent-kinases and Cdk Activity Is Required for v-Abl-dependent Induction of c-*Myc* Transcription.

The activity of E2F-DP heterodimers is modulated by association with Rb family proteins and the ability of Rb family proteins to associate is regulated by phosphorytion [38-41]. Rb family proteins are phosphorylated by cyclin-dependent kinases: cdk4-Cyclin D is active early in G1 and cdk2-CyclinE is active later in G1 [38]. Therefore we asked if cdk activity changed in response to v-Abl signaling.

We took advantage of the D5 cell line, a 3T3 subclone transformed with a temperature-sensitive form of v-Abl [42]. D5 cells were made quiesent by serum starvation at 39°C for 48 hr. Subsequently the temperature was shifted to 32°C to activate v-Abl and initiate v-Abl-dependent proliferation. Cdk2 was immunoprecipitated from the D5 cultures at various times following temperature shift and kinase activity was assayed *in vitro* using histone H1 as substrate. Cdk2 activity increased following activation of v-Abl upon temperature shift from 39°C to 32°C. An increase in cdk2 activity was observed at 2 hr and reached maximal level by 8 hr (Fig. 6). During this period, the amount of cdk2 protein, determined by immunoblot, did not change significantly. The D-type cyclin-associated kinase activity was also examined in this system by immunoprecipitation with cyclin D1 antibodies at various time following temperature shift, and the associated kinase activity was assayed by using GST-Rb substrates. Smaller but reproducible increases in kinase activity were observed (not shown). During this period, the amount of cdk4 protein, determined by immunoblot did not change significantly. Thus, we observe a v-Abl-dependent increase in cdk activity, especially for cdk2, which is consistent with the possiblity of v-Abl-dependent phosphorylation of Rb-family proteins and subsequent activation of E2F proteins.

To test directly if cdk activity is required for v-Abl-dependent induction of c-*myc* transcription, we expressed p21 in the co-transfection assay along with v-Abl and the reporter dependent on the *c-myc* promoter. p21 is a universal inhibitor of cdk activity [43]. v-Abl activated the -140/+340Luc c-*myc* promoter reporter approximately 6 fold

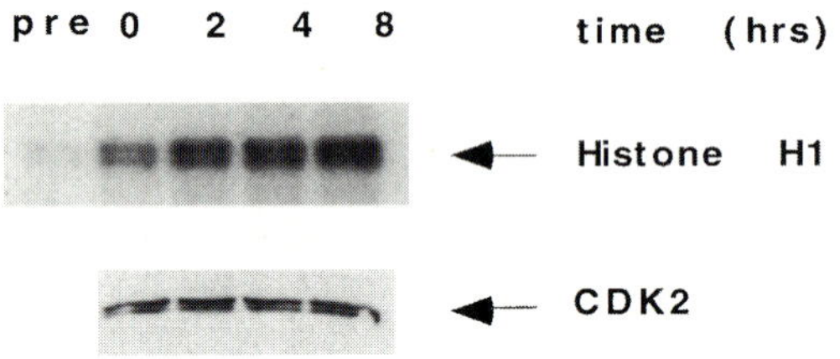

Fig. 6 v-Abl activates cdk2. D5 cells were made quiesent by serum starvation at 39°C for 48 hrs, then shifted to 32°C and harvested at indicated time points. Lysates (50μg of protein) were immunoprecipitated with an anti-cdk2 antibody or preimmune serum. Immune complexes were assayed for kinase activity using histone H1 as substrates. ^{32}P-labeled histone H1 was shown. Lower panel: The same protein lysates as in the upper panel were immunblotted with anti-cdk2 antibody.

(Fig. 7A); however, in the presence of p21, this activation was completely ablated. As a control, we examined the effect of p21 on v-Abl-dependent activation of a reporter dependent upon a SRE. Since v-Abl-dependent activation of a SRE requires Rac [44], it appears to proceed by a different signal transduction path. v-Abl activated SRE-Fluc more than 6 fold (Fig. 7B) and this activation was not affected by co-transfection of the p21 expression plasmid. Thus, inhibition of v-Abl-dependent induction by p21 expression is specific for c-*myc* transcription and is not required for SRE-dependent transcription. We conclude that cdk activity is required for transactivation of c-*myc* transcription by v-Abl.

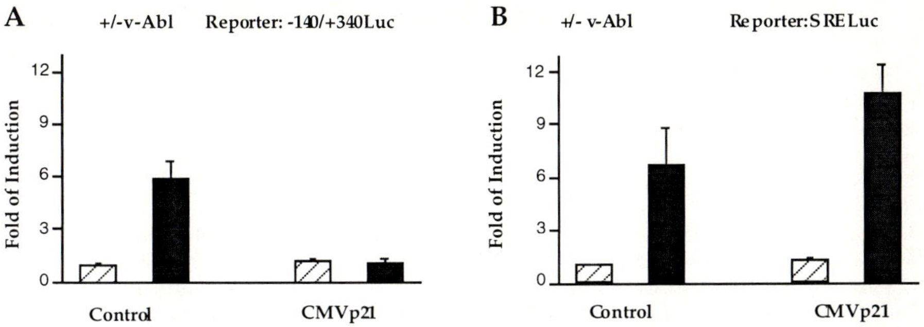

Fig. 7 Cdk Activity is Required for v-Abl-Dependent Activation of c-Myc Transcription. 4A2 cells were transfected with 5μg of a reporter containing the c-*myc* promoter (A) or a reporter dependent upon c-*fos* SRE site (B) and the control (hashed bars) or v-Abl (filled bars) expression plasmids. As indicated below, control or p21 expression plasmids were also included.

Rb-Family Proteins Are Hyperphosphorylated in Response to v-Abl Signalling and Rb Blocks Induction of c-*Myc* by v-Abl.

Since Rb family proteins are primary substrates of cdks, as well as regulators of E2F proteins, we examined the phosphorylation states of Rb, p107 and p130 in D5 cells by immunoblotting. Several forms of Rb were apparent prior to temperature shift; following temperature shift, the percentage of hyperphosphorylated ppRb increased from 40% at 0 hr to more than 80% at 8 hr (not shown). Similarly, p107 and p130 also became increasingly phosphorylated following v-Abl activation by temperature shift.

Association of E2F-DP heterodimers with pRb, p107 and/or p130 inhibits their ability to act as transcriptional activators and can create transcriptional repressors [41]. Thus our results are consistent with a model in which v-Abl signaling results in activation of cdks, phosphorylation of Rb-family proteins, release of Rb proteins from association with E2F-DP and, finally, activation of c-*myc* transcription via the E2F site. To further test this model, we used the cotransfection assay to test if overexpression of Rb could block v-Abl-dependent transactivation of c-*myc* transcription. Our results show that ectopic Rb does block c-*myc* transcription in this assay (Fig. 8). These results are consistent with the idea that c-*myc* transcription is sensitive to the levels of hypophosphorylated Rb and lend support to the suggestion that v-Abl activation via E2F sites depends upon phosphorylation of Rb-family proteins.

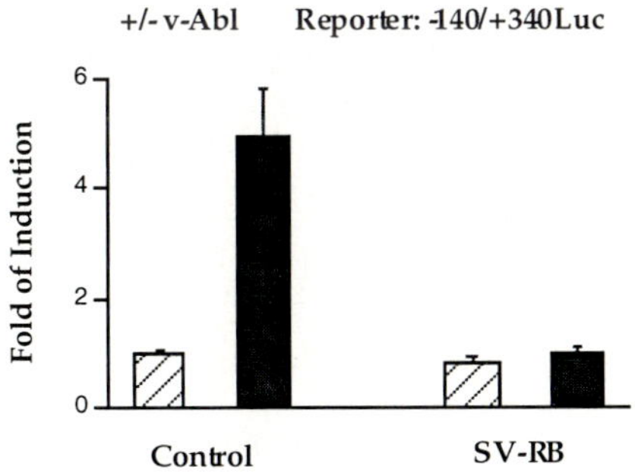

Fig. 8 Rb Inhibits the Ability of v-Abl to Induce c-*Myc* Transcription. 4A2 cells were transfected with 5μg of the c-*myc* reporter and the combination of v-Abl and pRB expression plasmids. Lanes: 1 and 2, control plasmid; 3 and 4, 5μg of pSV-RB, expression plasmid for Rb.

DISCUSSION

c-*Myc* as a Target Gene for Blimp-1, a Master Regulator of B-cell Terminal Differentiation. Our data identify the c-*myc* gene as an important target of the Blimp-1 transcriptional regulator and underscore the importance of repressing c-*myc* during terminal B-cell differentiation. This is consistent with previous studies showing that expression of c-*myc* is incompatible with terminal differentiation [3-12] and with the identification of Blimp-1 as a master regulator of terminal B-cell differentiation [26]. Although c-Myc's role in blocking terminal differentiation has been well-established, Blimp-1 is the first transcription factor shown to specifically repress c-*myc* transcription as part of a program of terminal differentiation. It will be particularly interesting to determine if Blimp-1 has other important target genes in B cells or if repression of c-*myc* is sufficient to trigger terminal differentiation.

The restricted pattern of Blimp-1 expression [25,26] suggests that the Blimp-1-mediated suppression of c-*myc* transcription may be a mechanism which is unique to B lymphocytes. However, the human homologue PRD1-BF1 is induced upon viral infection of fibroblasts [45] and preliminary results show that Blimp-1 deficient mice die during embryonic development (M. Davis, personal communication). Therefore, it will be important to determine if Blimp-1 also represses c-*myc* transcription in other lineages of terminally differentiated cells.

A Phosphorylation Cascade from v-Abl to Induction of c-*Myc* Transcription.

We have identified key components of the signaling pathway between v-Abl and activated E2F site binding proteins. Dominant negative as well as constitutively active forms of Ras, Raf1 and Rac were used in cotransfection assayes to show that E2F-activation requires Ras and Raf1 but is independent of Rac. Although we have no direct evidence for activation of cdc25A, we infer that it occurs. A role for cyclin dependent kinases was established by the inhibition of c-*myc* induction with cdk inhibitor p21 and the demonstration that v-Abl causes activation of cdk2 and cdk4. Finally, v-Abl-dependent induction of c-*myc* was shown to be accompanied by hyperphosphorylation of three pocket proteins, Rb, p107 and p130. Hyperphosphorylation of these proteins releases and thereby activates E2F transcription factors.

Based on our data, we propose that v-Abl induces c-*myc* transcription by the following pathway: v-Abl, Shc, Grb2/Sos, Ras, Raf1, cdc25A, cdk2/4-, hyperphosphorylated pRb family proteins, activated E2F proteins, activated c-*myc* transcription. This path may not be the only way v-Abl induces c-*myc*, and it is clearly not the only signaling pathway which v-Abl utilizes to carry out its full program of cell transformation. However, this represents the most complete understanding to date of a signaling pathway from v-Abl to a functionally important target gene.

There is evidence that Raf1 activates cdc25A which in turn activates cdks [46]. The regulation of E2F transription factors by cdk-mediated phosphorylation of Rb family proteins and the ability of E2F proteins to regulate c-*myc* transcription are also well-established [41,47]. This is all consistent with the pathway we propose and with our suggestion that cdc25 action ultimately regulates c-*myc* transcription. However, c-Myc/Max was recently shown to activate transcription of cdc25A at a time in G1 when c-Myc induction peaks [48]. This is consistent with previous work showing that c-Myc stimulates the activity of cyclin E- and cyclin D1-dependent kinases, possibly via cdc25, and leads to hyperphosphorylation of pRb [49]. c-Myc has also been reported to activate transcription of cylin A and D1 and there are binding sites for c-Myc/Max in the E2F1 promoter [50,51]. These data raise the possibility that in D5 cells v-Abl activates E2F proteins by another Ras/Raf-dependent path and the subsequent increase in c-Myc induces transcription of cdc25, Cyclin D1, Cyclin A and/or E2F1. Thus c-Myc would be the cause, rather than the result, of increased cdk2 and cdk4 activity, hyperphosphorylation pRB, p107 and p130 and altered E2F-binding proteins which we observe. However, this model is not consistent with our observation that p21 blocks the ability of v-Abl to transactivate c-*myc*, which establishes a requirement for cdk action in the path from v-Abl to c-*myc*. We favor the view that v-Abl, and probably normal mitogens, lead to a dynamic situation with multiple autoregulatory loops in which c-Myc, cdc25, cdks and E2F1 can be both regulators and subject to regulation.

REFERENCES

1. Ryan, K. M. and Birnie, G. D. (1996) Biochemical Journal, 314(Pt 3), 713-21.
2. Marcu, K., Bossone, S. and Patel, A. (1992) Ann Rev Biochem, 61, 809-860.
3. Lachman, H. M. and Skoultchi, A. I. (1984) Nature, 310(5978), 592-4.
4. Resnitzky, D., Yarden, A., Zipori, D. and Kimchi, A. (1986) Cell, 46, 31-40.
5. Westin, E. H., Wong, S. F., Gelmann, E. P., Dalla, F. R., Papas, T. S. and Lautenberger. (1982) Proc Natl Acad Sci U S A, 79(8), 2490-4.
6. Einat, M., Resnitzky, D. and Kimchi, A. (1985) Nature, 313(6003), 597-600.
7. Chisholm, O. and Symonds, G. (1992) Int J Cancer, 51(1), 149-58.
8. Selvakumaran, M., Liebermann, D. and Hoffman-Liebermann, B. (1993) Blood, 81(9), 2257-62.
9. Coppola, J. and Cole, M. D. (1986) Nature, 320, 760-763.
10. Prowchownik, E. V. and Kukowska, J. (1986) Nature, 322, 848-850.
11. Dimitrowsky, E., Kuehl, W., Hollis, G. F., Kirsch, I. R., Bender, T. P. and Segal, S. (1986) Nature, 322, 748-750.
12. Miner, J. H. and Wold, B. J. (1991) Mol Cell Biol, 11(5), 2842-2851.
13. La Rocca, S. A., Crouch, D. H. and Gillespie, D. A. (1994) Oncogene, 9, 3499-3508.
14. Yokoyama, K. and Imamoto, F. (1987) Proc Natl Acad Sci USA, 83, 6480-84.
15. Holt, J. T., Redner, R. L. and Nienhuis, A. W. (1988) Mol Cell Biol, 8, 963-73.
16. Wickstrom, E. L., Bacon, T. A., Gonzalez, A., Freeman, D. L., Lyman, G. H. and Wickstrom, E. (1988) Proc Natl Acad Sci USA, 85(4), 1028-1032.
17. Nguyen, H. Q., Selvakumaran, M., Liebermann, D. A. and Hoffman, B. (1995) Oncogene, 11(11), 2439-44.
18. Griep, A. E. and Westphal, H. (1988) Proc Natl Acad Sci USA, 85, 6806-6810.
19. Zhao, X., Wang, X., Zhou, C., Peng, R., Yan, S. and Wu, M. (1995) Science in China - Series B, Chemistry, Life Sciences & Earth Sciences, 38(5), 580-9.
20. Littlewood, T. D. and Evan, G. I. (1990) Adv Dent Res, 4, 69-79.
21. Evan, G., Wyllie, A., Gilbert, C., Littlewood, T., Land, H., Brooks, M., Waters, C., Penn, L. and Hancock, D. (1992) Cell, 69, 119-28.
22. Kaptein, J. S., Lin, C. K. E., Wang, C. L., Nguyen, T. T., Kalunta, C. I., Park, E., Chen, F. S. and Lad, P. M. (1996) J Biol Chem 271(31), 18875-84.
23. Wu, M., Arsura, M., Bellas, R., Fitzgerald, M., Lee, H., Schauer, S., Sherr, D. and Sonenshein, G. (1996) Mol Cell Biol, 16, 5015-25.
24. Kakkis, E. and Calame, K. (1987) Proc Natl Acad Sci U S A, 84(20), 7031-5.
25. Kakkis, E., Riggs, K. J., Gillespie, W. and Calame, K. (1989) Nature, 339(6227), 718-21.
26. Turner, C. A., Mack, D. and Davis, M. M. (1994) Cell, 77, 297-306.
27. Blackman, M., Tigges, M., Minie, M. E. and Koshland, M. E. (1986) Cell, 47, 609-617.
28. Matsui, K., Nakanishi, K., Cohen, D. I., Hada, T., Furuyama, J. I., Hamaska, T. and Higashino, K. (1989) J Immunol, *1*42, 2918-2923.
29. Raffel, G. D., Parmar, K. and Rosenberg, N. (1996) J Biol Chem, 271(9), 4640-5.
30. Sawyers, C., Callahan, W. and Witte, O. (1992) Cell, 70, 901-910.
31. Sawyers, C. L., McLaughlin, J. and Witte, O. N. (1995) J Exp Med, 181(1), 307-13.
32. Goga, A., McLaughlin, J., Afar, D. E., Saffran, D. C. and Witte, O. N. (1995) Cell, 82(6), 981-8.
33. Maru, Y. and Witte, O. (1991) Cell, 67, 459-68.

34. Clark, S. S., McLaughlin, J., Crist, W. M., Champlin, R. and Witte, O. (1987) Science, 235, 85-88.
35. Bruder, J. T., Heidecker, G. and Rapp, U. R. (1992) Genes & Dev, 6(4), 545-56.
36. Duyao, M. P., Kessler, D. J., Spicer, D. B. and Sonenshein, G. E. (1990) Curr Top Microbiol Immunol, 166, 211-20.
37. Duyao, M. P., Buckler, A. J. and Sonenshein, G. E. (1990) Proc Natl Acad Sci USA, 87(12), 4727-31.
38. Weinberg, R. A. (1995) Cell, 81, 323-330.
39. Chen, P. L., Riley, D. J. and Lee, W. H. (1995) Critical Reviews in Eukaryotic Gene Expression, 5(1), 79-95.
40. Adams, P. D. and Kaelin, W. G., Jr. (1995) Seminars in Cancer Biology, 6(2), 99-108.
41. Cobrinik, D. (1996) Current Topics in Microbiology and Immunology, 208, 31-61.
42. Renshaw, M., Kiipreos, E., Albrecht, M. and Wang, J. (1992) EMBO J, 11, 3941-51.
43. Kelliher, M. A., McLaughlin, J. and Witte, O. (1990) Proc Natl Acad Sci USA, 87, 6649-53.
44. Elefanty, A. G., Hariharan, I. K. and Cory, S. (1990) EMBO J., 9, 1069-//.
45. Keller, A. and Maniatis, T. (1991) Genes & Dev, 5, 868-79.
46. Galaktionov, K., Jessus, C. and Beach, D. (1995) Genes and Dev, 9, 1046-58.
47. Slansky, J. E. and Farnham, P. J. (1996) Current Topics in Microbiology & Immunology, 208, 1-30.
48. Cooper, J. (1991) Meth Enzymol, 201, 251-61.
49. (1988) Antibodies, A Laboratory Manual (Harlow, E., and Lane, D., Eds.), Cold Spring Harbor Laboratory, Cold Spring Harbor.
50. Jansen-Durr, P., Meichle, A., Steiner, P., Pagano, M., Finke, K., Botz, J., Wessbecher, J., Draetta, G. and Eilers, M. (1993) Proc Natl Acad Sci USA 90(8), 3685-9.
51. Boyle, W. J., van der Geer, P. and Hunter, T. (1991) Meth Enzymol, 201, 110-143.

Structure and Expression of the c-Myc/Pvt 1 Megagene Locus

D. Siwarski[1], U. Müller[2], J. Andersson[2], V. Notario[3],
F. Melchers[2], A. Rolink[2] and K. Huppi[1]
[1] Lab. of Genetics, NCI, Bethesda, MD, USA
[2] Basel Institute for Immunology, Basel, Switzerland
[3] Department of Radiation Medicine, Georgetown University Medical Center, Washington, D.C., USA

Abstract

A chromosomal translocation (Tx) that interrupts the transcription of either c-Myc or Pvt 1 is the principal lesion in many B cell malignancies including Burkitt's Lymphoma (BL), AIDs-NHL, mouse plasmacytoma (Pct) and possibly multiple myeloma (MM). There is a restriction associated with this Tx such that only the immunoglobulin (Ig) heavy chain gene is found juxtaposed to c-Myc and only the Ig light chain gene is found juxtaposed to Pvt 1. Over the past several years, our laboratory has been instrumental in the elucidation of the structure of the mouse Pvt 1 locus as a means of understanding the relationship between these two divergent Txs which, nevertheless, produce indistinguishable disease phenotypes. In the mouse, we have identified a uniform Pvt1/Ig Ck fusion product which is consistently found in all tumors harboring Pvt 1 associated Txs. We have recently constructed transgenic mice harboring a translocated Pvt 1/Ck segment in order to determine whether 1). these mice produce the Pvt 1/Ck fusion product 2). these mice are immunocompromised and 3). these mice develop tumors of a B cell origin.

Introduction

The *Pvt 1* locus was originally identified as a "plasmacytoma variant translocation" (1,2) due to the infrequency with which Txs were observed that involved a region located downstream of the the *c-Myc* locus. Unlike *c-Myc/Ig-H* associated Txs which are found in greater than 80% of mouse Pcts, the variant Txs, which constitute the other 20% of Pct associated Txs, are uniformly translocated with *Ig-L* genes. The *Pvt 1* region is conserved along with c-Myc among many species (3,4) and indeed, *Pvt 1* associated Txs have been found in BLs and in similar association with the Ig-L chain. Although T cell lymphomas with retroviral integration sites within the *Pvt 1* region have been found in rodents (5,6), no other Txs have consistently been found to involve the *Pvt 1* region in tumors of human, rat or mouse origin.

Among the models that have been considered for the role of Pvt 1 in these Txs, we have to entertain the issue of whether *Pvt 1* is a functional gene, whose expression is disrupted by Tx, or whether *c-Myc* is ultimately the long range target of Ig enhancers brought into proximity by *Pvt 1* Txs. The transcriptional accessibility hypothesis (7) has been particularly useful in predicting transcriptionally active regions and hence, provided the framework to assume that *Pvt 1* might actually represent a gene. To approach this issue, we and others searched for and identified cDNAs associated with sequences from the

Pvt1 region in mouse (8) and human (9). Unfortunately, no significantly long open reading frames (ORFs) were found that would indicate a coding region in any of the cDNAs examined. Discouraging as this result might have been, it was nevertheless, encouraging to realize that further investigation showed these precise transcripts to be truncated in mouse Pcts and BLs with Pvt 1 associated Txs (Fig. 1). The uniform presence of these truncated transcripts has raised the possibility that chimeric mRNAs containing Pvt 1/Ig-Ck might be the key to understanding Pvt 1 associated Txs and perhaps even c-Myc associated Txs. This paper focusses on our studies of the Pvt 1/Ig-Ck transcript in tumor bearing mouse Pcts and in transgenic mice.

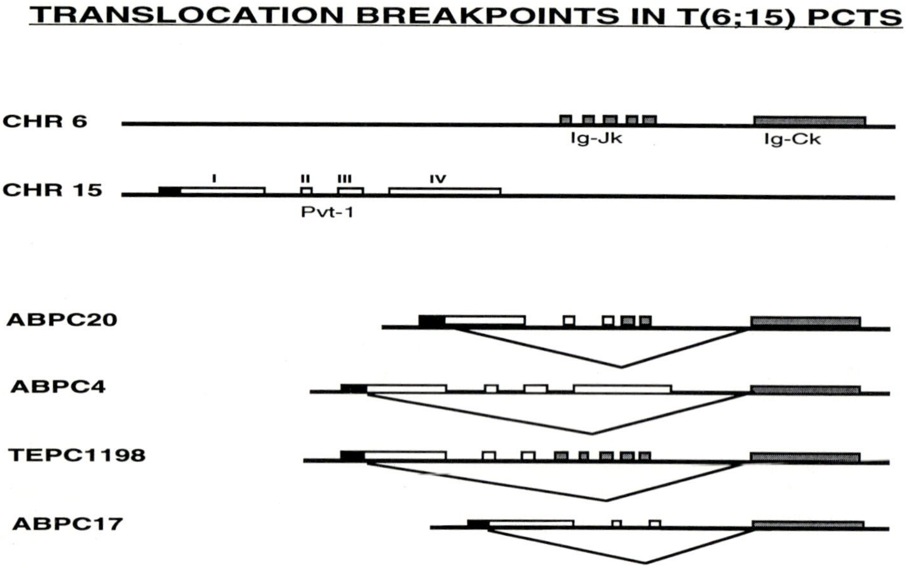

Fig. 1. The exon structures of the Ig kappa locus on mouse Chr. 6 (including Jk and Ck regions) and of the Pvt 1 locus on mouse Chr. 15 (Exons I, II, III, IV) are shown above. Depicted scematically below are four mouse Pcts (ABPC20, ABPC4, TEPC1198 and ABPC17) with t(6;15) breakpoints, the location of these breakpoints and the splice that generates the same Pvt-1a/Ig-Ck chimeric mRNA in each case.

Results and Discussion

A Pvt 1/Ig-Ck Chimeric mRNA is Produced in Pvt 1 Associated Txs

To elucidate the structure of the truncated Pvt 1 transcripts, we have cloned and sequenced multiple cDNA clones from a single mouse Pct, ABPC20 (10). The sequences revealed that a small segment of Pvt 1, referred to as Pvt-1a, was most often spliced directly to Ig-Ck (Fig. 1). We subsequently developed an RT-PCR assay using a primer from this 57bp Pvt-1a segment and a 3' primer from the Ig-Ck region to study mRNA from several Pcts with Pvt 1 associated Txs (11). Sequencing studies from these mouse Pcts again revealed that Pvt-1a was spliced directly to Ig-Ck (eliminating the Jk segment). This splicing event also generated a unique tryptophan codon between Pvt-1a and Ig-Ck as well as a continuous ORF in each of the tumors studied (9,10). The size of the Pvt-1a segment and its putative amino acid composition is very similar to that of leader peptides located at the amino-terminal end of Ig variable regions which are necessary for transport of Ig to the cell surface.

Pvt 1/Ig-Ck has no Transforming Activity in NIH/3T3 Cells
If the Pvt 1/Ig-CK chimera product is of importance in Pcts, one would expect that Ig-Ck plays the most significant role as the largest, and most complete gene. Ig genes (even truncated ones), however, have never shown transforming activity as assayed by NIH/3T3. To further test this, we introduced constructs of Pvt 1/Ig-Ck, Pvt 1 alone and Ig-Ck alone into NIH/3T3 cells in a focus forming assay to formally prove there was no transforming activity (Table 1). The few detectable foci that developed were only observed after prolonged incubation of the NIH/3T3 culture (see legend to Table 1) and can be considered to be due to spontaneous transformation events.

Table 1-Generation of foci in NIH/3T3 Cells

Construct	Foci/assay[a,b]
Pvt 1	8
Pvt/Ig-Ck	2
Ig-Ck	2
T24[c]	117

[a]20ug of DNA used per assay
[b]Foci observed after 5 weeks
[c]The T24 Bladder Carcinoma has an Hras-codon 12 mutation

The Search for a Pvt 1/Ig-Ck Protein
Although we have observed a Pvt 1/Ig-Ck transcript, any biological functionality to a product of this sort would require a translated product. We have searched for a Pvt 1/Ig-Ck protein product using antisera derived from either the Pvt 1a segment or Ig-kappa. For the generation of antisera to Pvt-1a, we synthesized a 18aa peptide corresponding to the amino-terminal sequence (MTIVMGSVEVGAAAKVKS) coupled to poly lysine (Research Genetics Inc.). Two rabbits were then inoculated and sera withdrawn after 6 weeks. As shown in Fig.2, we could not detect any bands unique to the post-immune sera indicative of a Pvt 1 product. Since there was no hint of any specific protein product using the anti-Pvt-1a peptide sera, we attempted to identify a chimeric Pvt 1/Ig-Ck protein using anti-kappa sera and lysates from tumors with Pvt associated Txs (data not shown. The data with the anti-kappa antisera is also inconclusive, probably due to the coincidence in size of the predicted 12kD product with normal Ig-kappa.

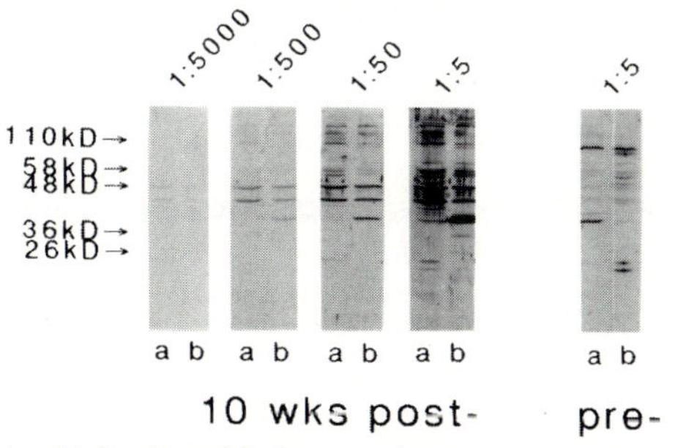

Fig. 2. Western Analysis with Pvt-1a and Ig-kappa antisera.
Varying dilutions (1/5000, 1/500, 1/50, 1/5) of cell lysates from the t(6;15) mouse Pct T1198 (a) and the mouse lymphoma AJ9 (b) were treated with post immune rabbit sera (10weeks) or pre-immune rabbit sera.

The Construction of a Pvt 1/Ig-Ck Transgenic Mouse

One way to bypass the dilemma of identifying a 12kD chimera among serum Ig would be to examine tumors with Pvt 1 associated Txs to Ig-Ck which also express Ig-λ as the immunoglobulin. Unfortunately, this scenario is extremely rare as Igλ is only expressed in 5% of normal mouse sera. We have turned to the generation of Pvt 1/Ig-Ck transgenic mice as the next most efficient means of directly elucidating the biological function of Pvt 1/Ig-Ck and possibly isolating the Pvt 1/Ig-Ck product as well for further study. The construct used for the generation of these mice was a silicone-induced mouse Pct with a Pvt 1 associated Tx. A 20kb Bam H1 genomic clone (Fig. 3) containing 14.8kb of genomic DNA from the Pvt 1 region (including exon 1 and 5' sequences) and 5.2kb of genomic DNA from the translocated Ig-Ck segment (including Jk and Ck sequences) was purified and inserted into the embryos of C57BL/6J mice. No positive transgenic mouse lines were successfully obtained by this approach possibly due to some lethality. Therefore, we repeated the introduction of the same constructs into (C57BL/6J x DBA/2)F_1 mice which were then backcrossed to C57BL/6 mice. As a control, the 18kb nonrearranged Pvt 1 clone was also injected into mouse embryos (Fig. 3). From this protocol, we obtained 6 transgenic mouse lines containing the Pvt 1/Ig-Ck and 2 transgenic mouse lines containing the Pvt 1 (only) construct. To examine whether Pvt 1/Ig-Ck is transcribed in immune organs, we isolated mRNA from spleen cells of three Pvt 1/Ig-Ck transgenic lines (15, 19 and 66) and assayed for the presence of the Pvt-1a/Ig-Ck transcript. Indeed, a transcript was found in each case confirming that we were able to re-introduce the chimeric transcript into these mice and obtain appropriate spleen cell expression (most likely as a result of the Ig-K enhancer). We also assayed these mice for enhanced levels of c-Myc expression (of which there was none) and looked for tumorigenicity (of which there was also none). Absence of tumors in these mice is not necessarily surprising since C57BL/6J and DBA/2 mice are quite resistant to the development of Pcts. A more appropriate experiment would be to transfer the Pvt 1/Ig-Ck transgene back onto a BALB/c (Pct susceptible) genetic background or to infect these mice with a potentially cooperating oncogene such as Bcl 2 or Abl. We have also investigated whether these transgenic mice show signs of B or T cell developmental defects as a consequence of this transgene (J.A. and A.R., data not shown). No gross obvious defects in the immune system have been found to date.

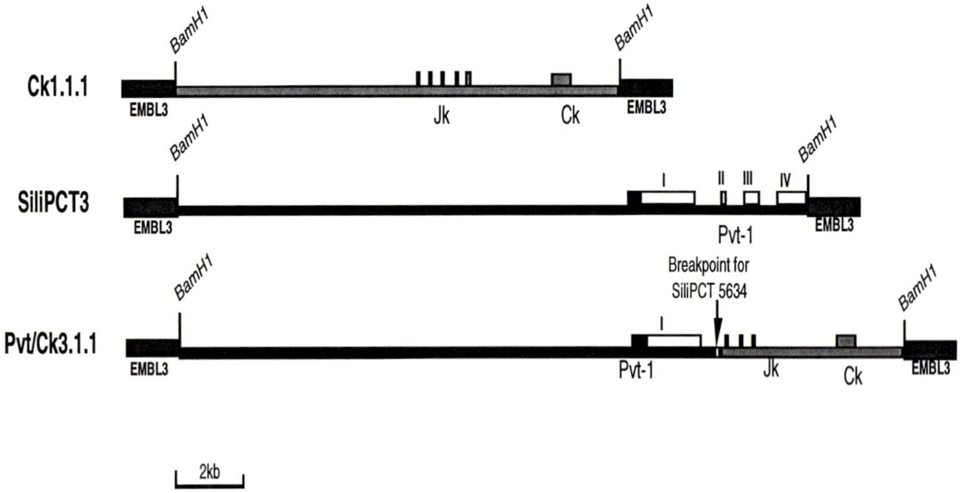

Fig.3. Three genomic clones were obtained from the SiPct 5634 mouse Pct that contained normal Ig-Ck (Ck1.1), Normal Pvt 1 (SiliPct3) or a translocated Pvt 1/Ig-Ck segment (Pvt/Ck3.1). All clones have EMBL3 vectors and were generated in the Bam H1 site.

In conclusion, we have found that Pvt 1/Ig-Ck is expressed in all Pvt 1 associated tumors, yet Pvt 1/Ig-Ck is not transforming. Since Pvt 1/Ig-Ck is very receptor-like in structure, it is this concept that we have proposed to explain how Pvt 1 may play a role in the genesis of B cell tumors. This hypothesis, obviously relies on the detection of such a receptor followed by proof of its function. We would predict that Pvt 1/Ig-Ck should be expressed at an early pre-B cell stage (pre-II) and then continues to be expressed in a dysregulated manner. In contrast, λ5 and v-preB are turned off before the pre-II stage (Fig. 4 and ref. 13).

We would also predict that similar PVT 1/Ig-Ck or Ig-Cλ products should be found in BLs with T(8:22) or T(2:8) Txs. Indeed, chimeric mRNAs of 0.8-1.0kb have been identified in 6 BL cell lines (BL21, BL64, LY91, LY66, PA682 and MWIKA) that are found to contain a small portion of the 5' end of PVT (termed RPS0.45) and the Ig Constant region gene (9). More detailed cloning and sequencing studies of the human chimeric mRNAs from BL21 revealed only a 14aa PVT segment joined in-frame to Ck from an AUG codon (14). This result lead the authors to attempt to precipitate the predicted 14kD sized product from BL21 with human kappa antisera, but without success. Recently, we have rexamined the sequence data originally obtained from the MWIKA cell line and we find a 16-17aa peptide that starts with an AUG codon, is hydrophobic in composition and is also in-frame with Cλ (minus the Jλ sequence). The omnipresence of chimeras of PVT in BL cells further supports the feasibility that these products indeed play a role in B cell neoplasia. Whether this role is as a receptor, as we have proposed, is quite dependent on the identification and isolation of the Pvt 1/Ig-Ck protein product.

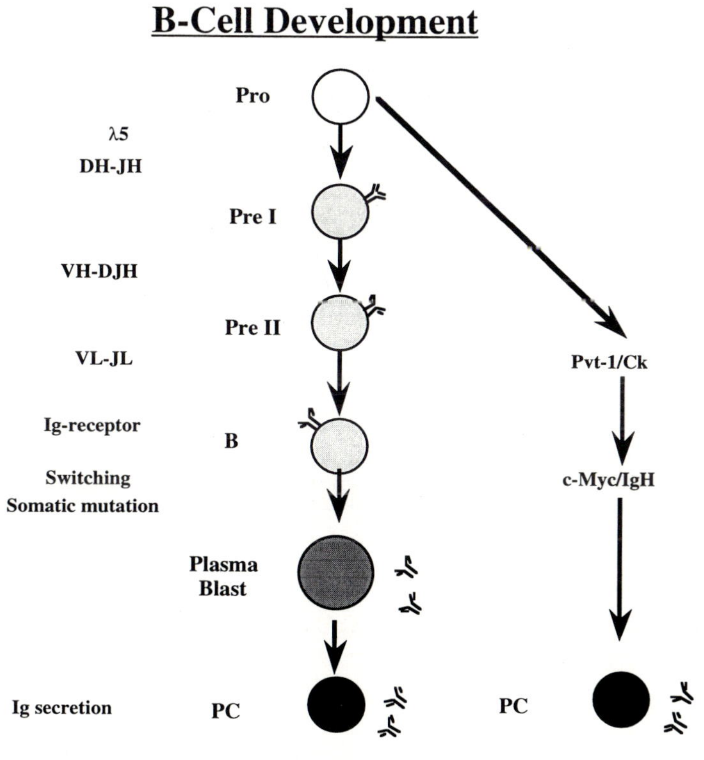

Fig. 4. A Schematic of B Cell development. Indicated on the left are stage specific events (ie. expression or rearrangement) characteristic of each stage (center) in the maturation of lymphocyte precursors. On the right side is the putative transgression that Pvt 1/Ig-Ck (or c-Myc/Ig-H) chimeras may follow in generating a transformed plasma cell.

References

1. Erickson J, Nishikura K, Ar-Rushdi A, Finan J, Emmanuel B, Lenoir G, Nowell P and Croce C (1983) Translocation of an immunoglobulin k locus to a region 3' of an unrearranged c-myc oncogene enhances c-myc transcription. Proc Natl Acad Sci USA 80: 7581-7585
2. Webb E, Adams JM and Cory S (1984) Variant (6;15) translocation in a murine plasmacytoma occurs near an immunoglobulin k gene but far from the myc oncogene. Nature 312:777-779
3. Graham M and Adams JM (1986) Chromosome 8 breakpoint far 3' of the c-myc oncogene in a Burkitt's lymphoma 2:8 variant translocation is equivalent to the murine pvt-1 locus. EMBO J 5: 2845-2851
4. Villeneuve L, Rassart E, Jolicoeur P, Graham M and Adams JM (1986) Proviral integration site Mis-1 in rat thymomas corresponds to the pvt-1 translocation breakpoint in murine plasmacytomas. Mol and Cell Biol 6:1834-1837
5. Cory S, Graham M, Webb E, Corcoran I and Adams JM (1985) Variant (6;15) translocations in murine plasmacytomas involve a chromosome 15 locus at least 72kb from the c-myc oncogene. EMBO J 4:675-681
6. Tsichlis PN, Lee JS, Bear S, Lazo PA, Patriotis C, Gustafson E, Shinton S, Jenkins NA, Copeland NG, Huebner K, Croce C, Levan G and Hanson C (1989) Activation of multiple genes by provirus integration in the Mlvi-4 locus in T-cell lymphomas induced by moloney murine leukemia virus. J Virol. 64: 2236-2244
7. Kirsch IR, Brown JA, Lawrence J, Korsmeyer SJ and Norton CC (1985) Translocations that highlight chromosomal regions of differentiated activity. Cancer Genet Cytogenet 18:159-171
8. Huppi K, Siwarski D, Skurla R, Klinman D and Mushinski J F (1990) Pvt-1 transcripts are found in normal tissues and are altered by reciprocal (6;15) translocations in mouse plasmacytomas. Proc Natl Acad Sci USA 87: 6964-6968
9. Shtivelman E, Henglein B, Groitl P, Lipp M and Bishop JM (1989) Identification of a human transcription unit affected by the variant chromosomal translocations 2;8 and 8;22 of Burkitt lymphoma. Proc Natl Acad Sci USA 86: 3257-3260
10. Huppi K, Siwarski D, Goodnight J, Skurla Jr RM and Mushinski JF (1992) Alternative splicing of Pvt-1 transcripts in murine B-lymphocytic neoplasms accompanies amplification and chromosomal translocation. Int J of Oncol 1:525-532
11. Huppi K and Siwarski D (1994) Chimeric transcripts with an open reading frame are generated as a result of translocation to the Pvt-1 region in mouse B-cell tumors. Int J Cancer 59:848-851
12. Axelson H, Panda CK, Silva S, Sugiyama H, Wiener F, Klein G and Sumegi J (1991) A new variant 15;16 translocation in mouse plasmacytoma leads to the juxtaposition of c-myc and immunoglobulin lambda. Oncogene 6: 2263-2270
13. Karasuyama H, Rolink A, Shinkai Y, Young F, Alt FW and Melchers F (1994) The expression of Vpre-B/l5 surrogate light chain in early bone marrow precursor B cells of normal and B cell-deficient mutant mice. Cell 77:133-143
14. Shtivelman E and Bishop JM (1990) Effects of Translocations on Transcription from PVT. Mol and Cell Biol 10:1835-1839

Murine and Human 3' IgH Regulatory Sequences

B. K. Birshtein, C. Chen, S. Saleque, J. S. Michaelson, M. Singh and R. D. Little
Department of Cell Biology, Albert Einstein College of Medicine, Bronx, NY 10461, USA

Mouse plasmacytomas and human Burkitt lymphomas are marked by characteristic chromosomal translocations involving the c-myc gene on one chromosome (murine chromosome 15, human chromosome 8) and the IgH locus on a second chromosome (murine chromosome 12, human chromosome 14). These result in the conversion of the c-myc gene from a normal cellular gene into the c-myc oncogene (reviewed in [1]). The formation of the myc oncogene is generally brought about by divorce of c-myc coding sequences, located in its exons 2 and 3, from exon 1 and upstream regulatory regions, coupled with the juxtaposition of myc coding sequences to immunoglobulin heavy chain (IgH) gene sequences (Fig. 1). (The reciprocal product, involving myc exon 1 and its upstream regulatory sequences, is not required for malignant transformation). Thus, the formation of the myc oncogene involves not only loss of its normal regulatory elements but also the acquisition of different regulatory influences associated with its new, immunoglobulin-associated, chromosomal environment. The focus of this paper is on the nature of IgH associated sequences that impact upon the c-myc oncogene in B cell malignancies.

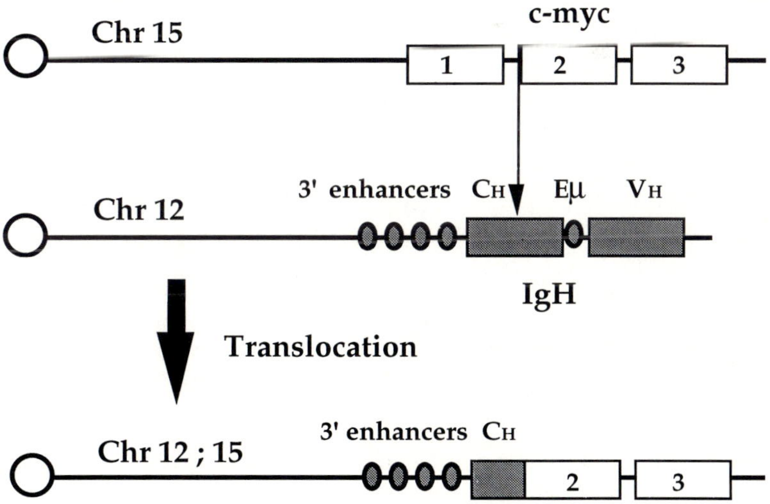

Fig. 1: The myc oncogene is juxtaposed to IgH 3' enhancers in mouse plasmacytomas

The Murine 3' IgH Regulatory Region

Sequences 3' of the murine IgH gene cluster are implicated in myc oncogenesis in mouse plasmacytoma cells

Various elements are involved in the regulation of the construction and expression of IgH genes (reviewed in [1]). These include not only the promoter elements upstream of each VH gene, but also the intronic enhancer, Eμ, and - as described primarily in mouse - a 3' regulatory region (Fig. 2). Chromosomal translocation breakpoints in mouse myelomas generally occur within switch sequences that lie upstream of each of the CH genes, with the exception of delta. In fact, many myelomas show translocations involving switch alpha (Sα) sequences. As shown in Fig. 1, the location of these breakpoints necessarily eliminates a potential role for the intronic enhancer, Eμ, in the formation of the myc oncogene, and instead implicates IgH sequences downstream of Sα. Hence, the 3' regulatory region is a prime candidate for influencing myc oncogenesis.

The murine 3' regulatory region

The existence of 3' regulatory sequences, located downstream of the Cα gene, at the terminus of the mouse IgH gene cluster, was first confirmed by the discovery of Pettersson et al of a 3' enhancer from rat [2]. This was followed by identification of a homologous element in mouse [3, 12]. Subsequently, additional enhancers have been located in an ~50 kb DNA segment using a variety of approaches [4-6]. These have included forthright screening of DNA segments for enhancer activity using transient transfection assays, as well as identification of putative regulatory elements by their DNase I hypersensitivity profiles [6, 7].

Currently, four enhancers have been identified in the 3' regulatory region, and they comprise two separate structural and functional units (Fig.2) [8]. The most 3' enhancer, hs4, appears to be the single enhancer within its unit. It is the only one of the four 3' enhancers that is DNase I hypersensitive early in B cell differentiation, i.e. in pre-B cells, as well as later, in plasma cell lines [5, 7]. Because hs4 contains a BSAP binding site [9], and because BSAP plays an essential role in B cell differentiation [10], we have proposed that hs4 might be a critical early target for BSAP, playing a role, perhaps, in the VDJ joining process [11].

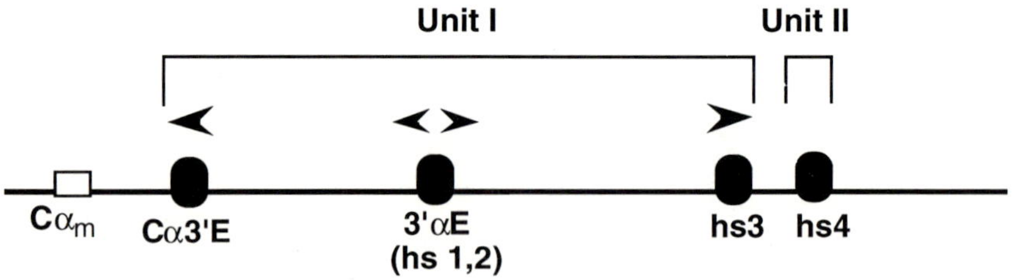

Fig. 2: The 3' IgH regulatory region is composed of two structural and functional units

As shown in Fig. 2, the three 5' enhancers constitute a separate unit of ~25 kb, characterized by extensive dyad symmetry [8]. The dyad symmetry is evidenced in several ways. First, the central enhancer, 3'αE(hs1,2) is closely flanked by inverted repeats [12]. Second, on both sides of 3'αE(hs1,2) are two families of repetitive sequences that are uniquely located only in this DNA region [7, 8, 13]. For example, one family consists of five distinct segments, two of which are located upstream of 3'αE(hs1,2) and three of which are located downstream.

Additionally, and of considerable interest, is the recent understanding that the other two enhancers located within this region, i.e. Cα3'E and hs3 (Fig. 2), are virtually identical to each other. While each enhancer had been separately identified and reported [4, 6], no data had been presented indicating their similarities. While carrying out genomic Southern analysis, we observed that hs3 hybridizing sequences were present in two positions, one corresponding to the published location of hs3, and a second, located in the general region in which Cα3'E had been localized. We compared the GenBank sequences of a 597 bp fragment reported for Cα3'E with that of hs3 and found that they were 97% identical except for an ~100 bp gap within Cα3'E. To identify the extent of sequence similarity, we determined additional sequences in the region around Cα3'E. These studies have revealed that except for the ~100 bp gap, these two enhancer regions are virtually identical throughout 1067 bp [8].

Furthermore, genomic Southern analysis and DNA sequence determination has shown that Cα3'E and hs3 are arrayed in inverted orientation with respect to each other (Fig. 2) [8]. Data published by Chaveau and Cogne have led to similar observations [14]. The general structure of this ~25 kb unit, which contains 3'αE(hs1,2) at the center and inverted repeats at the termini, is like that of a complex transposable element [8], raising intriguing questions about the evolutionary origin of this DNA segment. Data we have garnered about human IgH 3' sequences, as discussed later, lend support to this hypothesis.

These three enhancers-Cα3'E, 3'αE(hs1,2) and hs3- are each DNase I hypersensitive late in B cell differentiation, namely, in plasma cell lines and not in pre-B cells [7, 8, 12]. Transient transfection assays [3, 12, 15-17] and a transgenic mouse [18] have specifically documented activity of the central enhancer, 3'αE(hs1,2), at late stages of B cell differentiation, i.e. in plasma cell lines and in normal activated B cells. At earlier stages of B cell development, this enhancer is actively downregulated through the concerted interaction of several DNA binding proteins, including BSAP, octamer-binding proteins, kappa B binding proteins (p50), and a G-rich DNA binding protein [16, 17, 19]. As for the two "identical" flanking enhancers-Cα3'E and hs3, neither one of these shows significant enhancer activity as a monomer in either pre-B cells or in plasma cells [4, 6, 8]. However, when assayed as dimers, both enhancers show significant and synergistic activity in plasma cell lines, but not in 18-81 pre-B cells [6, 8]. Together, these data suggest that these three enhancers may indeed work together as a unit to affect later stage B cells, with the terminal enhancers capable of transcriptional synergy.

Functional impact of murine 3' regulatory region during normal B cell differentiation.

What are the roles of these enhancers in normal B cell differentiation? This question is gradually being approached through various transcriptional assay systems as well as through analysis of mice and cell lines in which individual or multiple enhancers have been deleted. The results of several experiments so far suggest roles for 3' regulatory enhancers in events throughout B cell differentiation, including VH gene assembly, class switching, somatic mutation and high levels of IgH gene expression in plasma cells. For example, an IgH heavy chain low-expressing phenotype identified in a variant of a plasmacytoma cell line is accompanied by deletion of the entire 3' regulatory region [5, 20]. Targeted substitution of 3'αE(hs1,2) with the neo gene in a plasma cell line [21] has implicated this specific enhancer as essential for high levels of IgH gene expression in this late stage cell, while a similar experiment in mouse [22] has implicated this same enhancer in class switching to some, but not all, isotypes. However, it has been shown that the phenotype that results from the introduction of an active neo gene into a regulatory locus might reflect derailed interactions between enhancers other than, or in addition to, the targeted enhancer [23]. Hence, experiments to specifically eliminate the neo gene from the final targeted locus and to examine the resulting phenotype are in progress in several laboratories.

Functional impact of murine 3' regulatory region on myc oncogenesis

Are these 3' regulatory enhancers the critical elements involved in dysregulation of the myc oncogene? Experiments by Madisen and Groudine [6] have shown that when assayed in plasmacytoma or the Raji Burkitt lymphoma cell lines, the amalgam of the three enhancers-3'αE(hs1,2), hs3 and hs4-has conferred upon the myc promoter the property of promoter bias that is generally evidenced in myc-transformed cells. Furthermore, this amalgam conferred upon stable transfectants the property of locus-independent, copy-number independent expression, properties which, if displayed in transgenic mice, have been associated with a locus control region. However, the recognition of the dyad symmetry of this 3' regulatory region (Fig. 2) [8, 14] suggests the possibility that thc in vivo locus control region might actually be more complex and involve all four enhancers. Nonetheless, the data are consistent with the identification of important roles for these 3' regulatory elements in the dysregulation of myc in malignant B cells.

Human 3' IgH Regulatory Sequences

Human Cα associated sequences

With the identification of the murine 3' regulatory region has come a natural interest in determining whether similar elements are present in the human IgH gene locus. The human locus is more complex than mouse, containing not one but two Cα genes, each one arrayed in a duplicated unit also containing two Cγ genes and an epsilon or epsilon-like gene. Hence, the question has been further specified: is there a 3' regulatory region downstream of Cα2, or Cα1, or both genes? A cloning obstacle has prevented answering this question until recently, when we [24] and others [25, 26] have implemented different approaches to be able to identify sequences immediately downstream of Cα membrane exons (Fig. 3). These sequences are characterized by lengths of 20 bp tandem repeats that flank a central ~500 bp non-repetitive sequence. The 20 bp tandem repeats bear homology to switch mu and switch alpha sequences, and we have speculated that they may play a role in stabilizing a switch recombination complex [24].

Interestingly, this region downstream of the human Cα1 gene has been shown to be the site of a rare integration of EBV sequences in the RGN1 human lymphoblastoid cell line by Gualandi and colleagues [25, 27]. This observation has provided one thought-provoking idea with respect to the evolutionary origin of the ~25 kb unit of the mouse 3' regulatory region as a transposable element. More cogent data have come from our observation of ~60% homologies between the human Cα1 20 bp repeat region (Fig. 3) and mouse IgH sequences which are located at both ends of the 25 kb unit, namely upstream of Cα3'E and downstream of hs3 (Fig. 2) [8]. In other words, sequences which, in mouse, are located ~25 kb from each other, are homologous to what is, in human, a collinear DNA segment of ~2 kb. Furthermore, this collinear DNA segment in human was the site of the EBV integration in one human lymphoblastoid cell line [25, 27]. While not conclusive, together, these observations are tantalizing with respect to the notion that a large segment of the murine 3' regulatory region may have entered as a transposable element sometime during evolution.

We have been successful in cloning additional sequences downstream of the 20 bp tandem repeat segments (Fig. 3). Both Cα1 and Cα2 associated sequences are highly homologous throughout the ~10 kb regions we have isolated. Associated with each Cα gene is a region of inverted repeats within which an enhancer element has been identified (C. Chen and B. K. Birshtein, manuscript in preparation). These enhancers are virtually identical to each other in sequence except for varying numbers of a 53 bp motif. Significantly, each enhancer bears a segment of ~177 bp that is homologous to a 191 bp segment of the murine enhancer 3'αE(hs1,2), within which the single octamer is located.

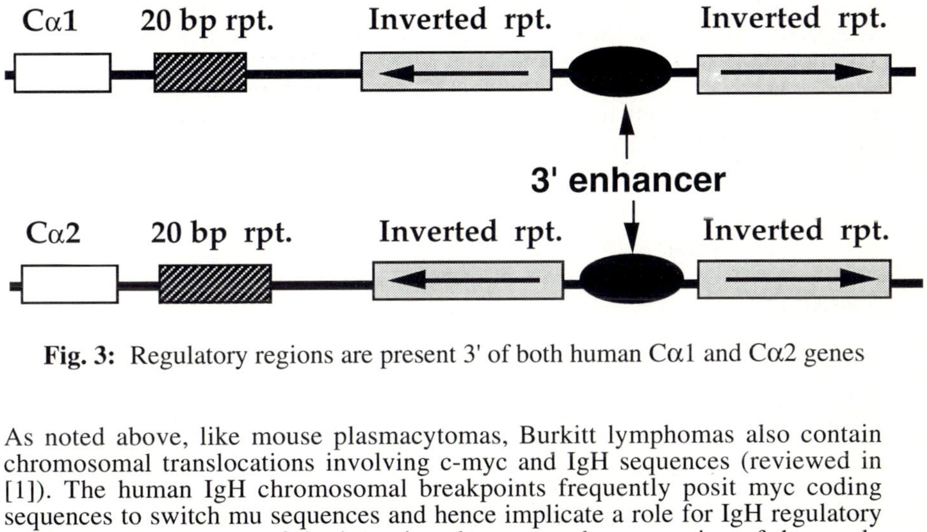

Fig. 3: Regulatory regions are present 3' of both human Cα1 and Cα2 genes

As noted above, like mouse plasmacytomas, Burkitt lymphomas also contain chromosomal translocations involving c-myc and IgH sequences (reviewed in [1]). The human IgH chromosomal breakpoints frequently posit myc coding sequences to switch mu sequences and hence implicate a role for IgH regulatory sequences downstream of the intronic enhancer on the expression of the newly generated myc oncogene. Our identification of human IgH 3' enhancers suggests that these may be one component of a 3' regulatory segment that influences myc oncogenesis.

It is interesting that mouse plasmacytomas and Burkitt lymphomas affect B cells at different stages of B cell differentiation, raising the speculation that if 3' enhancers are involved in myc oncogenesis, mouse and human enhancers may operate differently. In fact, this idea is consistent with our finding that the region of homology between the human enhancer, and that of rat and mouse encompasses only a portion of these enhancers and in mouse, we know that enhancer activity involves sequences outside this "core" segment [9, 19]. We predict that in humans, human-specific flanking sequences may impinge differently upon the conserved core.

Human myeloma DNA rearrangements

Unlike Burkitt lymphomas, human myeloma cells do not show consistent chromosomal DNA rearrangements, and hence, it has been an ongoing challenge to identify the nature of the chromosomal changes resulting in malignant transformation. Kuehl and colleagues have recently carried out a systematic and successful search for the involvement of switch sequences, and hence, switch recombination, in human myeloma [28]. Based on our identification of human 3' regulatory sequences (Chen and Birshtein, in preparation) and our observation of DNA rearrangements of murine 3' regulatory regions in mouse B cell lines [13], we have been interested in testing whether similar rearrangements of human 3' regulatory sequences might accompany malignant transformation. In collaboration with Dr. Kuehl, we have carried out genomic Southern analysis on a panel of human myeloma cell lines using probes for sequences 3' of human Cα genes, including segments containing 20 bp tandem repeats [24] and the Cα associated enhancers. In many samples of human DNA, both DNA segments identify the same Hind III fragments. However, in two myeloma cell lines, we have observed differences in hybridization patterns. Notably, two distinct Hind III fragments were identified in each sample, one with each probe, and each of a different size than we have previously observed. We have considered three interpretations: 1) Polymorphism, involving the introduction of a Hind III site; 2) DNA integration, similar to that previously observed in the EBV integration in a B lymphoblastoid cell line; and 3) Chromosomal translocation, involving a putative oncogene. To discriminate between these possibilities, we intend to carry out additional mapping and cloning to identify the nature of rearranged DNA sequences.

Summary

Both murine plasmacytomas and human Burkitt lymphomas contain chromosomal translocations involving the c-myc gene and the Ig gene cluster. As a result of the translocation in mouse plasmacytomas, the myc oncogene comes under the influence of regulatory sequences 3' of the murine IgH gene cluster. The murine 3' regulatory region contains four enhancers, three of which are located in a 25 kb unit of dyad symmetry [8, 14]. This unit contains a central enhancer, flanked by two identical enhancers at the termini, and we have speculated that this unit has entered the mouse genome during evolution as a transposable element. The fourth, and most downstream, enhancer comprises a separate structural and functional unit. Synergy among these enhancers has been documented and it has been suggested that these elements comprise a locus control region [6]. We have identified two virtually identical human enhancers 3' of the IgH locus, one downstream of the Cα1 gene and one downstream of the Cα2 gene. These bear a region of homology to one of the mouse 3' enhancers, and are predicted to play a role in myc oncogenesis. Preliminary evidence for DNA rearrangements of 3' regulatory sequences in human myeloma cell lines is presented.

Acknowledgments

This work was supported by grants from the National Institutes of Health, R37AI13509 and P30CA13330, and by the Council for Tobacco Research. J.S.M. was supported by a Howard Hughes Predoctoral Fellowship 9-526-4653 and by an NIH training grant CA09173.

References

1. Max EE (1993) Immunoglobulins: Molecular Genetics. In:Paul WE (ed) Fundamental Immunology. Raven Press, N. Y., pp315-383
2. Pettersson S, Cook GP, Brüggemann M, Williams GT and Neuberger MS (1990) A second B cell-specific enhancer 3' of the immunoglobulin heavy-chain locus. Nature 344:165-168
3. Lieberson R, Giannini SL, Birshtein BK and Eckhardt LA (1991) An enhancer at the 3' end of the mouse immunoglobulin heavy chain locus. Nucl Acids Res 19:933-937
4. Matthias P and Baltimore D (1993) The immunoglobulin heavy chain locus contains another B-cell specific 3' enhancer close to the α constant region. Mol Cell Biol 13:1547-1553
5. Michaelson JS, Giannini SL and Birshtein BK (1995) Identification of 3'α-hs4, a novel Ig heavy chain enhancer element regulated at multiple stages of B cell differentiation. Nucl Acids Res 23:975-981
6. Madisen L and Groudine M (1994) Identification of a locus control region in the immunoglobulin heavy-chain locus that deregulates c-myc expression in plasmacytoma and Burkitt's lymphoma cells. Genes Dev 8:2212-2226
7. Giannini SL, Singh M, Calvo C-F, Ding G and Birshtein BK (1993) DNA regions flanking the mouse Ig 3'α enhancer are differentially methylated and DNAse I hypersensitive during B cell differentiation. J Immunol 150:1772-1780
8. Saleque S, Singh M, Little RD, Giannini SL, Michaelson JS and Birshtein BK (1997) Dyad symmetry within the 3' IgH regulatory region includes two virtually identical enhancers (Cα3'E and hs3). J Immunol, Accepted in principle
9. Michaelson JS, Singh M, Snapper CM, Sha WC, Baltimore D and Birshtein BK (1996) Regulation of 3' IgH enhancers by a common set of factors, including κB binding proteins. J Immunol 156:2828-2839
10. Urbánek P, Wang Z-Q, Fetka I, Wagner EF and Busslinger M (1994) Complete block of early B cell differentiation and altered patterning of the posterior midbrain in mice lacking Pax5/BSAP. Cell 79:901-912
11. Michaelson JS, Singh M and Birshtein BK (1996) B cell lineage-specific activator protein (BSAP): a player at multiple stages of B cell development. J Immunol 156:2349-2351
12. Dariavach P, Williams GT, Campbell K, Pettersson S and Neuberger MS (1991) The mouse IgH 3'-enhancer. Eur J Immunol 21:1499-1504
13. Calvo C-F, Giannini SL, Martinez N and Birshtein BK (1991) DNA sequences 3' of the IgH chain cluster rearrange in mouse B cell lines. J Immunol 146:1353-1360
14. Chaveau C and Cogné M (1996) Palindromic structure of the IgH 3' locus control region. Nature Genet 14:15-16
15. Grant PA, Arulampalam V, Ährlund-Richter L and Pettersson S (1992) Identification of ets-like lymphoid specific elements within the immunoglobulin heavy chain 3' enhancer. Nucl Acids Res 20:4401-4408
16. Neurath MF, Strober W and Wakatsuki Y (1994) The murine Ig 3'α enhancer is a target site with repressor function for the B cell lineage-specific transcription factor BSAP (NF-HB, Sα-BP). J Immunol 153:730-742
17. Singh M and Birshtein BK (1993) NF-HB (BSAP) is a repressor of the murine immunoglobulin 3'α enhancer at early stages of B-cell differentiation. Mol Cell Biol 13:3611-3622
18. Arulampalam M, Grant PA, Samuelsson A, Lendahl U and Pettersson S (1994) Lipopolysaccharide-dependent transactivation of the temporally regulated immunoglobulin heavy chain 3' enhancer. Eur J Immunol 24:1671-1677

19. Singh M and Birshtein BK (1996) Concerted repression of an immunoglobulin heavy chain 3'α enhancer, 3'αE(hs1,2). Proc Natl Acad Sci USA 93:4392-4397
20. Gregor PD and Morrison SL (1986) Myeloma mutant with a novel 3' flanking region: loss of normal sequence and insertion of repetitive elements leads to decreased transcription but normal processing of the alpha heavy-chain gene products. Mol Cell Biol 6:1903-1916
21. Lieberson R, Ong J, Shi X and Eckhardt LA (1995) Transcription of an immunoglobulin γ2a gene ceases upon deletion of an enhancer region over 70 kilobases away. EMBO J 14:6229-6238
22. Cogné M, Lansford R, Bottaro A, Zhang J, Gorman J, Young F, Cheng H-L and Alt FW (1994) A class switch control region at the 3' end of the immunoglobulin heavy chain locus. Cell 77:737-747
23. Fiering S, Epner E, Robinson K, Zhuang Y, Telling A, Hu M, Martin DI, Enver T, Ley TJ and Groudine M (1995) Targeted deletion of 5'HS2 of the murine beta-globin LCR reveals that it is not essential for proper regulation of the beta-globin locus. Genes Dev 9:2203-2213
24. Chen C and Birshtein BK (1996) A region of 20 bp repeats lies 3' of human Ig Cα1 and Cα2 genes. Int Immunol 8:115-122
25. Gualandi G, Frezza D, Scotto d'Abusco A, Bianchi E, Gargano S, Giorgi S, Fruscalzo A and Calef E (1995) Integration of a Epstein-Barr virus episome into the gene encoding immunoglobulin heavy-chain alpha 1 in a lymphoblastoid cell line. Gene 166:221-226
26. Kang HK and Cox DW (1996) Tandem repeats 3' of the IgHA genes in the human immunoglobulin heavy chain gene cluster. Genomics 35:189-195
27. Gualandi G, Santolini E and Calef E (1992) Epstein-Barr virus DNA recombines via latent origin of replication with the human genome in the lymphoblastoid cell line RGN1. J Virol 66:5677-5681
28. Bergsagel PL, Chesi M, Nardini E, Brents LA, Kirby SL and Kuehl WM (1997) Promiscuous translocations into IgH switch regions in multiple myeloma. Proc Natl Acad Sci, in press

Negative Regulation of C-Myc

Receptor-specific Regulation of NF-κB, c-Myc and Fas-mediated Apoptosis in Primary B Cells

D. A. Francis[1], R. Sen[2] and T. L. Rothstein[3]

[1] Department of Pathology, Boston University Medical Center, Boston, MA, USA

[2] Department of Biology, Brandeis University, Waltham, MA, USA

[3] Department of Medicine and Microbiology, Boston University Medical Center, Boston, MA, USA

Introduction

The NF-κB transcription factor complex plays a role in directing the inducible expression of a number of genes involved in the immune response, importantly including c-*myc* [1]. NF-κB consists of homo- or hetero-dimers drawn from a family of proteins, the members of which share a conserved 300 amino acid sequence, the Rel homology domain, originally identified as the transforming agent of the avian reticuloendotheliosis virus. Mammalian Rel-related proteins include NF-κB1 (p50), NF-κB2 (p52), c-Rel, RelA (p65), and RelB. NF-κB1 and NF-κB2 are derived from larger precursor proteins (p105 and p100, respectively) that can inhibit NF-κB. c-Rel, RelA and RelB contain transactivation domains at their carboxyl terminal ends that are capable of activating gene transcription. Transcriptionally active dimers are those in which one of the proteins contains a transactivation domain (for review see [2-4]).

Mammalian NF-κB is regulated through protein-protein interactions that dictate intracellular location. In most cell types NF-κB is found in the cytoplasm bound to one or more inhibitor proteins of the IκB family that includes IκBα, IκBβ, IκBγ and the gene encoded by *bcl-3*. Inducible activation of NF-κB depends on phosphorylation of IκB, which targets the inhibitor for degradation via a ubiquinin-mediated proteasome pathway, after which NF-κB dimers are free to translocate to the nucleus and bind decameric κB sites.

During the past several years, links between lymphocyte surface receptors and nuclear transcription factor induction have been defined. We have studied two receptors of B lymphocytes, the surface immunoglobulin (sIg) antigen receptor, which is primarily responsible for T-independent B cell stimulation, and the CD40 receptor, a member of the TNF receptor family, that is primarily responsible for T-dependent B cell stimulation and is triggered by the T cell activation antigen, CD40 ligand or gp39. sIgM and CD40 are each fully competent mitogenic receptors, in that crosslinking of either receptor provides a stimulus capable of driving resting B cells through the cell cycle to S phase, although the intermediary pathways leading to this outcome differ in a receptor-specific fashion [5]. These receptors also trigger nuclear expression of some of the same transcription factor complexes, suggesting the possible existence of a final common transcriptional pathway leading to cell cycle progression [6 and unpublished observations].

Although nuclear NF-κB expression is developmentally regulated and is constitutively present in mature B cells, additional NF-κB is present in cytosolic fractions in a sequestered form bound to IκB. We and others have shown that despite baseline nuclear NF-κB expression, substantial additional nuclear NF-κB is induced in B cells following engagement of either the sIgM or CD40 receptors [6-10]. However, the intracellular signaling pathways leading from CD40 and sIgM to nuclear NF-κB differ, at least at the level of PKC-dependence, and as far as is known these pathways appear to share few elements in common [6,9]. This led us to question whether NF-κB induced by these two receptors is truly identical, particularly with respect to the Rel-related protein composition of induced κB-binding dimers. In fact, we found a distinct difference with respect to RelB expression that in turn suggests a new level of NF-κB regulation that is receptor- and Rel-related protein-specific.

Results

The nature of NF-κB was examined by obtaining high salt nuclear extracts from purified murine splenic B lymphocytes before and after stimulation with $F(ab')_2$ fragments of goat anti-mouse IgM antibody (anti-Ig) or a chimeric fusion protein consisting of the extracellular domains of murine CD40L and CD8α, crosslinked with anti-CD8 antibody (CD40L), as previously described [6,11]. Nuclear extracted protein was tested for DNA-binding activity by electrophoretic mobility shift assay (EMSA) using a radiolabeled oligonucleotide containing the consensus κB site from the κ light chain enhancer [7].

κB-Binding Nucleoprotein Complexes Induced by Anti-Ig and CD40L

As expected on the basis of previous work, nuclear extracted protein from unstimulated B cells expressed DNA-binding NF-κB, the level of which was substantially increased following B cell stimulation with anti-Ig or CD40L. Peak induction was observed about 2 hours following stimulation through either receptor, and consisted of two major nucleoprotein complexes. At the late time point of 24 hours, however, the nucleoprotein complex with the greatest electrophoretic mobility was lost from the κB-binding activity obtained from anti-Ig stimulated B cell nuclei, but remained present in the κB-binding activity obtained from CD40L-stimulated B cells. This suggested the possibility that NF-κB induced by these two receptors may be distinct, at least at late time points.

Rel Protein Composition of Receptor-stimulated NF-κB

A more careful analysis of receptor-stimulated NF-κB was then undertaken by utilizing Rel protein-specific antibodies (kindly provided by Dr. N.R. Rice, National Cancer Institute, Frederick, MD) in supershift EMSA. Constitutive nuclear κB-binding activity from primary B cells was shown to consist of p50, p52, c-Rel and RelB, but not RelA. Although it is impossible to be quantitative in such experiments because many characteristics of the antibodies are unknown, the largest supershifts were produced by anti-p50/p105 and anti-c-Rel.

Following B cell stimulation for 2 hours, nuclear extracted protein produced κB-binding complexes that were supershifted by antisera directed against all five of the mammalian Rel-related proteins, specifically including RelA. Thus, at the peak of induction, NF-κB produced by anti-Ig and by CD40L was similar in containing p50, p52, c-Rel, RelA and RelB. As before, the largest supershifts were produced by anti-p50/p105 and anti-c-Rel.

The pattern changed, however, when B cells were stimulated for 24 hours, and this change was receptor-specific. Nuclear extracts obtained from B cells stimulated with CD40L for 24 hours produced a pattern of supershifted κB-binding nucleoprotein complexes little different from that observed after B cell stimulation for 2 hours, indicating the continued presence of all five Rel-related proteins. In contrast, nuclear κB-binding activity from B cells stimulated with anti-Ig for 24 hours failed to be supershifted with anti-RelB. The other Rel-related proteins were expressed in anti-Ig-induced DNA-binding material, although there was a little less RelA than in CD40L-stimulated B cell nuclear extracts. These results suggest that DNA-binding NF-κB induced by anti-Ig, but not by CD40L, undergoes a change in which the RelB component is lost as a function of time, indicating receptor- and Rel-protein-specificity in the regulation of NF-κB in primary B cells.

Loss of RelB from Anti-Ig-Induced NF-κB

To confirm these results Shift-Western analysis was undertaken [12]. EMSA-shifted nucleoprotein complexes were electro-transferred to stacked nitrocellulose membranes and DE81 paper; during this process DNA and protein undergo dissociation, with protein binding to nitrocellulose and radiolabeled DNA binding to DE81. The DE81 paper was autoradiographed to mark the location of oligonucleotide-shifted protein, and the nitrocellulose membrane containing κB-binding protein was blotted with anti-RelB. As suggested by the supershift results, Shift-Western analysis indicated that RelB was present in nuclear κB-binding material obtained from unstimulated B cells and from B cells stimulated with anti-Ig or CD40L for 2 hours, as well as from B cells stimulated with CD40L for 24 hours, with more RelB at 24 hours than at 2 hours. The Western blotted RelB band coincided with the electrophoretic mobility of the more rapidly migrating, CD40L-induced nucleoprotein complex (observed by autoradiography of the DNA-binding DE81 paper) that is absent in EMSA using nuclear extracts obtained from B cells treated for 24 hours with anti-Ig. In keeping with this, Shift-Western analysis showed that RelB was completely absent from κB-binding material obtained from B cells stimulated with anti-Ig for 24 hours.

In control Shift-Western experiments, there was no Western blotted RelB that migrated in the position of the κB-binding activity when oligonucleotide was omitted from the EMSA using CD40L-stimulated B cell nuclear extracts ("no DNA control"). Further, detection of RelB in Shift-Western analysis of CD40L-stimulated B cell nuclear protein was blocked by pre-incubation of the RelB-specific antiserum with the RelB peptide against which the antiserum was raised, but not by pre-incubation with a nonspecific peptide.

Time course experiments indicated that the loss of RelB from anti-Ig induced nuclear κB-binding activity occurred between 6 and 9 hours of B cell stimulation. Remarkably, however, straight Western analysis indicated the presence of RelB protein in nuclear extracts obtained from B cells stimulated with anti-Ig for 9-24 hours (times when RelB is lost from κB-binding material) in amounts similar to those present in B cells stimulated with CD40L. These results suggest that the loss of RelB from the κB-binding material obtained from anti-Ig-stimulated (24 hours) B cells is not due to the absence of RelB protein (or its dimerizing partners, p50 and p52). Instead, the loss of κB-binding RelB appears to result from post-translational modification of RelB or the intervention of an inhibitory activity; considering the delay in the disappearance of RelB, synthesis of an inhibitory factor seems plausible. Regardless of the mechanism, these results point to a previously unrecognized level of Rel protein regulation, in which κB-binding is modulated in the nucleus in a manner that is specific for RelB and for the sIg receptor.

Table 1. Rel protein composition of constitutive and induced NF-κB

		Induced			
Rel protein	Constitutive	anti-Ig 2 hr	CD40L 2 hr	anti-Ig 24 hr	CD40 24 hr
p50/p105	++	++	++	++	++
p52/p100	+	+	+	+	+
c-Rel	++	++	++	++	++
RelA	-	+	+	+	+
RelB	+	+	+	-	++

Loss of IκB Induced by Anti-Ig and CD40L

The possibility that one of the recognized IκB family members might be involved was explored by Western analysis of these proteins in whole cell extracts. IκBα and IκBβ responded to B cell stimulation by either anti-Ig or CD40L with a decrease in protein levels followed by recovery. For IκBβ, the loss occurred more rapidly and was a little more long lasting after stimulation by CD40L than anti-Ig, over a 24 hour time course. However, inasmuch as IκB has greater affinity for Rel proteins other than RelB [13], it is unlikely that the small differences observed between anti-Ig- and CD40L-stimulated B cells could account for the disappearance of κB-binding RelB, although the presence of nuclear IκBα/IκBβ has not been examined to date. There was no change in Bcl-3 protein levels following B cell stimulation.

Regulation of Fas-mediated Apoptosis

In collaborative work with Dr. Gail Sonenshein and colleagues (Boston University School of Medicine, Boston, MA), we have demonstrated an association between the prolonged expression of NF-κB in CD40L-treated WEHI 231 B cells and resistance to apoptosis induced through sIg crosslinking of these immature B cells, which appears to mediated by prevention of the late fall in c-*myc* expression that typically follows anti-Ig treatment [14]. In mature B cells, we have shown that the CD40 and sIg receptors oppose each others' actions in terms of apoptosis mediated by engagement of the surface receptor, Fas (CD95). In this case, B cell stimulation with CD40L leads to enhanced Fas expression and susceptibility to Fas-mediated apoptosis, whereas treatment with anti-Ig (alone or with CD40L) leads to a state of Fas-resistance [15]. The possibility that RelB expression might determine the level of Fas-sensitivity in primary B cells was tested by examining c-*myc* expression and the dominance of the RelB phenotype.

Expression of c-Myc was induced by either anti-Ig or CD40L, but induction following anti-Ig was more long-lasting (Fig. 1). In preliminary experiments, anti-Ig induced renewed c-Myc expression in CD40L-treated B cells, which correlates with the induction of Fas-resistance by anti-Ig in CD40L-treated B cells. It is unclear whether this might relate to anti-Ig-induced Fas-resistance. However, in several situations in which anti-Ig-induced Fas-resistance dominates (sequential treatment of B cells with anti-Ig and CD40L, for example, as in [16]) the absence of RelB also dominated, and this was true whether the κB site was drawn from the κ light chain enhancer or from the c-*myc* promoter. These results suggest the possibility that receptor-specific regulation of RelB may be associated with receptor-specific alteration of the level of B cell sensitivity to apoptosis mediated by Fas engagement.

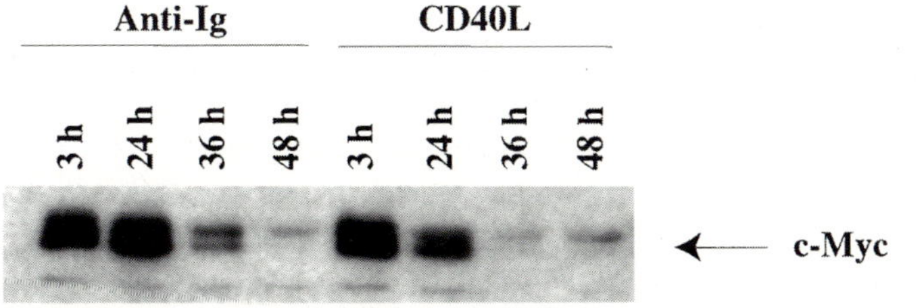

Fig. 1. Inducible expression of c-Myc protein. Primary B lymphocytes were stimulated with either anti-Ig or CD40L for various periods of time in hours (h), after which cellular proteins were size separated by SDS-PAGE and immunoblotted with a c-Myc-specific antiserum. The level of c-Myc in the medium control sample (0 h) was similar to that in the 48 h samples.

Discussion

In the present study we analyzed the composition of NF-κB induced by two mitogenic B cell receptors, sIg and CD40. Both receptors triggered nuclear expression of κB-binding material that contained all five mammalian Rel-related proteins, despite differences in the intracellular signaling pathways utilized by these receptors. The initial similarity in NF-κB induced by sIg and CD40 suggests that a final common pathway for nuclear NF-κB expression may be utilized by both receptors, at least early on. However, B cell nuclear κB-binding material induced by anti-Ig, but not by CD40L, changed with the loss of DNA-binding RelB during continued stimulation. Thus, the nature of inducible NF-κB may change as a function of time, which suggests a possible explanation for modulation of κB-dependent responses. Time-dependent alterations in the composition of induced NF-κB have previously been suggested on the basis of UV photocrosslinking experiments carried out in T cells [17].

The mechanism by which RelB is regulated remains to be clarified, but the observation that RelB protein is present in anti-Ig-induced nuclear extracts that have lost κB-binding RelB strongly suggests that it is the function, rather than the level, of RelB that is affected. This could be due to posttranslational modification of RelB or accumulation of a RelB inhibitor. The time required for RelB loss would seem to favor the latter explanation. It is remarkable, however, that whatever mechanism is involved appears to be specific for RelB, leaving closely related Rel proteins unperturbed. Thus, our results suggest that individual Rel-related proteins may be separately regulated, and that this regulation may be directed in a manner that depends on specific receptor engagement, rather than the general state of B cell activation.

Constitutive nuclear RelB expression is developmentally controlled in the B cell lineage, appearing in mature B cells and immunoglobulin producing plasma cells [18]. However, the complete loss of RelB by gene targeting produces mice in which B lymphocyte populations develop normally [19,20]. Despite the many and complex pathological abnormalities found in RelB deficient mice, isotype switching proceeds normally as does the induced expression of NF-κB regulated genes such as IFNγ, TNFα, and IL-2, although B cell proliferative responses are diminished in vitro [19-21]. Thus, the way in which the loss of RelB from κB-binding activity induced through sIgM as opposed to CD40 might distinguish the later effects of signaling through these two receptors remains unknown. However, on the basis of previous work in the WEHI 231 system it seems plausible that receptor-specific differences in NF-κB composition may play a role in setting the sensitivity point of B cell targets for Fas-mediated apoptosis, in which CD40L stimulation induces susceptibility to Fas killing and anti-Ig treatment produces a state of Fas-resistance. Future work will explore the validity of this concept.

The loss of κB-binding RelB is not the only example of receptor-specific differences in the composition of DNA-binding transcription factor complexes induced in primary B cells through sIg and CD40. Thus, B cell stimulation with anti-Ig leads to expression of the AP-1 proteins JunB, JunD, c-Fos and Fra-1, whereas B cell stimulation with CD40L leads to expression of the same Jun/Fos proteins plus FosB [22-24]. B cell stimulation with anti-Ig leads to nuclear expression of STAT1, STAT3, STAT5, and STAT6, whereas B cell stimulation with CD40L leads to nuclear expression only of STAT5 and STAT6 [25,26, and unpublished observations]. Taken together, these results suggest that the fine regulation of inducible responses depends on receptor-specific features of transcription factor complex composition, rather than the simple presence or absence of a sequence-specific DNA-binding complex, which may be preferentially responsible for lineage commitment and developmental switches.

Acknowledgments

This work was supported by United States Public Health Service grant CA66626 awarded by the National Institutes of Health.

References

1. Lee H, Arsura M, Wu M, Duyao M, Buckler AJ, and Sonenshein GE (1995) Role of Rel-related factors in control of c-*myc* gene transcription in receptor mediated apoptosis of the murine B cell WEHI 231 line. J Exp Med 181:1169-1177
2. Baeuerle PA, and Henkel T (1994) Function and activation of NF-κB in the immune system. Annu Rev Immunol 12:141-179
3. Thanos E, and Maniatis T (1995) NF-κB: A lesson in family values. Cell 80:529-532
4. Baeuerle PA, and Baltimore D (1996) NF-κB: Ten years later. Cell 87:13-20
5. Kawakami K, and Parker DC (1993) Antigen and helper T lymphocytes activate B lymphocytes by distinct signaling pathways. Eur J Immunol 23:77-84
6. Francis DA, Karras JG, Ke X-Y, Sen R, and Rothstein TL (1995) Induction of the transcription factors NF-κB, AP-1 and NF-AT during B cell stimulation through the CD40 receptor. Intl Immunol 7:151-161
7. Liu J, Chiles TC, Sen R, and Rothstein TL (1991) Inducible nuclear expression of NF-κB in primary B cells stimulated through the surface Ig receptor. J. Immunol. 146:1685-1691
8. Rooney JW, Dubois PM, and Sibley CH (1991) Crosslinking of surface IgM activates NF-κB in B lymphocytes. Eur J Immunol 21:2993-2998
9. Lalmanach-Girard A-C, Chiles TC, Parker CD, and Rothstein TL (1993) T cell-dependent induction of NF-κB in B cells. J. Exp. Med. 177:1215-1219.
10. Berberich I, Shu GL, and Clark EA (1994) Cross-linking CD40 on B cells rapidly activates nuclear factor-κB. J Immunol 153:4357-4366

11. Lane P, Brocker T, Hubele S, Padovan E, Lanzavecchia, A, and McConnell, F (1993) Soluble CD40 ligand can replace the normal T-cell derived CD40 ligand signal to B cells in T cell dependent activation. J Exp Med 177:1209-1213
12. Demczuk S, Harbers M, and Vennström B (1993) Identification and analysis of all componenets of a gel retardation assay by ccombination with immunoblotting. Proc Natl Acad Sci USA 90:2574-2578
13. Dobrzanski P, Ryseck RP, and Bravo R (1994) Differential interactions of Rel-NF-κB complexes with IκBα determine pools of constitutive and inducible NF-κB activity. EMBO J 13:4608-4616
14. Schauer SL, Wang Z, Sonenshein GE, and Rothstein TL (1996) Maintenance of nuclear factor-kB/Rel and c-myc expression during CD40 ligand rescue of WEHI 231 early B cells from receptor-mediated apoptosis through modulation of IkB proteins. J Immunol 157:81-86
15. Rothstein TL, Wang JKM, Panka DJ, Foote LC, Wang Z, Stanger B, Cui H, Ju S-T, and Marshak-Rothstein A (1995) Protection against Fas-dependent Th1-mediated apoptosis by antigen receptor engagement in B cells. Nature 374:163-165
16. Foote LC, Schneider TJ, Fischer GM, Wang JKM, Rasmussen B, Campbell KA, Lynch DH, Ju S-T, Marshak-Rothstein A, and Rothstein TL (1996) Intracellular signaling for inducible antigen receptor-mediated Fas resistance in B cells. J Immunol 157:1878-1885
17. Molitor JA, Walker WH, Doerre S, Ballard DW, and Greene WC (1991) NF-kB: a family of inducible and differentially expressed enhancer-binding proteins in human T cells. Proc Natl Acad Sci USA 87:10028-10032
18. Liou H-C, Sha WC, Scott ML, and Baltimore D (1994) Sequential induction of NF-κB/Rel family proteins during B-cell terminal differentiation. Mol Cell Biol 14:5349-5359
19. Weih F, Carrasco D, Durham SK, Barton DS, Rizzo CA, Ryseck R-P, Lira SA, and Bravo R (1995) Multiorgan inflammation and hematopoietic abnormalities in mice with a targeted disruption of RelB, a member of the NF-κB/Rel family. Cell 80:331-340
20. Burkly L, Hession C, Ogata L, Reilly C, Marconi LA, Olson D, Tizard R, Cate R, and Lo D (1995) Expression of relB is required for the development of thymic medulla and dendritic cells. Nature 373:531-536
21. Snapper CM, Rosas FR, Zelazowski P, Moorman MA, Kehry MR, Bravo R, and Weih F (1996) B cells lacking RelB are defective in proliferative responses, but undergo normal B cell maturation to Ig secretion and Ig class switching. J Exp Med 184:1537-1541
22. Chiles TC, and Rothstein TL (1992) Surface Ig receptor-induced nuclear AP-1 dependent gene expression in B lymphocytes. J Immunol 149:825-831
23. Huo L, and Rothstein TL (1995) Receptor-specific induction of individual AP-1 components in B lymphocytes. J Immunol 154:3300-3309
24. Huo L, and Rothstein TL (1996) Isolation and characterization of murine *fra-1*. Induction mediated by CD40 and surface Ig is protein kinase C dependent. J Immunol 157:3812-3818
25. Karras JG, Wang Z, Coniglio SJ, Frank DA, and Rothstein TL (1996) Antigen-receptor engagement in B cells induces nuclear expression of STAT5 and STAT6 proteins that bind and transactivate an IFN-γ activation site. J Immunol 157:39-47
26. Karras JG, Huo L, Wang Z, Frank DA, Zimmet J, and Rothstein TL (1996) Delayed tyrosine phosphorylation and nuclear expression of STAT1 following antigen receptor stimulation of B lymphocytes. J Immunol 157:2299-2309

c-Myc Promotes Survival of WEHI 231 B Lymphoma Cells from Apoptosis

M. Wu[1], W. Yang[1], R. E. Bellas[1], S. L. Schauer[2], M. J. FitzGerald[1], H. Lee[1] and G. E. Sonenshein[1]

[1] Department of Biochemistry, Boston University School of Medicine, Boston, MA 02118, USA

[2] Department of Microbiology, Boston University School of Medicine, Boston, MA 02118, USA

Introduction

The c-*myc* oncogene has been implicated in control of cell proliferation, differentiation, as well as neoplastic transformation. More recently, overexpression or inappropriate time of expression of the c-*myc* gene has been found to promote apoptosis. Cleveland and coworkers observed that addition of a vector expressing c-Myc protein accelerated apoptosis following IL-3 deprivation of the 32D IL-3-dependent myeloid cell line [3]. Similarly Evan and coworkers [10] found that transfection of 3T3 fibroblast cells with c-*myc* expression vectors led to enhanced levels of apoptosis upon growth arrest either by serum or isoleucine deprivation, or a thymidine block. These findings have been further extended using c-*myc* antisense oligonucleotides. Green and coworkers have shown that addition of these oligonucleotides to immature T cells and some T cell hybridomas, inhibited c-*myc* expression and prevented T cell receptor mediated apoptosis [23]. Together these results strongly suggest that inappropriate overexpression of c-*myc* promotes apoptosis in some cell systems.

The WEHI 231 lymphoma cell line has been characterized as an immature B cell on the basis of surface markers and biological properties [7,19]. Growth of these cells can be arrested within 24 hours by interaction with an antibody against the expressed surface immunoglobulin chains [19]. Boyd and Schrader [7] proposed this system as a model for self-induced B cell tolerance. In support of this hypothesis, it was demonstrated that anti-IgM treatment causes apoptosis of WEHI 231 cells within 18 hours [6]. Treatment of WEHI 231 cells with anti-IgM antiserum results in dramatic changes in c-*myc* expression. As we first showed several years ago, an initial 5-10-fold increase in c-*myc* mRNA levels between the first and second hours after treatment is followed by a rapid decline in c-*myc* expression [19]. By 6 to 8 hrs of treatment, c-*myc* RNA and protein levels fall well below control values [18,19]. Several lines of evidence suggest that it is the drop in c-*myc* expression following anti-Ig treatment that results in apoptosis of WEHI 231 cells, in contrast to the findings discussed above. Mutants of WEHI 231 resistant to anti-IgM induced apoptosis display only a transient increase in c-*myc* RNA following antiserum treatment [13], whereas, treatment of WEHI 231 cells with TGF-β1 induces a drop in c-*myc* expression and subsequently apoptosis [2,26]. More recently, Fischer et al. [11] have found that addition of an antisense oligonucleotide specific for c-*myc* prevented apoptosis of WEHI 231 cells but surprisingly led to stabilization of c-*myc* expression. Although, the mechanism for this stabilization was not determined, these results also suggest that it is the drop in c-*myc* expression below levels seen in exponentially growing cells that signals apoptosis.

Antigen receptor-mediated apoptosis in WEHI 231 B cells has been reported to be reversed by engagement of surface CD40 [25], a member of the TNFR family [rev. in 4]. CD40 plays a critical role in B cell function as evidenced by the absence of germinal centers and secondary immune responses in CD40-deficient mice and the association of mutations in CD40 ligand with the human disease, X-linked Hyper-IgM Syndrome [rev. in 4]. The reversal of WEHI 231 apoptosis by CD40 ligand (CD40L) provided the means to further probe the relationships between c-*myc* and B cell apoptosis. Addition of a soluble form of CD40L to anti-IgM treated WEHI 231 cells resulted in maintenance of elevated levels of c-Myc expression associated with sustained NF-κB binding to the c-*myc* NF-κB sites and reversal of anti-IgM-induced apoptosis [22]. Thus as described here, we next assessed the effects of CD40L on TGF-β1-mediated apoptosis and found similar maintenance of c-*myc* expression. These findings led us to test the effects of enforced c-*myc* gene expression, as well as inhibition of c-Myc levels. Our results demonstrate a drop in c-*myc* expression induces apoptosis of WEHI 231 B cells.

Results

CD40 Ligand Prevents Apoptosis and Induces c-Myc Expression

We first explored whether CD40L rescue from apoptosis mediated by treatment with TGF-β1 affected the levels of c-*myc* expresion. As seen in Fig. 1, the normal drop in c-Myc nuclear protein levels following treatment with TGF-β1 were abrogated in cells treated with a combination of TGF-β1 and CD40L. In fact an increase in c-Myc protein levels that were maintained above basal levels for up to 9 hrs were seen in the dual treated cells (Fig. 1). Similarly, the drop in c-*myc* expression normally seen following anti-IgM treatment was also blocked upon cotreatment with anti-IgM and CD40L [22]. Thus, rescue of WEHI 231 cells from apoptosis upon CD40L co-stimulation leads to the maintenance of elevated levels of c-*myc* expression.

Ectopic c-Myc expression ablates apoptosis mediated by anti-IgM or TGF-β1

We next assessed whether ectopic c-Myc expression protects WEHI 231 cells against anti-IgM receptor mediated cell killing. Stable transfectants were made with the c-*myc* expression vector pM21, which is driven by the MoMLV LTR

[27], and clonal lines were isolated by limiting dilution. As controls, pSV2neo transfected clones were similarly prepared. Two pSV2neo control (S8, S10) and two c-Myc expressing (P14, P17) lines were treated with anti-IgM. Cell death, monitored after 24 and 48 hours using conversion of MTS to its formazan product or trypan blue exclusion, was signficantly ablated in lines ectopically expressing c-*myc* compared to the neo controls (Fig. 2). Furthermore, continued cell proliferation was noted [27], similar to the effects of CD40L.

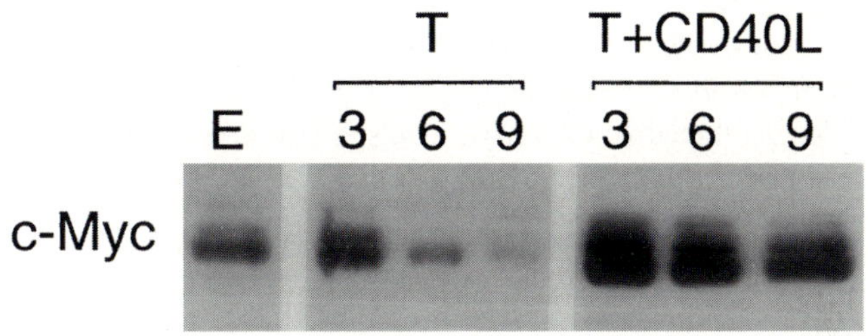

Fig. 1. CD40L treatment overrides TGF-β1 downmodulation of c-Myc expression. Nuclear proteins were isolated from WEHI 231 cells in exponential growth (E) or following treatment with either TGF-β1 alone (T) or in combination with CD40L (T + CD40L).

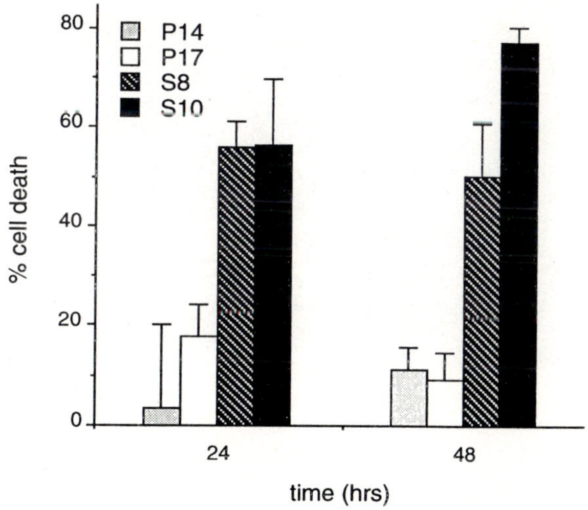

Fig. 2. Ectopic expression of c-Myc prevents apoptosis of WEHI 231 cells induced by anti-IgM treatment. Stable WEHI 231 clones transfected with either pSV2neo (S8 and S10) or pM21 c-*myc* expression vector (P14 and P17) were treated in duplicate with anti-IgM for 24 or 48 hrs and analyzed for cell viability by conversion of MTS dye to its formazan product. Data are plotted as percent viable cells relative to untreated control cultures.

The role of c-Myc in apoptosis induced by TGF-β1 was similarly tested. Two clones ectopically expressing c-*myc* displayed significant protection from apoptosis, as judged by the absence of DNA fragmentation, was observed. The S5 (neo) cells remained sensitive to TGF-β1 driven apoptosis (Fig. 3). As expected an elevated level of c-Myc protein was retained for up to 20 hrs following TGF-β1 treatment. These findings are in marked contrast to the downregulation of c-Myc observed in the control S5 cells (Fig. 3) and in the parental WEHI 231 cells (data not shown). In addition, the pM21 clones displayed extensive survival and were proliferating even after 48 hrs of TGF-β1 treatment (data not shown). Following TGF-β1 treatment of P17, an elevated level of c-Myc protein was retained for up to 20 hrs in marked contrast to the down-regulation observed in the neo control cells (Fig. 3, inset). These results indicate that the maintenance of c-Myc levels is sufficient to override the effects of TGF-β1 or anti-IgM treatment on viability of WEHI 231 cells.

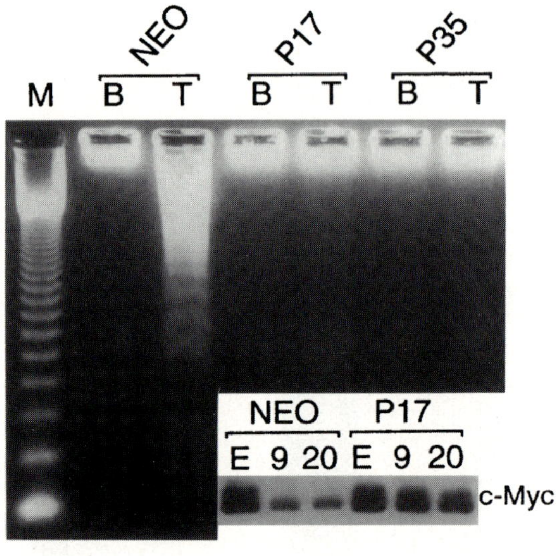

Fig. 3. Ectopic expression of c-Myc prevents apoptosis of WEHI 231 cells exposed to TGF-β1. Two stable c-Myc WEHI 231 clones P17 and P35 and a pSV2neo control were treated with TGF-β1 for 20 hrs and a DNA fragmentation assay performed. Alternatively, a stable WEHI 231 line expressing Bcl-XL was similarly analyzed. M, 123 marker DNA. Inset, The P17 and control neo lines were incubated in the absence (E) or presence of TGF-β1 for 9 and 20 hrs. Nuclear proteins (40ug) were subjected to immunoblotting for c-Myc.

TPCK Treatment Reduces c-*myc* mRNA and Induces Apoptosis of WEHI 231 Cells

The murine c-*myc* gene contains two functional NF-κB elements, which we termed the upstream and internal regulatory elements (URE and IRE, respectively) [8,15]. Recently we demonstrated that the NF-κB/Rel family of transcription factors plays a major role in the control of c-*myc* gene expression in WEHI 231 cells [17]. Exponentially growing WEHI 231 cells express a large amount of nuclear NF-κB/Rel factors, in part due to the rapid rate of turnover in these cells of the specific inhibitory protein IκB-α [17,20], and cotransfection of an IκB-α expression vector decreases c-*myc* promoter activity in these cells [17]. To test directly whether the decrease in c-*myc* expression promotes apoptosis of WEHI 231 cells, we treated WEHI 231 cells with the protease inhibitor N-Tosyl-L-phenylalanine chloromethyl ketone (TPCK), which inhibits IκB-α turnover in WEHI 231 cells [12,20]. Incubation with 25 uM TPCK resulted in a dramatic decline in NF-κB/Rel binding activity and c-*myc* expression (data not shown). The levels of c-Myc protein were measured by immunoblotting. The drop in c-Myc protein levels was noted by 2 hours of TPCK treatment and the levels continued to decline over the time course. Apoptosis as monitored by DNA fragmentation was easily detectable by about 4 hours of treatment (Fig. 4). To confirm the role of c-Myc in cell death, the P14 and P17 WEHI 231 lines ectopically expressing c-*myc* were similarly treated with TPCK; these lines displayed significant protection from apoptosis [28].Thus, induction of apoptosis in WEHI 231 cells correlates with the drop in c-*myc* RNA levels mediated by TPCK treatment.

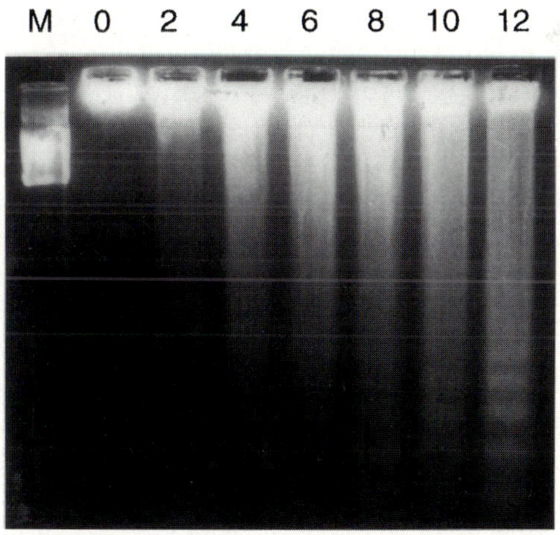

Fig. 4. TPCK treatment induces apoptosis of WEHI 231 cells. Control or TPCK-treated cells (1.5 x 10^6 cells/sample) were subjected to the DNA fragmentation assay of apoptosis.

Inhibition of NF-κB/Rel via microinjection of its specific inhibitor IκB-α induces apoptosis of WEHI 231 cells

To directly test the role of the inhibition of NF-κB/Rel binding, individual WEHI 231 cells were microinjected with either IκB-α-GST or GST protein or affinity purified NF-κB/Rel subunit antibodies. Introduction of IκB-α-GST induced apoptosis of WEHI 231 cells, as judged by increased appearance of chromatin condensation [28] and trypan blue exclusion (Fig. 5). As a control, WEHI 231 cells were similarly microinjected with GST protein alone, which had little effect on cell death. The most abundant transactivating Rel-related subunit expressed in WEHI 231 cells is c-Rel, whereas only lower levels of p65 subunit have been detected [17]. Significant levels of apoptosis were induced upon microinjection of a c-Rel antibody (Fig. 5), which was specific as judged by the dramatically reduced the extent of apoptosis upon microinjection of the c-Rel antibody in the presence of its cognate peptide. Microinjection of an affinity purified antibody against p65 led to only a slight increase in apoptotic cells. This finding might relate to the low level of this subunit in WEHI 231 cells [17] or to the observation that p65 positively regulates transcription of IκB-α. Therefore, a decrease in synthesis of the inhibitor IκB-α would compensate for an initial drop in the level of p65. Thus, a reduced level of NF-κB/Rel activity, and therefore c-*myc* expression, induces death of WEHI 231 B lymphoma cells. This was confirmed with the finding that induction of a vector expressing the antisense exon 2 and 3 c-*myc* RNA led to apoptosis of WEHI 231 cells. Thus a drop in c-*myc* expression mediates signals activating apoptosis of WEHI 231 B cells.

c-Myc Transactivation Through E-box is Not Apparent in WEHI 231 Cells

The differential effect of c-*myc* in apoptosis raised key questions about its functional role in these diverse cells. The c-Myc protein has been found to regulate gene expression through multiple mechanisms. Expression of c-*myc* activate genes containing an E-box element [5,9,16]. Thus, we tested for transactivation of an E-box driven heterologous promoter CAT reporter construct via contransfection analysis. Surprisingly, we were unable to detect any induction of CAT activity upon cotransfection of a c-*myc* expression vector (data not shown), in contrast to our findings with NIH 3T3 fibroblasts [1]. We next tested for expression of two genes that contain E-box elements and are controlled by c-Myc, ornithine decarboxylase (ODC) and α-prothymosin [5,9]. The changes in mRNA expression of these genes upon treatment of WEHI 231 cells with either TGF-β1 or anti-IgM failed to follow the increases or decreases in parallel with the changes in c-*myc* expression. Several groups have found that c-Myc inhibits expression of genes with an initiator (Inr) element [21]. Thus, we asked whether c-Myc expression in WEHI 231 cells down-regulates Inr driven transcription. An adeno promoter construct containing either two wild type or mutant copies of its Inr element was employed in transient transfection assays. WEHI 231 cells in exponential growth or following treatment with anti-IgM for 16 hours were transfected. An approximate 2.5-fold increase in CAT activity was seen. The activation of Inr mediated transcription is likely due in part to the drop in c-*myc* expression.

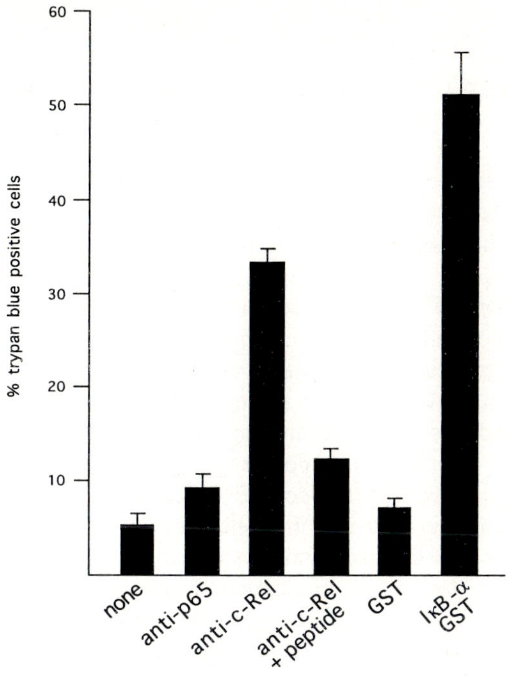

Fig. 5. Microinjection of IκB-α-GST or an affinity-purified c-Rel antibody promotes cell death of WEHI 231 cells. WEHI 231 cells were microinjected in duplicate with 1 mg/ml purified GST or I κB-α-GST fusion protein, or 4 mg/ml affinity-purified antibody against RelA (p65) or c-Rel proteins in the absence or presence of 4 mg/ml cognate peptide. Data are plotted as the mean percentage of cells stained positive for trypan blue and cell viability measured by dye exclusion. Data are plotted as the mean percentage of cells stained positive for trypan blue.

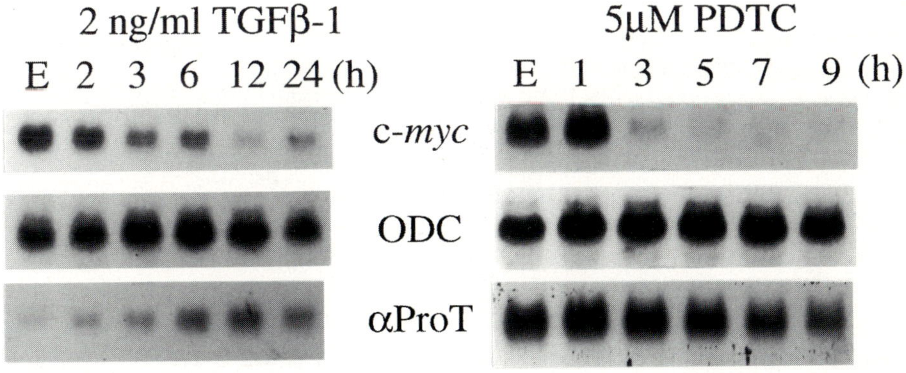

Fig. 6. ODC and α-prothymosin mRNA expression fails to parallel c-*myc* levels. RNA, isolated from WEHI 231 in exponential growth or following treatment with 2 ng/ml TGF-β1 or 5 uM PDTC, was analyzed for c-*myc*, ODC, and α-prothymosin mRNA levels by Northern blotting.

Discussion

Treatment of WEHI 231 cells with the CD40L protected against TGF-β1 induced apoptosis and led to maintenance of very high levels of c-Myc expression. Similarly, we found that CD40L protection from anti-IgM mediated apoptosis of WEHI 231 cells resulted in maintenance of elevated levels of c-Myc expression [22]. The finding that ectopic c-Myc expression led to enhanced survival of WEHI 231 B cells from the apoptosis induced by treatment with anti-IgM, TGF-β1, or TPCK [2,27] suggests that the c-*myc* gene plays an important role in this protection. Treatment of WEHI 231 cells with the protease inhibitor TPCK caused a significant reduction in NF-κB/Rel activity, which induced a dramatic decrease in c-*myc* mRNA and protein levels. Extensive apoptosis of these cells resulted from the TPCK treatment. Taken together these results demonstrate that the drop in c-*myc* expression mediates signals leading to induction of physiologic cell death of WEHI 231 B cells. Similar conclusions were drawn by Kaptein and coworkers who used antisense c-*myc* oligonucleotides which diminished c-Myc expression in EBV$^-$ Burkitt lymphoma lines and induced apoptosis [14]. As discussed above, treatment of other B cell lines at a similar stage of development, such as CH31 or CH33, with agents that result in decreased c-*myc* expression correlate with induction of apoptosis [2,26]. In this regard then B cells appear to differ in their regulation of apoptosis and the role of c-*myc* expression from some other cell types studied [3,5,10], in that the extent of drop in c-Myc expression, rather than its overexpression, appears responsible for the signalling that triggers induction of the apoptotic pathway.

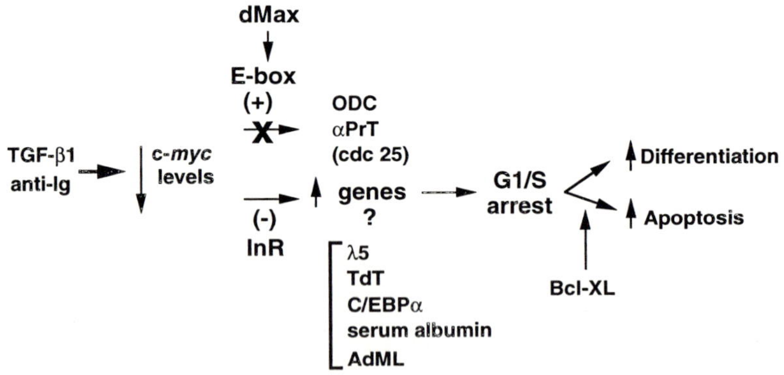

Fig. 7. Model of the functional role of c-Myc in apoptosis of WEHI 231 cells induced by treatment with anti-IgM or TGF-β1.

These differences can be reconciled by a model in which the ability of c-*myc* to function as either a positive or negative regulator is controlled in a cell-type specific fashion. As discussed above, both positive (E box) and negative (Inr) pathways of c-Myc action have been elucidated [16]. In WEHI 231 cells, our data argue that the positive pathway through E-box is turned off, as illustrated in Fig. 6. This may relate to the expression of dMax, which binds to c-Myc but prevents interaction with E-box and thus represents a naturally occurring dominant negative inhibitor of c-Myc transactivation through this element [1], although, additional negative regulators may also exist. Our data indicate that in WEHI 231 cells, c-Myc function is directed to the negative pathway. Thus, a drop in c-Myc expression can lead directly to the activation of expression of Inr-regulated gene through de-repression. Additional levels of control may also be mediated through YY1 [24]. If the regulation of pathway selection is differentially controlled, then this model would explain many of the apparent contradictory results on the role of this oncogene in control of gene expression and apoptosis.

Acknowledgments

We thank U. Siebenlist and S. Hann for generously providing protein and cloned DNAs, and antibody preparations, respectively. This work was supported by grants from the National Institutes of Health CA36355 (G.E.S.).

References

1. Arsura M, Deshpande A, Hann SR, Sonenshein GE (1995) Variant Max protein, derived by alternative splicing, associates with c-Myc in vivo and inhibits transactivation. Mol Cell Biol 15:6702-6709
2. Arsura M, Wu M, Sonenshein GE (1996) TGF-β1 inhibits NF-κB/Rel activity inducing apoptosis of B cells: transcriptional activation of IκBα. Immunity 5:31-40
3. Askew DS, Ashmun R, Simmons B, Cleveland J (1991) Constitutive c-myc expression in IL-3-dependent myeloid cell line suppresses cycle arrest and accelerates apoptosis. Oncogene 6:1915-1922
4. Banchereau J, Bazan R, Blanchard D, Briere F, Galizzi JP, van Kooten C, Liu YJ, Rousset F, Saeland S (1994) The CD40 antigen and its ligand. Annu Rev Immunol 12:881-922
5. Bello-Fernandez C, Packham, G, Cleveland JL (1993) The ornithine decarboxylase gene is a transcriptional target of c-myc. Proc. Natl. Acad. Sci. USA 90:7804-7808.

6. Benhamou L, Cazenave P, Sarthou P (1990) Anti-immunoglobulins induce death by apoptosis in WEHI-231 B lymphoma cells. Eur J Immunol 20: 1405-1407
7. Boyd A, Schrader J (1981) The regulation of growth and differentiation of a murine B-cell lymphoma. II. The inhibition of WEHI 231 by anti-immunoglobulin antibodies. J Immunol 126:2466-2469
8. Duyao MP, Buckler AJ, Sonenshein GE (1990) Interaction of an NF-κB-like factor with a site upstream of the c-myc promoter. Proc Natl Acad Sci USA 87:4727-4731
9. Eilers M, Schirm S, Bishop JM (1991) The Myc protein activates transcription of the alpha-prothymosin gene. EMBO J 10:133-141
10. Evan G, Wyllie A, Gilbert C, Littlewood T, Land H, Brooks M, Waters C, Penn L, Hancock D (1992) Induction of apoptosis in fibroblasts by c-myc protein. Cell 69:119-128.
11. Fischer G, Kent S, Joseph L, Green D, Scott D (1994) Lymphoma models for B cell activation and tolerance. X. anti-u-mediated growth arrest and apoptosis of murine B cell lymphomas is prevented by the stabilization of myc. J Exp Med 179:221-228
12. Henkel T, Machleidt T, Alkalay I, Kronke M, Ben-Niriah Y, Baeuerle P (1993) Rapid proteolysis of IκB-α is necessary for activation of transcription factor NF-κB. Nature 365:182-185
13. Hibner U, Benhamou L, Haury M, Cazenave PA, Sarthou P (1994) Signalling of programmed cell death induction in WEHI-231 B lymphoma cells. Eur J Immunol 4:1993-1999
14. Kaptein JS, Lin CK, Wang CL, Nguyen TT, Kalunta C, Park E, Chen FS, Lad PM (1996) Anti-IgM-mediated regulation of c-myc and its possible relationship to apoptosis. J Biol Chem 271:18875-18884
15. Kessler DJ, Spicer D, La Rosa F, Sonenshein GE (1992) A novel NF-κB element within exon 1 of the murine c-myc gene. Oncogene 7:2447-2453
16. Kretzner L, Blackwood EM, Eisenman RN (1992) Myc and Max proteins possess distinct transcriptional activities. Nature 359:426-429
17. Lee H, Arsura M, Wu M, Duyao MP, Buckler AJ, Sonenshein GE (1995) Role of Rel-related factors in control of c-myc gene transcription in receptor mediated apoptosis of the murine B cell WEHI 231 line. J Exp Med 181:1169-1177
18. Levine RA, McCormack JE, Buckler AJ and Sonenshein GE (1986) Transcription and posttranscriptional control of c-myc gene expression in WEHI 231 cells. Mol Cell Biol 6:4112-4116
19. McCormack JE, Pepe VH, Kent RB, Dean M, Marshak-Rothstein A, Sonenshein GE (1984) Specific regulation of c-myc oncogene expression in a murine B-cell lymphoma. Proc Natl Acad Sci USA 81:5546-5550
20. Miyamoto S, Chia P, Verma I (1994) Enhanced IκBα degradation is responsible for constitutive NF-κB activity in mature B-cell lines. Mol Cell Biol 14:3276-3282

21. Roy AL, Carruthers C, Gutjhar T, Roeder RG (1993) Distinct role for Myc in transcription initiation mediated by interactions with TFII-I. Nature 365:359-361
22. Schauer SL, Wang Z, Sonenshein GE, Rothstein TL (1996) Maintenance of Nuclear factor-κB/Rel and c-myc expression during CD40 ligand rescue of WEHI 231 early B cells from receptor-mediated apoptosis through modulation of IκB proteins. J Immunol 157:81-86
23. Shi Y, Glynn J, Guilbert L, Cotter T, Bissonnette R, Green D (1992) Role for c-myc in activation induced apoptotic cell death in T-cell hybridoma. Science 257:212-215
24. Shrivastava A, Saleque S, Kalpana GV, Artand S, Goff SP, Calame K (1993) Inhibition of transcriptional regulator Yin-Yang-1 by association with c-Myc. Science 262:1889-1892
25. Tsubata T, Wu J, Honjo T (1993) B-cell apoptosis induced by antigen receptor crosslinking is blocked by a T-cell signal through CD40. Nature 364:645-648
26. Warner GL, Ludlow J, Nelson DO, Gaur A, Scott D (1992) Anti-immunoglobulin treatment of B cell lymphomas induces active TGF-β but pRB hypophosphorylation is TGF-β independent. Cell Growth and Diff 3:175-181
27. Wu M, Arsura M, Bellas RE, FitzGerald MJ, Lee H, Schauer SL, Sherr DH, Sonenshein GE (1996) Inhibition of c-myc expression induces apoptosis of WEHI 231 murine B cells. Mol Cell Biol 16:5015-5025
28. Wu M, Lee H, Bellas RE, Schauer SL, Arsura M, Katz D, FitzGerald MJ, Rothstein TL, Sherr DH, Sonenshein GE (1996) Inhibition of NF-κB/Rel induces apoptosis of murine B cells. EMBO J 15:4682-4690

Role of c-myc and p27 in Anti-IgM Induced B-Lymphoma Apoptosis

D. W. Scott*, D. Donjerković, B. Maddox, S. Ezhevsky and T. Grdina
Department of Immunology, Holland Laboratory for the Biomedical Sciences, American Red Cross, Rockville, MD 20855, USA

Abstract

Crosslinking membrane IgM receptors on a set of murine B cell lymphomas leads to a rapid increase in c-myc, followed by a decrease in its expression to undetectable levels by 8-24 hours. These cells die soon thereafter via apoptosis. IgD receptor crosslinking also leads to an increase in c-myc expression, but it remains above baseline levels for more than 24 hours; these cells continue to proliferate and do not die. We previously reported that antisense oligonucleotides for c-myc prevented growth arrest and cell death in these lymphomas, independent of the presence of mitogenic CpG motifs. Indeed, antisense for c-myc actually led to a stabilization of c-myc message and protein. Growth arrest in these cells is dependent on the increased synthesis of the p27 cyclin kinase inhibitor (Kip1) normally induced after anti-IgM crosslinking. Consistent with its biologic effects, anti-IgD does not cause an increase in p27. Since dexamethasone causes a loss of myc and synergizes with the anti-IgM signal, we suggest that accelerated cell death with this steroid in the presence of anti-IgM is due to a more rapid degradation of this oncogene product. Finally, we propose that c-myc drives the transcription or activation of an inhibitor of the p27 Kip (Kipi). Hence, loss of c-myc in response to anti-IgM signals in these B-cell lymphomas leads to upregulation of p27, growth arrest and apoptosis. It follows that maintenance of c-myc in these B-cell lymphomas should lead to survival and no increase in p27.

Introduction

For more than a decade, we have used the growth arrest and cell death induced by crosslinking of membrane IgM on murine and human B-cell lymphomas as a model for tolerance. Our results have shown that any reagent which can crosslink IgM receptors is effective in this process. This includes polyclonal and monoclonal anti-Ig reagents of any domain specificity and affinity [1-3]; intact IgG antibodies are not required, indicating the lack of a role for Fc receptor downregulation as part of the

* To whom correspondence should be addressed.

signal transduction cascade. These results have been confirmed in several labs and have led to the observation that cell death is due to apoptosis in this model [4-6]. Moreover, crosslinking the IgD receptor on these lymphoma cells fails to induce growth arrest or apoptosis [7,8], despite the sharing of many initial tyrosine phosphorylation events [7,9]. We know that initial signals via these receptors require ITAM sequences in Igα and Igβ [10, 11] and lead to an evanescent increase and subsequent loss of c-myc transcription, originally observed by McCormack et al [12]. Therefore, we have investigated the relationship between c-myc, growth arrest and apoptosis [13].

Basically, we have found that IgM crosslinking, which must occur in early G_1, causes an inactivation of the cyclin (A)-Cdk-2 kinase complex that is responsible for the phosphorylation of the retinoblastoma gene product, pRB [14,15]. This is mediated primarily by the increase in the levels of the $p27^{Kip1}$ kinase inhibitor [16,17] and the sequestration of virtually all cyclin A in complexes with an excess of p27. Interestingly, the upregulation of p27 occurs in unsynchronized cells after the levels of myc protein and message are well below baseline levels. Our hypothesis is that c-myc either is necessary for the transcription of an inhibitor of p27 (which we call Kipi) or that myc transcriptionally represses the synthesis of p27. However, our recent data suggest that myc levels *per se* can not account for the regulation of p27 but must be coupled with other signals initiated by the IgM receptor.

Results and Discussion

Kinetics of signaling via IgM: Regulation of cell cycle progression and myc expression

As noted above, we have shown that antibodies against IgM, but not IgD, induce growth arrest and apoptosis in CH33, in its IgD transfected derivative called ECH408 [8], and in a similarly transfected clone of the WEHI-231 lymphoma [7]. A typical dose response curve for growth arrest and apoptosis in WEHI-231 with anti-IgM is shown in **figure 1** (at 24 hours). Interestingly, growth arrest occurs after a significant lag, based on thymidine incorporation and cell cycle analyses [17, 18]. This is illustrated for the CH31 lymphoma in **figure 2**, which mirrors results seen with WEHI-231 [18], except that the former cells are more sensitive to anti-IgM arrest. We now know that this reflects the exquisite sensitivity of both of these cell lines to signals in G_1, after which they are insensitive to anti-IgM until the cells recycle back to early G_1 [2]. These kinetics are also explained by the fact that pRB becomes phosphorylated by mid-G_1, after which the regulatory events induced by anti-IgM are ineffective (see below). It is curious that the changes in c-myc appear to precede the events described above.

Thus, it is interesting that anti-IgM treatment of these B-cell lymphomas leads to a rapid but evanescent increase in the transcription of c-myc within 30-60 minutes (with a drop to undetectable levels within 5-24 hours)[12,13]. Moreover, anti-IgD crosslinking, which does not lead to growth arrest or apoptosis, also causes an increase in c-myc levels above background steady state levels, but this mRNA does not decrease to below background synthesis as it does with anti-IgM ([11,12]. An example of these patterns is shown in schematic form as **figure 3**. It is noteworthy that TGF-β, which also causes growth arrest and apoptosis of these B-cell lymphomas, also induces a loss of c-myc in our hands [14]. Interestingly, CAT assays with c-myc P1 and P2 promoter constructs (provided by Dr. Ken Marcu) showed that anti-IgM led to transcriptional upregulation of c-myc, whereas TGF-β caused a loss of CAT activity (data not shown).

Several years ago, we began to investigate the role of the products of the *c-myc* oncogene in growth arrest and apoptosis of these lymphomas. While we suspected that loss of myc was a crucial event for cell cycle progression and survival, data in T cells from Green's group suggested that overexpression of c-myc, especially at cell

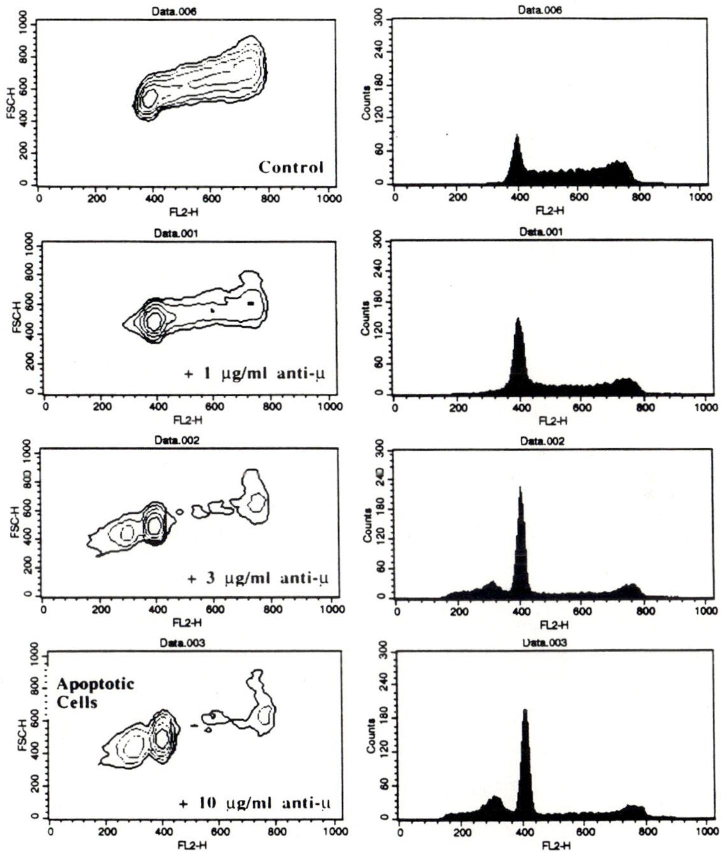

Fig. 1. Growth arrest and apoptosis induction by anti-IgM in the WEHI-231 B-cell lymphoma. Data in this figure are from propidium iodide analysis of WEHI-231 cells at 24 hours with increasing concentrations of anti-IgM. Forward scatter plots versus PI are shown on the left, whereas PI versus cell numbers are represented on the right. In both cases, anti-IgM causes a loss of cells in S and an increase in the G_1 peak. Hypodiploid cells, verified as apoptotic appear at the left in both plots.

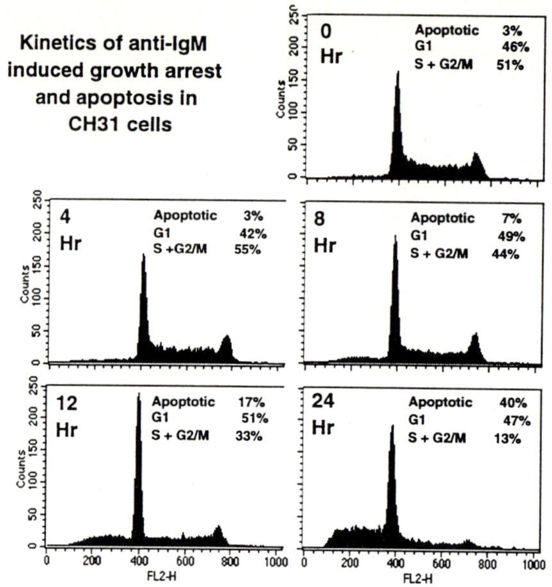

Fig. 2. Kinetics of growth arrest and apoptosis induction by anti-IgM in the CH31 B-cell lymphoma. Data plotted as in figure 1 (right) from propidium iodide analysis of CH31 cells at 0-24 hours with 1 μg/ml of anti-IgM. Note that CH31 is considerably more sensitive to anti-IgM than is WEHI-231 (*cf.* figure 1).

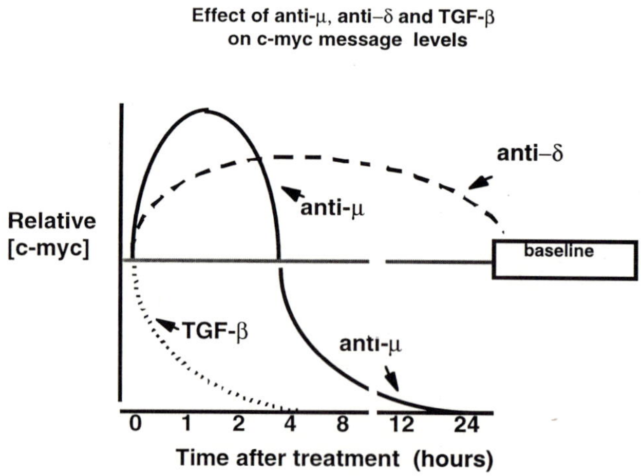

Fig. 3. Scheme for representative increases and decreases in c-myc message and protein levels induced by anti-IgM (solid line), anti-IgD (dashed line) and TGF-b (dotted line). Data are modified from refs. [7], [12] and [13].

cycle restriction points, could cause apoptosis [19]. Therefore, we treated CH31 and WEHI-231 cells with antisense S-oligonucleotides (directed at the first translational start site in exon 2) or scrambled nonsense oligos, as well as oligos against c-jun and fos, for their effects on anti-IgM-driven apoptosis. The results in **Table 1** indicate that antisense for c-myc effectively protected both of these B lymphomas from anti-IgM driven cell death (data summarized from ref. 13). When we examined the levels of myc protein and message in these cells, we were surprised to observe that antisense c-myc actually caused an increase in myc, rather than a block in its transcription and/or translation. Moreover, antisense myc protected against the anti-IgM-induced disappearance of this oncogene message and protein! These results, demonstrating a stabilization of myc, were soon confirmed by Sonenshein and colleagues [20] using nuclear run-ons, for example. Antisense for c-myc had no effect on the anti-IgD signal (Scott, unpublished).

Table 1

Effect of antisense and nonsense c-myc oligonucleotides on anti-IgM induced apoptosis in CH31

Anti-IgM	Oligos added	Per cent apoptosis*
-	None	6
+	None	46
-	Antisense c-myc	7
+	Antisense c-myc	5
-	Nonsense c-myc	7
+	Nonsense c-myc	48

* Per cent of cells with apoptotic bodies as identified microscopically with acridine orange staining. Representative data modified from ref. 13. See also ref. 23.

A note of caution that must be mentioned is that Krieg and colleagues [21] recently reported that oligonucleotides that contain a unmethylated CpG motif, usually flanked by a pyrimidine dimer, are particularly mitogenic for resting B cells and can prevent anti-IgM-induced apoptosis in WEHI-231 [22]. Since our antisense c-myc contained such a motif, it was important to establish whether mitogenicity of these oligos might account for the prevention of growth arrest and apoptosis. Fortunately, this does not appear to be the case since antisense oligos downstream from the translational start site (and lacking the mitogenic CpG motif) were also effective and several other CpG containing oligos failed to reverse the effects of anti-IgM [13, Maddox and Scott, unpublished and see ref. 23]. Moreover, methylated cytosine containing oligos were also effective at blocking apoptosis. Thus, the effects of antisense oligos for c-myc appear to be specific, although the reasons why myc message is stabilized by them are not known. More recent data from Sonenshein's lab [24 and *vide infra*] reiterate the fact that stabilization of myc is more important in the prevention of apoptosis in these lymphoma cells. The possible link between myc stabilization and cell cycle control is considered next.

Role of p27 in the regulation of cell cycle progression and apoptosis

We know that anti-IgM treatment of WEHI-231 and CH31 lymphoma cells leads to an accumulation of these cells in late G_1, after which they are committed to apoptosis during the next 24 hours [1, 2, 13, 18]. As noted above, delivery of the negative signal must occur in early G_1 since delaying crosslinking fails to block cell cycle progression. This correlates with the lag in the kinetics of growth arrest as well as the dynamics of the phosphorylation of the retinoblastoma growth suppressor (pRB). We and others [14,15,22] have shown that growth arrest by anti-IgM treatment was due to the accumulation of the hypophosphorylated form of the retinoblastoma gene product, pRB, and not a dephosphorylation event. A nuclear phosphoprotein, which undergoes cell-cycle dependent phosphorylation and dephosphorylation, hypophosphorylated pRB is growth-suppressive and is tightly associated with the nucleus [25]. It is assumed that hypophosphorylated pRB regulates cell cycle progression by binding a number of proteins, including E2F. Once pRB is phosphorylated, E2F is released and the cells progress into S phase.

This phosphorylation process occurs on serine and threonine residues of pRB during G_1 and is dependent on the formation of an active cyclin-Cdk complex that we now know to contain Cdk-2, cyclin A and a stoichiometric amount of the p27 kinase inhibitor in these B-cell lymphomas [15-17]. Our most recent data suggest that the kinetics of growth arrest mirrors the state of phosphorylation of pRB and the activity associated with a kinase of cyclin A (or E) and Cdk-2 [see refs. 15,17 for details]. Key to this result is the fact that virtually all of the cellular cyclin A is associated with p27 in arrested WEHI-231 cells, whereas in growing cells, less than half of the cyclin complex is p27-associated. An example of this is shown in **figure 4**.

Since both anti-IgM and anti-IgD crosslinking drive many of the same initial signals (PTK activation, phosphatidyl inositol breakdown, early c-myc upregulation) but have different biological results (death *versus* life), it was important to determine whether they had the differential effects on pRB via p27. We found that anti-IgD treatment did not lead to a prevention of the phosphorylation of pRB (L. Joseph and D. W. Scott, unpublished), as anti-IgM crosslinking does. Western blots for p27 were then performed on extracts of an IgM+, IgD+ lymphoma called ECH408 (a derivative of CH33), which had been treated with either anti-IgM or anti-IgD reagents. A

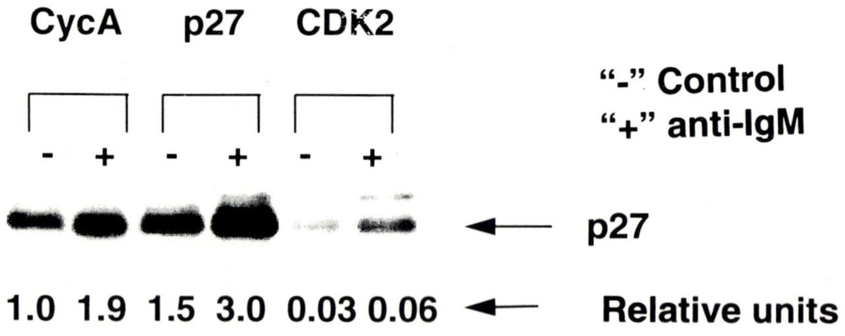

Fig. 4. The p27 kinase inhibitor protein increases and becomes associated with both cyclin A and Cdk-2 in anti-IgM arrested B-lymphoma cells. After 24 hours with anti-IgM, S^{35} labeled lysates from WEHI-231 cells were immunoprecipitated with anti-cyclin A (left), anti-p27 or anti-Cdk-2, electrophoresed and the gels exposed to reveal the ~27 kDa bands. This figure shows that there is a twofold increase in the amount of p27 associated in these complexes, which were independently immunoblotted to verify identity with $p27^{Kip1}$.

sample of these data is shown in **figure 5** (Donjerkovic' and Scott, in preparation). As shown earlier [17], anti-IgM consistently caused an upregulation of p27, while anti-IgD treatment does not.

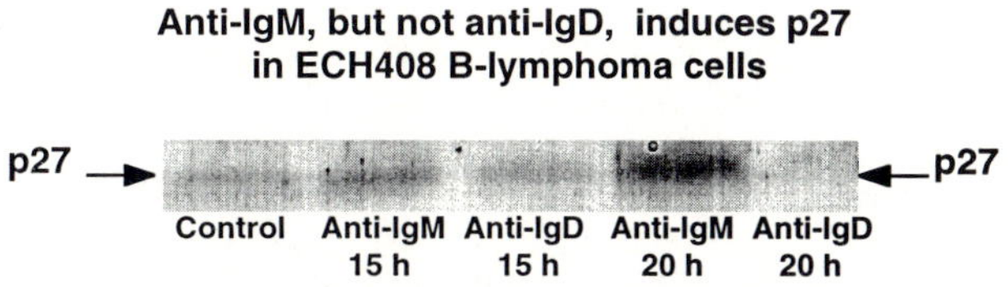

Fig. 5. Anti-IgM treatment induces p27 in ECH408 B-lymphoma cells whereas anti-IgD does not. Shown is an immunoblot of ECH408 B-lymphoma cells treated with anti-IgM or anti-IgD for up to 20 hours, and probed with rabbit anti-p27 (from Dr. Tony Hunter).

Thus, regulation of p27 synthesis may be critical in the control of B-lymphoma growth and apoptosis. To test this hypothesis further, we used the antisense oligo approach employed with c-myc. In these experiments, B-lymphoma cells were cultured with antisense oligos for p27 simultaneously with anti-IgM. We found that this antisense caused a complete blockade of growth arrest and apoptosis, and blocked the upregulation of p27 by anti-IgM [26]. However, this oligonucleotide also contained the consensus mitogenic CpG motif, suggesting that the effects were secondary to the antisense design. Alternative oligos, lacking the motif or containing methylated cytosine, were variable in blocking apoptosis. While these experiments do not prove a critical role of p27 in cell cycle blockade and apoptosis, they suggest a causal linkage. Examination of myc over-expressing WEHI-231 cells will be useful in dissecting the role of p27. We predict that ectopically expressed myc will prevent the increase in p27; moreover, we expect that antisense c-myc will likewise block p27 upregulation. Preliminary results suggest that this is true.

Relation between p27 and c-myc in B-lymphoma apoptosis

Our data are consistent with the hypothesis anti-IgM induces an increase in the levels of available p27 (subsequent to the loss of c-myc expression), and that the relative binding of p27 to a cyclin:Cdk kinase complex inactivates it in early G_1, thus preventing pRB phosphorylation and cell cycle progression. These arrested cells soon are committed to undergo apoptosis. Thus, the sequence of events is the loss of c-myc, the increase in p27, inactivation of kinase activity, growth arrest and apoptosis. The pathway by which p27 upregulation via anti-IgM regulates B-cell growth and apoptosis is illustrated in the **figure 6**. It is not clear whether the levels of c-myc regulate the expression of p27 directly or the synthesis or activity of p27 via an inhibitor of this Kip protein (*i.e.*, via a Kipi). One possibility is that c-myc is a negative regulator of p27 transcription. Hence, the loss of c-myc may lead to a change in the composition of heterodimers involved in p27 transcription, or alternatively, to an excess of max:max (or other) homodimers that may transcriptionally repress a novel Kipi. While the effects of anti-IgM on max levels are minimal, it is not known how crosslinking of the Ig receptor affects levels of YY1, mnt or other myc or max binding proteins, respectively. Although data in non-lymphoid cells is consistent with translational regulation of p27 [27,28], Han *et alia* [29] recently reported that anti-IgM induced a 2X increase in p27 message in WEHI-231 lymphoma cells. They also found that anti-CD40 treatment, which prevents growth arrest and apoptosis, prevented this rise in p27 message. Whether this is purely transcriptional control or via effects on message stability is not known.

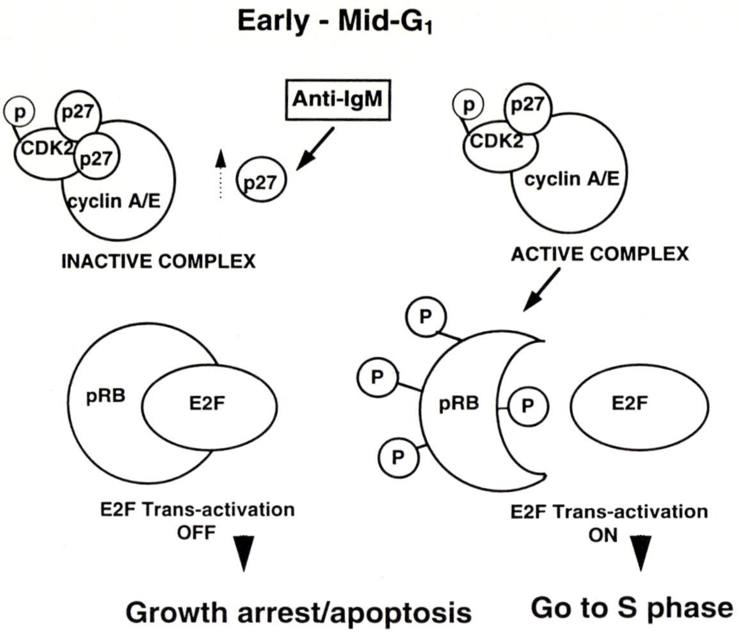

Fig. 6. Theoretical scheme for the role of p27 in growth arrest and apoptosis. See text for explanation.

Clearly, a decrease in the level of c-myc *per se* does not directly lead to an increase in p27 since reagents such as TPCK and TGF-β can cause a dramatic loss of c-myc with only minor effects on p27 levels (Donjerkovic´ and Scott, in preparation). We propose that an unknown second signal downstream of ITAM-regulated tyrosine phosphorylation is necessary for the ultimate effects of anti-IgM (and c-myc) on growth arrest and apoptosis in these lymphoma cells. It is interesting in this context that treatment of B-cell lymphomas with dexamethasone augments apoptosis induced by receptor crosslinking [30], whereas it blocks anti-TCR-mediated apoptosis in T cells [31]. We propose that c-myc is also downregulated by dexamethasone in these B cells, a process which leads to a more rapid loss of c-myc than Ig-receptor crosslinking alone. Preliminary experiments to reduce c-myc levels coupled with anti-Ig signals in "resistant" lymphomas are in progress to identify these anti-Ig-regulated steps.

Acknowledgments

This is publication #16 of the Holland Lab Immunology Department, American Red Cross and was supported by USPHS grants, CA55644 and AI29691 (DWS). The authors thank Dr. Achsah Keegan for a critical reading of the manuscript.

References

1. Pennell, CA and Scott, DW (1986) Lymphoma models for B-cell activation and tolerance IV. Growth inhibition by anti-Ig of CH31 and CH33 B lymphoma cells. Eur J Immunol 16:1577-1583.
2. Scott, DW, Livnat, D, Pennell, CA, and Keng, P (1986) Lymphoma models for B-cell activation and tolerance III. Cell cycle dependence for negative signalling of WEHI-231 B lymphoma cells by anti-μ. J Exp Med 164: 156-164.
3. Scott, DW, Chace, J, Warner, G, O'Garra, A, Klaus, GGB and Quill, H (1987) Role of T cell-derived lymphokines in two models of B-cell tolerance. Immunol Rev 99: 153-171.
4. DeFranco, A L, Gold, MR and Jakway, JP (1987) B-lymphocyte signal transduction in response to anti-immunoglobulin and bacterial lipopolysaccharide. Immunol Rev 95: 161-176.
5. Benhamou, LE, Cazenave PA and Sarthou P (1990) Anti-immunoglobulins induce death by apoptosis ir WEHI-231 B-lymphoma cells. Eur J Immunol 20: 1405-1407.
6. Hasbold J and Klaus GGB (1990) Anti-immunoglobulin antibodies induce apoptosis in immature B-cell lymphomas Eur J Immunol 20:1685-1690.
7. Tisch, R, Roifman, CM, and Hozumi, N (1988) Functional differences between immunoglobulins M and D are expressed on the surface of an immature B-cell line. Proc Natl Acad Sci USA 85: 6914-6918.
8. Alés-Martínez, J, Warner, G and Scott, DW (1988) IgM and IgD mediate signals which are qualitatively different in B cells with an immature phenotype Proc Nat Acad Sci (US) 85: 6919-6923.
9. Alés-Martínez JE, Scott, DW, Phipps, RP, Casnellie, J, Kroemer, G, Martinez-AC and Pezzi, L (1992) Cross-linking of surface IgM and IgD causes differential biological effects in spite of overlap of tyrosine (de)phosphorylation profiles Eur J Immunol 22: 845-850.
10. Reth, M (1989) Antigen receptor tail clue. Nature 338: 383-384.
11. Yao, X-r, Flaswinkel, H, Reth M and Scott DW (1995) Immunoreceptor tyrosine-based activation motif is required to signal pathways of receptor-mediated growth arrest and apoptosis in murine B-lymphoma cells. J Immunol 155: 652-661.
12. McCormack, JE, Pepe, VH, Kent, RB, Dean, M, Marshak-Rothstein, A and Sonenshein, GE (1984) Specific regulation of c-myc oncogene expression in a murine B-cell lymphoma. Proc Natl Acad Sci USA 81: 5546-5550.
13. Fischer, G, Kent, S, Joseph, L, Green, DR and Scott, DW (1994) Lymphoma models for B-cell activation and tolerance X Anti-μ-mediated growth arrest and apoptosis of murine B-lymphomas is prevented by the stabilization of myc. J Exp Med 179: 221-228.
14. Warner, GL, Nelson D, Ludlow, J, and Scott, DW (1992) Anti-immunoglobulin treatment of murine B-cell lymphomas induces active TGF-b but pRB-hypophosphorylation is TGF-b-independent. Cell Growth and Different 3: 175-181.
15. Joseph, L, Ezhevsky, S, and Scott, DW (1995) Lymphoma Models for B-cell Activation and Tolerance. XI. Anti-IgM Treatment Induces Growth Arrest by Preventing the Formation of an Active Kinase Complex which Phosphorylates pRB in G_1 Cell Growth and Different 6: 51-57.
16. Toyoshima, H and T Hunter T (1994) p27, a novel inhibitor of G_1 cyclin-Cdk protein kinase activity, is related to p21. Cell 78: 67-74.
17. Ezhevsky, S, Toyoshima, H , Hunter, T and Scott, DW (1996) Role of cyclin A and p27 in anti-IgM-induced G_1 growth arrest of murine B-cell lymphomas, Molec Biol of the Cell 7: 553-564.
18. Scott, DW, Tuttle, J, Livnat, D, Haynes, W, Coggswell, J and Keng, P (1985) Lymphoma models for B-cell activation and tolerance II Growth inhibition by anti-mu of WEHI-231 and the selection of properties of resistant mutants Cell Immunol 93: 124-131,
19. Shi, Y., Glynn, M, Guilbert, LJ, Cotter, TG, Bissonette, RP, and Green, DR (1992) Role for c-myc in activation induced apoptotic cell death in T-cell hybridoma. Science 257: 212-214.
20. Maheswaran, S, JE McCormack and GE Sonenshein (1991) Changes in phosphorylation of myc oncogene and RB anti-oncogene protein products during growth arrest of the murine lymphoma WEHI 231 cell line. Oncogene 6: 1965-1971.
21. Krieg, A, Yi, A-K, Matson, S, Waldschmidt TJ, Bishop, GA, Teasdale, R, Koretsky, G, and Klinman, D (1995) CpG motifs in bacterial DNA trigger B-cell activation Nature 374: 546-549.
22. Yi, A-K, Hornbeck P, Lafrenz D, and Krieg, A (1996) CpG DNA rescue of murine B lymphoma cells from anti-IgM-induced growth arrest and programmed cell death is associated with increased expression of c-myc and bcl-x_L. J. Immunol 157: 4918-4925.
23. Scott, DW, Lamers, M, Köhler, G, Sidman, C, Maddox, B, Wang, R, and Carsetti, R (1996) Regulation of spontaneous and anti-receptor induced apoptosis in adult murine B-cells by c-Myc. Internat Immunol 8: 1375-1385.

24. Wu M, Arsura M, Bellas R, Fitzgerald M, Lee H, Schauer S, Sherr D, Sonenshein G (1996) Inhibition of c-myc expression induces apoptosis of WEHI 231 B cells. Mol Cell Biol 16: 5015-5025.
25. Mittnacht, S and Weinberg, RA (1991) G1/S phosphorylation of the retinoblastoma protein is associatec with an altered affinity for the nuclear compartment. Cell 65:381-393.
26. Scott, DW, Brunner, T, Donjerkovic´, D, Ezhevsky, S, Grdina, T, Green, D, Shi, Y and Yao, X (1997) Murder and suicide: A tale of T and B cell apoptosis In: YB Shi, Y Shi, DW Scott and X Yu (eds) Programmed Cell Death, Plenum Press, New York.
27. Hengst L and Reed SI (1996) Translational control of $p27^{Kip\ 1}$ accumulation during the cell cycle. Science 271: 1861-1864.
28. Pagano, M, SW Tam, AM Thedoras, P Beer-Romero, G Del Sal, V Chau, PR Yew, GF Draetta and M Rolfe (1995) Role of the ubiquitin-proteasome pathway in regulating abundance of the cyclin-dependent kinase inhibitor p27. Science 269: 682-685.
29. Han, H, Nomura T, Honjo T, and Tsubata T (1996) Differential modulation of cyclin-dependent kinase inhibitor $p27^{Kip\ 1}$ by negative signaling via the antigen receptor of B cells and positive signaling via CD40. Eur J. Immunol 26: 2425-2432.
30. Zacharchuk, CM , Mercep, M, Chakraborti, PK, Simons, SS, and Ashwell, JD (1990) Programmed T lymphocyte death. Cell activation- and steroid-induced pathways are mutually antagonistic. J Immunol 145, 4037-4045.
31. Scott, DW, Grdina, T and Shi, Y (1996) T cells commit suicide but B cells are murdered. J Immunol 156: 2352-2356.

C-Myc Protein Interactions

Mnt: A Novel Max-interacting Protein and Myc Antagonist

P. J. Hurlin, C. Qúeva and R. N. Eisenman
Division of Basic Sciences, Fred Hutchinson Cancer Research Center, Seattle, Washington 98104, USA

Summary

We have identified a novel Max-binding protein, Mnt, which belongs to neither the Myc nor the Mad families (Hurlin et al. 1997). Mnt interacts with Max in vivo and functions as a transcriptional repressor of reporter genes containing promoter-proximal CACGTG sites. Mnt:Max complexes also efficiently suppress Myc-dependent activation from the same promoter. Transcription repression by Mnt maps to a 13 amino acid N-terminal region related to the Sin3 interaction domain (SID) of Mad proteins. This region of Mnt mediates interaction with mSin3 corepressor proteins and its deletion converts Mnt from a repressor to an activator and from a suppressor of Myc-dependent transformation to a cooperating oncogene. This latter result suggests that Mnt and Myc regulate an overlapping set of target genes *in vivo*. Expression of *mnt* RNA is observed in many tissues and in both proliferating and differentiating cells. Likewise, Mnt protein is expressed in many proliferating cell types in culture where both Myc:Max and Mnt:Max complexes are detected. An exception is P19 embryonal carcinoma cells, where Mnt is expressed and in a complex with Max, but Myc proteins are not detected. Mnt is likely to be a key regulator of Myc activities *in vivo* and, in addition, may possess Myc-independent functions.

Introduction

The Myc family of basic-helix-loop-helix-leucine zipper (bHLHZip) transcription factors are thought to play a fundamental role as positive regulators of cell proliferation (for recent review see Henricksson and Lüscher, 1996). The potent influence of Myc proteins on cell proliferation is revealed by their well documented role in tumorigenesis. Oncogenic activation of Myc proteins is thought to occur by events such as chromosomal translocations, gene amplification and viral insertion, resulting in their deregulated overexpression. In some cases, mutations in the Myc coding region may also contribute to their oncogenic activation, possibly by affecting their transactivation functions. However, both coding region mutations and overexepression of Myc in tumors are thought to contribute to an increase in the expression of target genes whose protein products promote cell proliferation.

The severe consequences of deregulated overexpression of Myc proteins raise the question of whether there exist factors in cells that naturally counter or modulate the transcriptional activities of Myc. Proteins that are candidates for such factors are the Mad family of bHLHZip proteins (Ayer et al. 1993; Zervos et al. 1993; Hurlin et al. 1995). Like Myc, Mad family proteins heterodimerize with Max and recognize Myc:Max binding sites (Blackwell et al. 1990; Blackwood and Eisenman, 1991; Pendergast et al. 1991; Blackwood et al. 1992). In contrast to Myc:Max complexes which activate transcription (Kretzner et al. 1992; Amin et al. 1993; Gu et al. 1993), Mad proteins are transcriptional repressors capable of suppressing the oncogenic activities of Myc (Ayer et al. 1993; Zervos et al. 1993; Chen et al. 1994; Lahoz et al. 1994; Koskinen et al. 1995; Hurlin et al. 1995). However, it is not clear whether Mad proteins normally function to modulate Myc activities. This is because, based on both RNA *in situ* analysis and protein expression studies,

Myc and Mad expresseion are typically reciprocally regulated. For example, studies of Mad1 show that its levels are very low in proliferating cells where Myc proteins are expressed, and that it is induced during cell differentiation, when Myc is typically downregulated (Ayer et al. 1993b; Hurlin et al. 1994; Hurlin et al. 1995a). The reciprocal regulation of Myc and Mad1 suggests that they fulfill complementary roles during differentiation involving the downregulation and subsequent (or concomitant) active repression of Myc target genes. Although RNA expression studies of the other members of the mad family indicate that they are induced during differentiation, it does appear that they may also be coexpressed with myc genes in some proliferating cell types (C.Q., P.J.H. and R.N.E.). However, these RNA studies have yet to be confirmed by examination of Mad proteins other than Mad1.

Whereas mad gene and protein expression is clearly induced in cells undergoing growth arrest associated with differentiation, another recently identified Max-interactor, Mnt, was found to be expressed in a wide variety of both proliferating and differentiating cell types (Hurlin et al. 1997). Mnt has a bHLHZip region that is most similar to Max and contains a repression domain (SID- Sin3 Interaction Domain) that has sequence and functional homology with Mad family proteins. Although Mnt and Mad proteins share conserved SID and bHLHZip domains, they otherwise show little or no sequence homology. The Mnt repression domain, like the Mad repression domain, mediates interaction with Sin3 corepressor proteins and transcriptional repression (Ayer et al. 1995; Hurlin et al. 1995; Schrieber-Agus et al. 1995; Hurlin et al. 1997). Deletion of the SID abolishes the transcriptional repression function of these proteins and converts them into weak activators. Whereas expression of wild-type Mnt and Mad proteins suppress Myc-dependent transformation of rat embryo fibroblasts (REFs), expression of mutants lacking the SID fail to suppress transformation. Furthermore, the Mnt mutant lacking the SID cooperates with Ras in transformation of REFs. This latter result provides evidence to suggest that Myc and Mnt regulate an overlapping set of target genes *in vivo.*

The expression of Mnt in proliferating cells suggested that it might be coexpressed with Myc. Indeed, Mnt was found to be coexpressed with Myc proteins in a wide variety of cell types and both Myc:Max and Mnt:Max complexes were identified in several different proliferating cell types (Hurlin et al., 1997). These results suggest that Mnt may normally fulfill a negative regulatory role on Myc functions *in vivo.* To examine this question further, Mnt was expressed in mice as a transgene under the control of the beta-actin promoter. *mnt* transgenic animals died *in utero*, primarily between day 9 and day 11 of embryonic development. Interestingly, the time of death of mnt transgenic mice and c-myc and N-myc knockout mice was very similar (Charron et al. 1992; Davis et al. 1993; Moens et al. 1992; Moens et al. 1993; Sawai et al. 1993; Stanton et al. 1992). In addition, several of the *mnt* transgenic embryos appeared to be delayed in development and suffered proliferative defects that may reflect a potential negative regulatory function of Mnt on Myc activities.

In this report we show that, like Myc and Mad proteins, Mnt is a rapidly degraded protein in vivo. We also show that Mnt and Mnt:Max complexes exist in at least one proliferating cell type in which Myc proteins can not be detected. These results suggest that Mnt expression in the absence of Myc is compatible with cell proliferation and that Mnt may have Myc-independent activities.

Results and Discussion

mnt expression

The results of experiments examining the affects of Mnt on transcription and on cell transformation suggest that the relative levels of Myc and Mnt in cells may be an important element for maintaining an appropriate level of proliferation (Hurlin et al. 1996, in press). Therefore, it was of interest to determine the expression pattern of mnt to identify possible model systems to test this idea. To examine *mnt* RNA expression, mRNA was isolated from a variety of mouse tissues, as well as from human keratinocytes and rat PC12 cells and hybridized with a ^{32}P-labelled *mnt* cDNA probe (Figure 1). In each tissue and in the cultured cells, an mRNA species on approximately 4.8 kb was detected. This size is very near to the size of the *mnt* cDNA (4.650 kb) identified in cDNA library screens. Due to variation in the amount of RNA loaded, it is difficult to make accurate estimates of the relative levels of *mnt* in these tissues. However, *in situ* hybridization analysis of mouse embryos at various stages of development and in various adult tissues (Hurlin et al. 1996 in press; C.Q. P.J.H. and R.N.E. unpublished) suggest that *mnt* levels are at fairly uniform levels in most cell types. In addition, these latter studies indicate that *mnt* is expressed in both proliferating and non-proliferating cells (e.g. differentiating cells, C.Q., P.J.H. and R.N.E., unpublished). Taken together, the results of experiments examining *mnt* expression suggested that Mnt and Myc proteins are likely to be coexpressed in a wide variety of cell types. Although, in general this notion appears to be correct, there are cell types which show exclusive expression of Myc or Mnt proteins (Hurlin et al. 1996, in press, and see below)

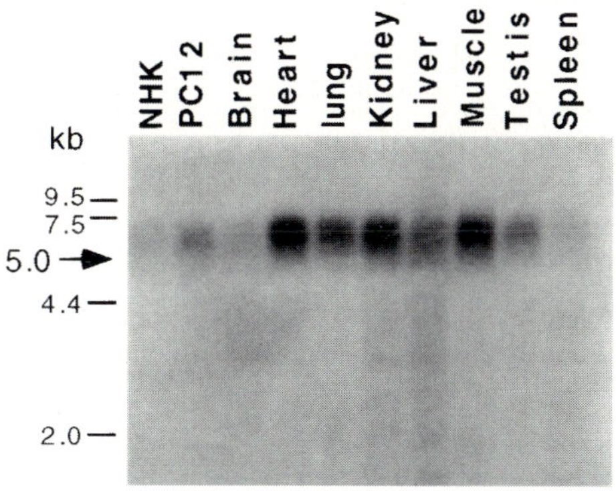

Figure 1. Expression of mnt in adult mouse tissues. The approximately 5 kb mnt message is indicated.

Mnt is rapidly degraded

As mentioned above, the relative levels of Mnt and Myc in cells (and of Myc:Max and Mnt:Max complexes) may influence the proliferative status of cells. One factor affecting the level of these proteins in cells is their half-lives. Previous studies have shown that Myc and Mad1 are both rapidly degraded *in vivo* (Hann et al. 1984; Ayer et al. 1993b). Because Max is a very stable protein, synthesis of Myc and Mad proteins is thought to be rate-limiting for formation of active Max heterodimeric complexes (Blackwood et al. 1992). However, unlike Mad1, Mnt appears to be frequently coexpressed with Myc, suggesting that it's half life might be an importnat factor influencing the ratio of Myc:Max to Mnt:Max in cells. To determine Mnt stability, human 293 cells, transfected with a Mnt expression vector, were used. Transfected cells were labeled with medium containing ^{35}S-methionine for 30 minutes, washed free of labeling medium and chased with medium containing "cold" methionine. As seen in Figure 2, the Mnt protein is initially observed as a 72 kd band that is chased into a 74 kd protein. The nature of the modification of the Mnt protein that gives rise to the slower migrating species is currently unknown. The estimated half-life of the Mnt proteins is 30 - 45 minutes, which is similar to the half-lives of Myc and Mad proteins (Hann et al. 1984; Ayer et al. 1993b). However, a low level of Mnt protein can still be detected following the two hour chase, suggesting that a fraction of the Mnt protein may possess a longer half-life.

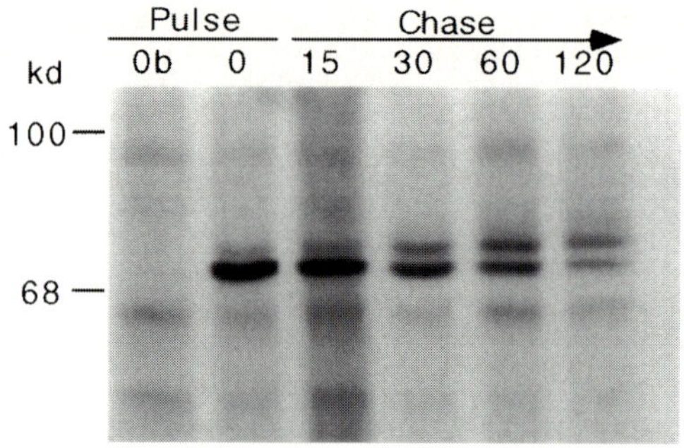

Figure 2. Mnt is rapidly degraded. mnt transfected 293 cells were pulsed labeled with ^{35}S-methionine for 30 minutes then chased in "cold" medium for the indicated times. b indicates serum preincubated (blocked) with GST-Mnt immunogen.

Mnt:Max complexes in proliferating cells

In order to determine whether endogenous Mnt and Max proteins interact *in vivo*, we initially used the MCF-7 human breast carcinoma and the HLF human neuroblastoma cell lines (Hurlin et al. 1997). The results from these experiments indicated that Mnt does interact with Max in these cells. Furthermore we showed that both Mnt:Max and Myc:Max heterocomplexes are present in proliferating MCF-7 and HLF cells. A number of other cell lines were tested to determine whether any differed from this pattern. Of the cell lines tested, their were several which either Mnt or Myc were not detected. For example, in K562 human erythroleukemia cells, Myc proteins could be detected, but Mnt could not (data not shown), and in P19 mouse embryonic carcinoma cells Mnt was detected, but Myc proteins were not (Figure 3). Furthermore, in P19 cells the Mnt protein was identified in a complex with Max (Figure 3).

The identification of Mnt and Mnt:Max complexes in proliferating P19 cells, but not Myc proteins, raises several important issues. One is the possibility that Myc expression may not be required for active proliferation of certain cell types. However, it is possible that a low level of Myc is expressed in P19 cells and that very long autoradiographic exposure periods are necessary to identify them. It should be noted that two Myc antisera were used in these experiments; antisera recognizing c-Myc and antisera recognizing c-Myc, N-Myc and L-Myc (see Materials and methods). In side by side experiments using MCF-7 breast carcinoma and NLF neuroblastoma cells, these antisera recognized c-Myc and N-Myc respectively. Therefore, the lack of detectable Myc is likely not due to the efficacy of the antiserum used.

A related issue raised by this result is why Mnt expression, in the absence of Myc expression, is not growth inhibitory. Although Mnt inhibits Myc + Ras transformation of rat embryo fibroblasts, additional experiments are consistent with the notion that Mnt overexpression is not growth inhibitory. For example, Mnt does not inhibit transformation of NIH3T3 cells by Ras oncogenes (i.e., Myc-independent transformation, Hurlin et al.1997). Furthermore, Mnt overexpression had no affect on colony forming efficiency of a variety of cell lines (P.J.H., unpublished). One interpretation of these results is that Mnt functions to restrict proliferation pathways that require Myc. It is possible that the lack of Myc expression (and the lack of activation of proliferative pathways that require Myc) is important in pluripotent cells such as P19 cells, and that expression of Mnt in these cells functions to ensure that Myc target genes are in a repressed state. It will be important to test this notion by determining the affects of overexpression of Myc in P19 cells.

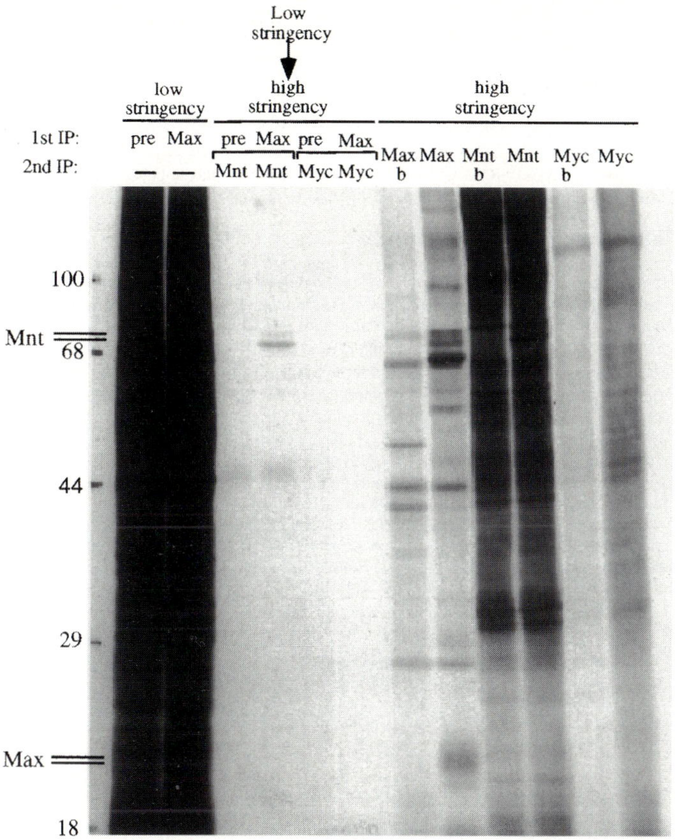

Figure 3. Identification of Mnt and Mnt:Max complexes in P19 cells. Max antiserum or preimmune (pre) serum (from the same Max antiserum-producing rabbit) was used in low stringency (LS) immunoprecipitations from ^{35}S-methionine-labeled, logarithmically growing P19 cells. Associated proteins were eluted under high stringency conditions and reimmunoprecipitated using Mnt or Myc antisera (Hurlin et al., in press; and see Materials and methods section). Max, Mnt and Myc proteins were also immunoprecipitated under high stringency conditions from cell lysates to examine levels of expression. b (blocked) indicates the use of antiserum preincubated with immunogen.

Materials and methods

Northern Blot Analysis

Tissues were collected from adult mice, and whole RNA isolated using TRIzol reagent (GibcoBRL) as described by the manufacturer. Poly(A)$^+$ RNA was then affinity purified using oligo dT cellulose (New England Biolabs). Four micrograms poly(A)$^+$ RNA was electrophoresed on 1.4% agarose gel and transfered to nylon membrane (N+, Amersham). For probe, a ^{32}P-labeled full-length mnt cDNA fragment was used.

Antibodies and Immunoprecipitations

To generate Mnt antiserum (serum #6823H), the GSTMntBHLHZip fusion protein (see above) was used as immunogen for immunizing a New Zealand white rabbit. The immunogen was used to control for specificity in immunoprecipitations by preincubation with the Mnt antiserum. Max (serum #8711) and Myc (serum #1537 for c-Myc and serum #1096 for N-Myc) antiserum have been described previously (Blackwood et al. 1992). For detection of Mnt in transfected cells for the pulse-chase experiments, 5×10^6 cells were metabolically labeled for 30 min using 250mCi ^{35}S-methionine (Amersham). Cells were washed two times with PBS and complete DMEM medium added. Cells were harvested at timed intervals and immunoprecipitated with the Mnt antibody. Immunoprecipitations on non-transfected cells were performed using $1\text{-}5 \times 10^7$ cells labeled with 400mCi ^{35}S-methionine. In experiments to detect Max, cells were metabolically labeled for 1-2 hrs to increase the specific activity of Max polypeptides (Blackwood et al. 1992). Low stringency (LS) immunoprecipitations, were performed in LS buffer (20mM HEPES (pH 7.5), 100mM KCl, 10mM MgCl2, 5mM dithiothreinol (DTT) and 0.2% NP40) containing 0.5% aprotinin and 0.2mM phenylmethysulfonyl fluoride (PMSF). For the detection of Max-associated proteins, LS Max immunoprecipitations were collected on protein A-Sepharose beads and washed 3 times with LS buffer. LS washed proteins were either eluted and analyzed directly or the Protein A-Sepharose beads were incubated in high stringency (HS) buffer (20mM Tris-HCl (pH 7.4), 50mM NaCl, 1mM EDTA, 0.5% NP-40, 0.5% deoxycholate, 0.5% SDS, 0.5% aprotinin and 0.2mM PMSF), centrifuged briefly and the supernatant reimmunoprecipitated with anti-Mnt or anti-Myc serum. High stringency immunoprecipitations and washing conditions were carried out as described previously (Blackwood et al. 1992).

References

Amin, C., A.J. Wagner and N.Hay. 1993. Sequence-specific transcriptional activation by Myc and repression by Max. *Mol. Cell. Biol.* **13**: 383-390.

Ayer, D.E., L. Kretzner and R.N. Eisenman. 1993a. Mad: A heterodimeric partner for Max that antagonizes Myc transcriptional activity. *Cell* **72**: 211-222.

Ayer, D.E. and R.N. Eisenman. 1993b. A switch from Myc:Max to Mad:Max heterocomplexes accompanies monocyte/macrophage differentiation. *Genes & Dev.* **7**: 2110-2119.

Ayer, D.E., Q. A. Lawrence and R.N. Eisenman. 1995. Mad-Max transcriptional repression is mediated by ternary complex formation with mammalian homologs of the yeast repressor Sin3. *Cell* **80**: 767-776.

Blackwell, T.K., L. Kretzner, E.M. Blackwood, R.N. Eisenman and H. Weintraub. 1990. Sequence-specific DNA-binding by the c-Myc protein. *Science* **250**: 1149-1151.

Blackwood, E.M. and R.N. Eisenman. 1991. Max: A helix-loop-helix zipper protein that forms a sequence-specific DNA-binding complex with Myc. *Science* **251**: 1211-1217.

Blackwood, E.M., B. Lüscher and R.N. Eisenman. 1992. Myc and Max associate *in vivo*. *Genes and Dev.* **6**:71-80.

Charron, J., B.A. Malynn, P. Fisher, V. Stewart, L. Jeanotte, S.P. Goff, E.J. Robertson and F.W. Alt. 1992. Embryonic lethality in mice homozygous for a targeted disruption of the N-*myc* gene. *Genes Dev.* **6**:2248-2257.

Davis, A. C., M. Wims, G.D. Spotts, S.R. Hann and A. Bradley. 1993. A null c-myc mutation causes lethality before 10.5 days of gestation in homozygous and reduced fertility in heterozygous female mice. *Genes Dev.* **7**: 671-682.

Gu, W., K. Cechova, V. Tassi and Dalla-Favera, R. 1993. Opposite regulation of gene transcription by c-Myc and Max. *Proc. Natl. Acad. Sci.* USA **90**: 2935-2939.

Henriksson, M. and B. Lüscher. 1996. Proteins of the Myc network: essential regulators of cell growth and differentiation. *Adv. Cancer Res.* **68**: 109-182.

Hurlin, P.J., Queva, C. and R.N. Eisenman. 1997. Mnt, a Novel Max-Interacting Protein is Coexpressed with Myc in Proliferating Cells and Mediates Repression at Myc Binding Sites. 1997. Genes & Dev. in press.

Hurlin, P.J., D.A. Ayer, C. Grandori and R.E. Eisenman, 1994. The Max transcription network: involvement of Mad in differentiation and an approach to identification of target genes. Cold Spring Harbor Symposium, Cold Spring Harbor Press, NY.

Hurlin, P.J., K.P. Foley, D.E. Ayer, R.N. Eisenman, D. Hanahan and J.M. Arbeit. 1995a. Regulation of Myc and Mad during epidermal differentiation and HPV-associated tumorigenesis.*Oncogene* **11**: 2487-2501.

Hurlin, P.J., C. Quéva, P.J. Koskinen, E. Steingrímsson, D.E. Ayer, N.G. Copeland, N.A. Jenkins and R.N. Eisenman. 1995b. Mad3 and Mad4: Novel Max-interacting transcriptional repressors that suppress c-Myc-dependent transformation and are expresed during neural and epidermal differentiation. *EMBO J.* **14**: 5646-5659.

Koskinen, P.J., D.G. Ayer and R.E. Eisenman. 1995. Repression of Myc-Ras cotransformation by Mad is mediated by multiple protein-protein interactions. *Cell Growth and Differ.* **6**: 623-629.

Kretzner, L., E.M. Blackwood, R.N. Eisenman. 1992. The Myc and Max proteins possess distinct transcriptional activities. *Nature* **359**: 426-429.

Lahoz, E.G., L. Xu, N. Schreiber-Agus and R.A. DePinho. 1994. Suppression of Myc, but not E1a transformation activity by Max-associated proteins, Mad and Mxi1. *Proc. Natl. Acad. Sci.* USA **91**: 5503-5507.

Moens, C.B., A.B. Auerbach, R.A.Conlon, A.L. Joyner and Rossant, J. 1992. A targeted mutation reveals a role for N-myc in branching morphogenesis in the embryonic mouse lung. *Genes & Dev.* **6**:691-704.

Moens, C. B., B. R. Stanton, L. F. Parada and J. Rossant. 1993. Defects in heart and lung development in compund heterozygotes for two different targeted mutations at the N-myc locus.*Development* **119**: 485-499. Prendergast, G. C., D. Lawe and E. B. Ziff. 1991. Association of Myn, the murine homolog of Max, with c-Myc stimulates methylation-sensitive DNA binding and Ras cotransformation. *Cell* **65**: 395-407.

Sawai, S., A. Shimono, Y. Wakamatsu, C. Palmes, K. Hanaoka and H. Kondoh. 1993. Defects of embryonic organogenesis resulting from targeted disruption of the N-*myc* gene in the mouse. *Development* **117**: 1445-1455.

Schreiber-Agus, N., L. Chin, K. Chen, R. Torres, G. Rao, P. Guida, A.I. Skoultchi, and R. DePinho. 1995. An amino-terminal domain of Mxi1 mediates anti-Myc oncogenic activity and interacts with a homolog of the yeast transcriptional repressor SIN3. *Cell* **80**: 777-786.

Stanton, B.R., A.S. Perkins, L. Tessarollo, D.A. Sassoon and L.F. Parada. 1992. Loss of N-*myc* function results in embryonic lethality and failure of the epithelial component of the embryo. *Genes Dev.* **6**: 2235-2247.

Zervos, A. S., J. Gyuris, and R. Brent. 1993. Mxi1, a protein that specifically interacts with Max to bind Myc-Max recognition sites. *Cell* **72**: 223-232.

Acknowledgements

We thank Pei-Feng Cheng for expert technical assistance and members of the Eisenman laboratory for support and encouragement. This work was supported by NCI grant RO1CA20525 (R.N.E.). P.J.H. was supported by an NIH fellowship during the initial phases of this work.

Regulation of Cell Growth by the Myc-Max-Mad Network: Role of Mad Proteins and YY1

M. AUSTEN, C. CERNI[1], M. HENRIKSSON, S. HILFENHAUS, J. M. LÜSCHER-FIRZLAFF, A. MENKEL, C. SEELOS[1], A. SOMMER and B. LÜSCHER
Institut für Molekularbiologie, Medizinische Hochschule Hannover, 30623 Hannover, Germany
[1] Institut für Tumorbiologie, Universität Wien, Austria

Introduction

Since the discovery of the c-Myc dimerization partner Max (Blackwood and Eisenman 1991; Prendergast et al. 1991) a startling number of proteins capable to interact directly or indirectly with c-Myc and/or Max have been described (for review see Marcu et al. 1992; Henriksson and Lüscher 1996). It has become evident that at the center of this network lies Max which on one hand forms heterodimers with the Myc family of proteins, including c-, N-, and L-Myc and on the other hand heterodimerizes with proteins of the Mad family, including Mad1, Mxi1 (or Mad2), Mad3, and Mad4. In addition Max has also the ability to form homodimers. Thus Max is the true center of this array of proteins which we will refer to as the Myc/Max/Mad network.

All the members of the Myc/Max/Mad network are proteins of the basic region/helix-loop-helix/leucine zipper (bHLHZip) class of transcriptional regulators. The dimerization is specified by the HLHZip domains whereas the basic region determines specific DNA-binding. Importantly both Myc and Mad proteins cannot homodimerize and appear to require Max as their essential interaction partner (Amati et al. 1992, 1993; Ayer et al. 1993; Zervos et al. 1993; Hurlin et al. 1995a). The different dimeric complexes of the Myc/Max/Mad network bind to the E-box sequence 5'-CACGTG and to certain related sequences (for review see Lüscher et al. 1996).

The functional analysis of the different complexes of the Myc/Max/Mad network has revealed that Myc/Max dimers are positive regulators of cell growth whereas the evidence presently available regarding the Mad/Max complexes suggests a role of these proteins in negatively regulating cell growth. This is based on the functional analyses of Myc, Max, and Mad proteins in various experimental systems. Whereas Myc proteins stimulate transformation, promote S-phase entry and inhibit differentiation, Mad proteins appear to induce opposite effects (for review see Henriksson and Lüscher 1996). Specifically Mad proteins inhibit transformation and cell growth (Lahoz et al. 1994; Cerni et al. 1995; Koskinen et al. 1995; Chen et al. 1995; Roussel et al. 1996). The expression patterns of the different Mad proteins suggests a role in differentiation (Ayer et al. 1993; Zervos et al. 1993; Larsson et al. 1994; Hurlin et al. 1995a, b; Västrik et al. 1995). In addition c-Myc in close association with its capability to stimulate S-phase entry has also been reported to activate an apoptotic pathway in a number of cellular systems (for review see Packham and Cleveland 1995). Presently it is unclear whether Mad proteins can inhibit apoptosis.

At least part of the effects described above are mediated by the ability of the Myc/Max/Mad network to regulate gene transcription. Whereas Myc proteins possess a transactivation domain (TAD) and can positively regulate transcription, both Max and Mad proteins do not contain a TAD and appear to inhibit transcription. In the case of Mad proteins this repression is mediated by the Sin3-interaction domain (SID). Sin3 proteins contain four protein-protein interaction domains, so called paired amphipathic helices (PAH). Whereas PAH2 interacts with Mad proteins, the other PAH motifs have been suggested to mediate binding to corepressors and histone deacetylases. Thus an interesting model is that Sin3 represents a platform for gene regulatory proteins and, in addition, connects to transcription factors thereby regulating the expression of specific genes.

Recently also several proteins interacting with c-Myc have been described, including the pocket protein p107 and Bin1 which bind to the TAD and YY1 which binds to the C-terminal half of c-Myc (Shrivastava et al. 1993; Gu et al. 1994; Beijersbergen et al. 1994; Sakamuro et al. 1996). p107 inhibits c-Myc-specific transactivation of reporter gene constructs whereas Bin1 interferes negatively with Myc-specific transformation. Less clear is the role of YY1 in regulating Myc functions. Since the interaction domain includes the dimerization domain in Myc it is possible that YY1 also negatively regulates Myc, e.g. by interfering with Myc/Max dimer formation (see below).

It is now evident that numerous proteins have to be taken into account when analyzing the functional properties of the Myc/Max/Mad network. This is the case for the Mad-side of the network where the available evidence suggests that Mad family members by themselves have little direct activity regarding gene expression but are recruiting several proteins directly or indirectly to build a repressing complex. Additional proteins are likely to bind to this complex which will potentially reveal new activities associated with Mad proteins. The complexity of interactions is also increasing on the Myc-side of the network. Interestingly Myc interacting proteins in general appear to inhibit c-Myc function. Together with additional regulatory aspects such as the tight control over c-Myc expression as well as other transcription factors binding to the same DNA consensus sequence, thereby competing with Myc/Max complexes for binding, these findings suggest very stringent regulation of the function of c-Myc. A major task for future studies will be to unravel the functional properties of the extended Myc/Max/Mad network.

Functional Consequences of the Interaction of c-Myc with YY1

Inhibition of YY1 Function by c-Myc

YY1 is a Zn-finger transcription factor which has been implicated in a wide variety of regulatory events (for review see Hahn 1992; Shrivastava and Calame 1994). Depending on the promoter analyzed and on the cellular context YY1 either stimulates or represses gene transcription. In addition it has also been implicated in initiator function.

The interaction of c-Myc with YY1 was originally discovered using a yeast two-hybrid screen (Shrivastava et al. 1993). Recently this interaction has been confirmed by coimmunoprecipitation experiments (Shrivastava et al. 1996; MA et al. manuscript in preparation). Interestingly overexpression of c-Myc inhibits both the transcriptional activation as well as the repression function of YY1 suggesting that the observed interaction between the two proteins is functionally relevant (Shrivastava et al. 1993). Since a bacterially expressed C-terminal fragment of c-Myc results in a supershift of DNA-bound YY1 it appears unlikely that Myc's effect on YY1 function is due to inhibition of its DNA binding activity (Shrivastava et al. 1996). One possibility is that Myc may interfere with YY1 connecting to the basal transcriptional machinery (Fig. 1A). This may be due to direct competition of c-Myc with other YY1 binding partners such as the TATA binding protein (TBP), TBP-associated factors (TAFs), or coactivators of the p300/CBP class. However we think that this is unlikely since the binding of TBP, $TAF_{II}55$, TFIIB, or CBP to YY1 does not correlate with its transcriptional activity (Austen et al. 1997). An additional possibility worth considering is an indirect effect of c-Myc on YY1 function (Fig. 1B). This seems of particular interest since YY1 is much more abundant than c-Myc. We estimated that YY1 must be at least 100 times more abundant than c-Myc in several cell lines in which no overexpression of c-Myc was observed (MA unpublished observation). Thus an indirect mechanism could provide the amplification required to efficiently modulate YY1 function by c-Myc. Detailed mapping of the interaction domains and the functionally relevant regions will be required to address this question. Presently little evidence has been obtained to distinguish between these two models.

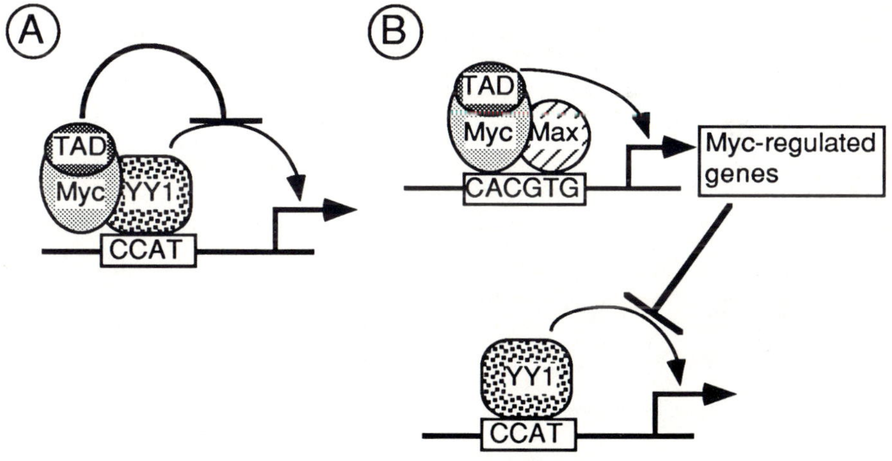

Fig. 1. Models for the inhibition of YY1 function by c-Myc.

A. c-Myc can directly interact with YY1 and inhibit its function both as a transcriptional activator and repressor. Only the activation is schematically shown.

B. The effect of c-Myc on YY1 function may occur indirectly. In such a model proteins encoded by Myc/Max-regulated target genes could alter YY1 function.

Negative Regulation of c-Myc by YY1

We have been interested in addressing whether YY1 could affect functional properties of c-Myc. This seemed a relevant question to us also in view of the large excess of YY1 over c-Myc. Therefore we analyzed the effect of YY1 on c-Myc-dependent transformation and transactivation. We observed that YY1 was able to inhibit the transformation of primary rat embryo cells (REC) by c-Myc and Ha-Ras. In addition in transient transfection experiments YY1 inhibited the c-Myc-specific activation of an ornithine decarboxylase reporter gene construct (MA et al. manuscript in preparation). Together these findings indicated that YY1 interfered negatively with two major functions attributed to c-Myc.

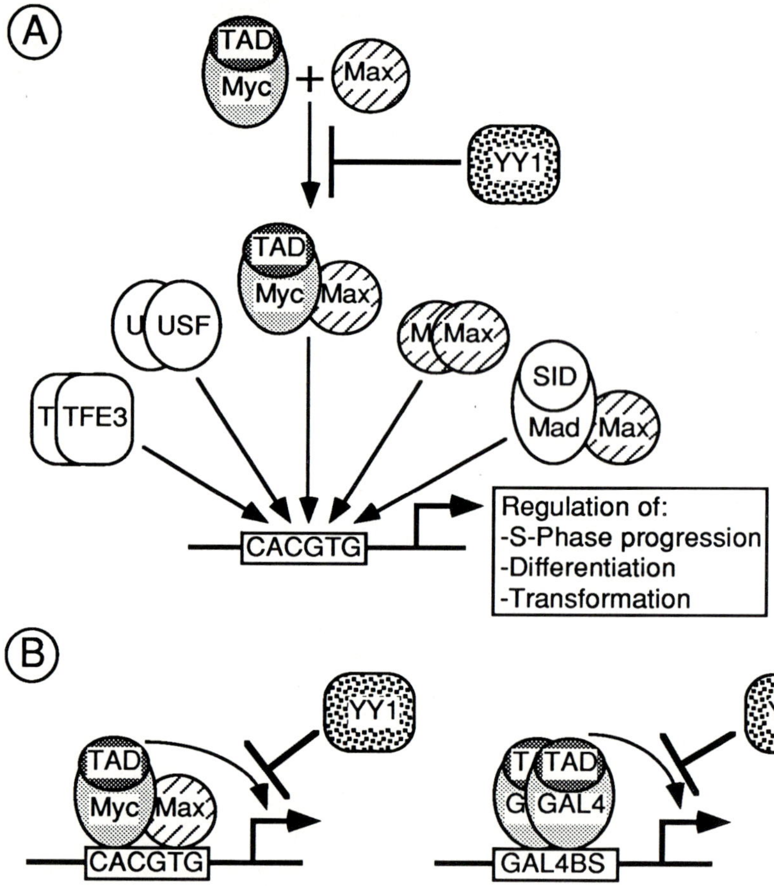

Fig. 2. Models for effects of YY1 on c-Myc function.

A. Competition model. YY1 and Max compete for binding to Myc. By interfering with c-Myc/Max dimer formation, YY1 leads to a reduction of functional Myc/Max complexes and thus may affect the accessibility of other transcriptional regulators (such as USF, TFE3, and other Max containing complexes) to the CACGTG consensus sequence. These factors may result in altered regulation of c-Myc-responsive genes.

B. Signaling model. YY1 activates a pathway which results in the negative regulation of the c-Myc TAD.

A possible explanation for the above described observations is that YY1 inhibits c-Myc/Max dimer formation (Fig. 2A) since YY1 interacts with the C-terminal half of c-Myc, including the bHLHZip domain (Shrivastava et al. 1993). However overexpression of YY1 did not affect c-Myc/Max DNA binding. Neither the formation of specific c-Myc/Max-oligonucleotide complexes was inhibited nor did YY1 alter the mobility of such complexes. This suggested that the effect of YY1 on Myc function may be indirect. To further evaluate such a concept we employed a panel of YY1 deletion mutants and compared their Myc binding capacity to their effect on c-Myc/Ha-Ras-dependent transformation of REC. Surprisingly no correlation could be observed further supporting the argument that YY1 modifies c-Myc function indirectly (Fig. 2B; MA manuscript in preparation). In addition to wild type c-Myc, the transactivating activity of GAL4-MycTAD fusion proteins was also inhibited by YY1. Together these findings argue for a pathway which can be stimulated by YY1 and which regulates c-Myc activity by interfering specifically with the function of the TAD.

At present it is unclear whether this postulated YY1-regulated pathway directly modifies c-Myc, e.g. by modulating the phosphorylation pattern of the TAD, or by altering the interaction to proteins binding to the TAD. In this respect the binding of p107 to c-Myc is of interest since the former is regulated by cyclin-dependent kinases (CDK). Thus it is attractive to postulate a role for YY1 in the regulation of CDKs. In addition YY1 may also modulate the function of Bin1. These possibilities are currently being investigated.

Inhibition of the progression from G0 into S-phase by Mad1

Mad proteins have received considerable attention since their discovery and several lines of evidence suggested that they may function as tumor suppressors (for review see Lüscher et al. 1996). Three findings have implicated Mad1 in negative regulation of cell cycle progression. First the expression of Mad1 is confined mainly to differentiating cells (Ayer et al. 1993; Larsson et al. 1994; Hurlin et al. 1995b; Bahram et al. manuscript in preparation). Second Mad1 is an efficient inhibitor of transformation (Lahoz et al. 1994; Cerni et al. 1995; Koskinen et al. 1995; Västrik et al. 1995). Third cell clones obtained after transfection of c-Myc, Ha-Ras, and Mad1 expressing plasmids grew very slowly whereas clones obtained in parallel without Mad1 did not show this phenotype (Cerni et al. 1995). To study a possible effect of Mad1 on cell cycle progression in more detail we employed a microinjection protocol. Fibroblasts were made quiescent by serum starvation prior to microinjection with Mad1-expressing plasmids. After the injection cells were stimulated with serum and the progression into S-phase of cells expressing Mad1 was determined. We found that Mad1 very efficiently inhibited entry into S-phase and that both the N-terminal as well as the C-terminal domains were required for this effect (AM et al. manuscript in preparation).

To analyze this S-phase block in more detail, time course experiments were performed which showed that Mad1 was capable to inhibit serum-induced S-phase entry until late in the G1-phase of the cell cycle (AM et al. manuscript in preparation). It is therefore possible that Mad1 may function near the restriction point (Fig. 3). A different result was obtained by injecting exponentially growing cells with Mad1 expressing plasmids. In these cells Mad1 was very inefficient in inhibiting S-phase progression. This was somewhat unexpected since infection of growing cells with Mad1-expressing retroviruses or recombinant adenoviruses was shown to result in an increase of cells in the G0/G1-phase of the cell cycle. Similarly in transiently transfected cells an enrichment in G0/G1 was observed in Mad1-expressing cells (Chen et al. 1995; Roussel et al. 1996). Nevertheless our findings indicate that Mad1 is more potent in inhibiting S-phase progression when cells are originating from a G0-state rather than from a previous cell cycle. Thus we propose a role for Mad1 in arresting cells in G0 rather than driving them into G0. This could be important to inhibit reentry of differentiating cells into the cell cycle.

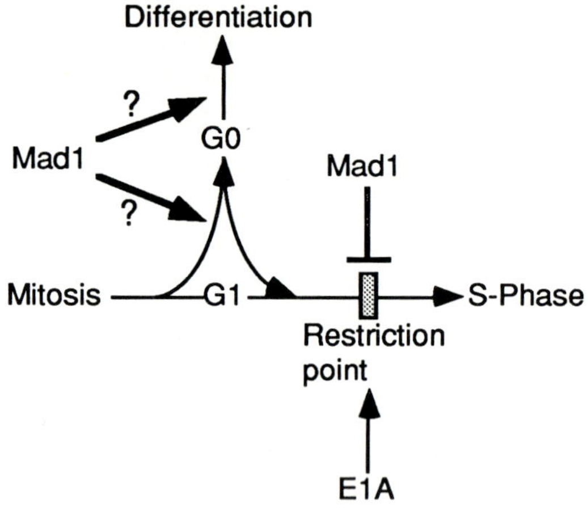

Fig. 3. Mad1 inhibits progression into S-phase until late in G1.
Three possible points of action for Mad1 are indicated. Our data show that Mad1 can block S-phase progression. In addition Mad1 could be relevant for the induction of differentiation pathways and/or for arresting cells in a G0-like state.

In order to test whether proteins known to potently stimulate the transition through the restriction point could overcome the block to S-phase progression, plasmids encoding the adenovirus E1A protein or c-Myc were coinjected with Mad1 expressing plasmids. We observed that neither E1A nor c-Myc were able to overcome the Mad block (AM et al. manuscript in preparation). Since E1A inactivates the p105RB tumor suppressor protein, it seems unlikely that Mad1 regulates RB function. This finding is also consistent with our observation that Mad1 can not only inhibit c-Myc/Ha-Ras but also E1A/Ha-Ras transformation of RECs (Cerni et al. 1995). A possible explanation could be that Mad1 affects an additional rate limiting event at or near the restriction point.

The consequences of the expression of Mad1 as well as the other Mad family members are still not very well understood. The induction of Mad1 and Mad4 expression upon stimulation of differentiation in several model systems (Ayer and Eisenman 1993; Larsson et al. 1994; Bahram et al. manuscript in preparation; AS et al. unpublished observation) suggests that these proteins are somehow involved in cell growth arrest and/or in the differentiation process (Fig. 3). However no satisfactory answer has been obtained thus far regarding the role of Mad proteins in these processes. This is in part due to the difficulties encountered in establishing cellular model systems with inducible mad constructs. Such systems will be important to determine the effects of Mad expression under specific circumstances, e.g. at different points in the cell cycle or during differentiation. Thus clearly more work is required to define more precisely the roles of Mad proteins in cell growth control.

Acknowledgment

This work was supported by grants from the Deutsche Krebshilfe (to BL), the Deutsche Forschungsgemeinschaft (to BL and JMLF), the Fonds der Chemischen Industrie (to BL), and the Herzfelder'sche Familienstiftung (to CC). SH is a recipient of a predoctoral fellowship of the Cusanus Werk.

References

Amati, B., Brooks, M. W., Levy, N., Littlewood, T. D., Evan, G. I., and Land, H. (1993). Oncogenic activity of the c-Myc protein requires dimerization with Max. Cell 72, 233-245.

Amati, B., Dalton, S., Brooks, M. W., Littlewood, T. D., Evan, G. I., and Land, H. (1992). Transcriptional activation by the human c-Myc oncoprotein in yeast requires interaction with Max. Nature 359, 423-426.

Austen, M., Lüscher, B., and Lüscher-Firzlaff, J. M. (1997). Characterization of the transcriptional regulator YY1: the bipartite transactivation doamin is independet of interaction with TBP, TFIIB, $TAF_{II}55$, or CBP. J. Biol. Chem. in press.

Ayer, D. E., and Eisenman, R. N. (1993). A switch from Myc:Max to Mad:Max heterocomplexes accompanies monocyte/macrophage differentiation. Genes Dev. 7, 2110-2119.

Ayer, D. E., Kretzner, L., and Eisenman, R. N. (1993). Mad: a heterodimeric partner for Max that antagonizes Myc transcriptional activity. Cell 72, 211-222.

Beijersbergen, R. L., Hijmans, E. M., Zhu, L., and Bernards, R. (1994). Interaction of c-Myc with the pRb-related protein p107 results in inhibition of c-Myc-mediated transactivation. EMBO J. 13, 4080-4086.

Blackwood, E. M., and Eisenman, R. N. (1991). Max: A helix-loop-helix zipper protein that forms a sequence-specific DNA-binding complex with Myc. Science 251, 1211-1217.

Cerni, C., Bousset, K., Seelos, C., Burkhardt, H., Henriksson, M., and Lüscher, B. (1995). Differential effects by Mad and Max on transformation by cellular and viral oncoproteins. Oncogene 11, 587-596.

Chen, J., Willingham, T., Margraf, L. R., Schreiber-Agus, N., DePinho, R. A., and Nisen, P. D. (1995). Effects of the Myc oncogene antagonist, Mad, on proliferation, cell cycling and the malignant phenotype of human brain tumor cells. Nature Medicine 1, 638-643.

Gu, W., Bhatia, K., Magrath, I. T., Dang, C. V., and Dalla Favera, R. (1994). Binding and suppression of the Myc transcriptional activation domain by p107. Science 264, 251-254.

Hahn, S. (1992). The yin and the yang of mammalian transcription. Curr. Biol. 2, 152-154.
Henriksson, M., and Lüscher, B. (1996). Proteins of the Myc network: Essential regulators of cell growth and differentiation. Adv. Cancer Res. 68, 109-182.
Hurlin, P. J., Quéva, C., Koskinen, P. J., Steingrímsson, E., Ayer, D. E., Copeland, N. G., Jenkins, N. A., and Eisenman, R. N. (1995a). Mad3 and Mad4: Novel Max-interacting transcriptional repressors that suppress c-Myc-dependent transformation and are expressed during neural and epidermal differentiation. EMBO J. 14, 5646-5659.
Hurlin, P. J., Foley, K. P., Ayer, D. E., Eisenman, R. N., Hanahan, D., and Arbeit, J. M. (1995b). Regulation of Myc and Mad during epidermal differentiation and HPV-associated tumorigenesis. Oncogene 11, 2487-2501.
Koskinen, P. J., Ayer, D. E., and Eisenman, R. N. (1995). Mad repression of Myc-Ras cotransformation is mediated by multiple protein-protein interactions. Cell Growth Diff., 6, 623-629.
Lahoz, E. G., Xu, L., Schreiber-Agus, N., and DePinho, R. A. (1994). Suppression of Myc, but not E1a, transformation activity by Max-associated proteins, Mad and Mxi1. Proc. Natl. Acad. Sci. USA 91, 5503-5507.
Lüscher, B., Austen, M., Sommer, A., Hilfenhaus, S., and Henriksson, M. (1996). Transcriptional regulation by the Myc-Max-Mad network. In: Papavassiliou AG (ed) Transcription factors in Eukaryotes. RG Land Company, in press.
Marcu, K. B., Bossone, S. A., and Patel, A. J. (1992). *myc* function and regulation. Annu. Rev. Biochem. 61, 809-860.
Packham, G., and Cleveland, J. L. (1995). c-Myc and apoptosis. Biochem. Biophys. Acta 1242, 11-28.
Prendergast, G. C., Lawe, D., and Ziff, E. B. (1991). Association of Myn, the murine homolog of Max, with c-Myc stimulates methylation-sensitive DNA binding and Ras cotransformation. Cell 65, 395-407.
Roussel, M. F., Ashmun, R. A., Sherr, C. J., Eisenman, R. N., and Ayer, D. E. (1996). Inhibition of cell proliferation by the Mad1 transcriptional repressor. Mol. Cell. Biol. 16, 2796-2801.
Sakamuro, D., Elliott, J., Wechsler-Reya, R., and Prendergast, G. C. (1996). Bin1 is a novel Myc-interacting protein with features of a tumour suppressor. Nature Genet. 14, 69-77.
Shrivastava, A., and Calame, K. (1994). An analysis of genes regulated by the multi-functional transcriptional regulator Yin Yang-1. Nucl. Acids Res. 22, 5151-5155.
Shrivastava, A., Saleque, S., Kalpana, G. V., Artandi, S., Goff, S. P., and Calame, K. (1993). Inhibition of transcriptional regulator Yin-Yang-1 by association with c-Myc. Science 262, 1889-1892.
Shrivastava, A., Yu, J., Artandi, S., and Calame, K. (1996). YY1 and c-Myc associate in vivo in a manner that depends on c-Myc levels. Proc. Natl. Acad. Sci. USA 93, 10638-10641.
Västrik, I., Kaipainen, A., Penttilä, T.-L., Lymboussakis, A., Alitalo, R., Parvinen, M., and Alitalo, K. (1995a). Expression of the mad gene during cell differentiation in vivo and its inhibition of cell growth in vitro. J. Cell Biol. 128, 1197-1208.
Zervos, A. S., Gyuris, J., and Brent, R. (1993). Mxi1, a protein that specifically interacts with Max to bind Myc-Max recognition sites. Cell 72, 223-232.

C-Myc Transrepression and Cell Transformation

L. A. LEE and C. V. DANG[1]
Department of Medicine, and [1]The Johns Hopkins Oncology Center, The Johns Hopkins University School of Medicine, Baltimore, MD, USA

The c-Myc oncoprotein affects cell differentiation, cell proliferation, apoptosis, and cell transformation. Many studies have ultimately centered on the ability of c-Myc to transactivate through the E-box as the mechanism underlying all of these Myc functions. It is so widely accepted that c-Myc transactivation is necessary for cell transformation, that the authentication of putative target genes requires the presence of E-boxes within these genes that can be transactivated by c-Myc in transient transfection assays. However, several examples exist where mutations of c-Myc result in the disassociation of c-Myc transformation from transactivation, suggesting the existence of other mechanisms that confer its transforming properties. Recently, c-Myc mediated transrepression, a poorly understood function of c-Myc, has been the focus of increased interest as several genes have been reported to be down-regulated by c-Myc. Evidence now suggests that transrepression may contribute to cell transformation.

The genes repressed by c-Myc comprise a diverse group, but the majority are highly expressed in differentiated cells (Table 1). Of particular interest are the genes that encode for proteins that affect cell adhesion such as thrombospondin-1 [1], LFA-1 [2], N-CAM [3], and collagen genes [4]. Since overexpression of c-Myc transforms cells, thus allowing cells to grow in a cell contact independent manner, perhaps down-regulation of cell adhesion molecules by c-Myc is required for the transformed phenotype. Interesting implications surround the down-regulation of MHC class I as well; the down-regulation of MHC class I described in melanoma and neuroblastoma cells may enhance survival of transformed cells by allowing escape from detection by the immune surveillance system.

The only viral gene on the list, the adenoviral major late (adML) gene, may not be a physiologic target of Myc, but it has nevertheless proven useful in our understanding of both c-Myc mediated transactivation and transrepression. Prior to the identification of definitive Myc target genes, the adML promoter was a natural alternative to artificial reporter constructs in the study of c-Myc transactivation because it contains two E-boxes. c-Myc clearly transactivates this promoter, but at

Table 1. Genes that are down-regulated by c-Myc

LFA-1[2]	thrombospondin-1[1]	C/EBPα[5,6]
N-CAM [3]	neu[7]	MT-1 [8]
collagen a2(I)[4]	adML[9]	MHC class I[10]

high concentrations of exogenous Myc, repression of this promoter occurs [11, 12]. Various control experiments confirmed that this repression was not a squelching phenomenon. An answer to this unexplained observation would soon become apparent.

Interest in c-Myc mediated repression grew when it was observed in *in vitro* transcription assays that Myc could inhibit TFII-I mediated transactivation using from part of the adML promoter [13]. Using gel-shift assays and mutational analysis, Roeder and colleagues demonstrated that TFII-I transactivation requires direct interaction of this protein with a promoter element called the initiator (Inr). The Inr element encompasses the initiation site of transcription (reviewed in [14, 15]). At least four types of initiators exist. The initiator found in the adenoviral major late promoter follows a consensus sequence YAYTCYYY where Y is a pyrimidine. The Inr is most commonly found in housekeeping genes which are TATA-less. In these genes it determines the start site of transcription. In promoters with TATA boxes, the Inr augments basal transcription. The Inr recruits elements of the basal transcriptional machinery much in the way the TATA box does, but in a different sequential order. Roeder found that Myc interacts directly with the initiator element of the adML promoter but only in the presence of TFII-I [13].

Ziff and colleagues took the observation that Myc could inhibit TFII-I transactivation through the Inr one step further. They recognized that the majority of genes reported to be repressed by c-Myc contain a weak consensus sequence for the adML initiator element [16]. To address whether transrepression of the adML promoter depends on the Inr, they compared transregulation of the wild-type adenoviral major late promoter with that of mutant adML promoters that bore nucleotide substitutions within the Inr [16]. Mutation of the Inr abolished c-Myc transrepression of the adML promoter.

In concurrent experiments, our laboratory also determined that high concentrations of c-Myc transrepressed the adML promoter [12]. To determine which domains were required for transrepression, we studied the properties of two non-transforming mutants that contain either a deletion of amino acids 106-143 of the transactivation domain or a deletion of the helix-loop-helix (HLH) dimerization motif. Within the 106-143 region lies Myc Box II, a highly conserved sequence of amino acids that are essential for cell transformation. Neither mutant resembled the pattern of activity observed with wild-type Myc; the mutant Δ106-143 caused a seven-fold activation of adML promoter, whereas the HLH mutant failed to activate or repress at all. These observations imply that both the transactivation and the dimerization domains are necessary for c-Myc transrepression through the Inr. We refer to the amino acids 106-143 as the transrepression domain (Fig. 1).

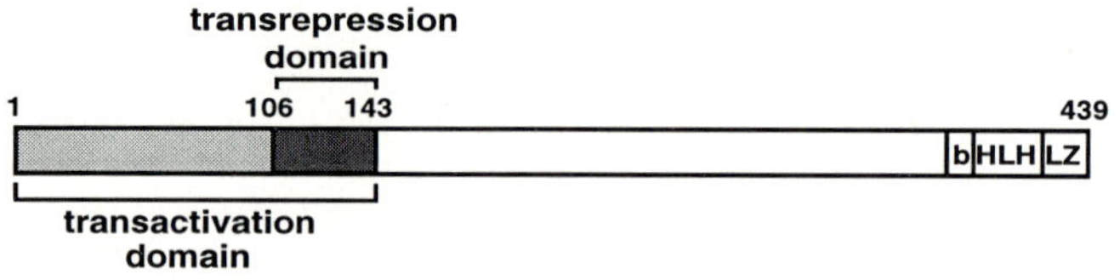

Fig. 1. Schematic diagram of the functional domains of the c-Myc oncoprotein. b = basic domain, HLH = helix-loop-helix motif, LZ = leucine zipper. Numbers designate amino acids.

c-Myc transrepression of Inr-containing promoters other than adML also occurs. C/EBPα, albumin, terminal deoxynucleotidyl transferase (tdt), and λ5 have each been reported to be repressed by c-Myc in an Inr-dependent manner [16, 17].

The physiologic significance of c-Myc transrepression of albumin, tdt and λ 5 have not yet been established.

An even more critical question is whether c-Myc transrepression contributes to cell transformation. Since it had been previously determined that amino acids 106-143 of the transactivation domain were necessary for transrepression, the biological activity of a Burkitt lymphoma-derived mutant, designated MycB2, that contains a point mutation within this region at position 115 (gift of T. Yano and M. Raffeld) was examined. In addition to the chromosomal translocation involving the Myc locus on chromosome 8, seventy percent of Burkitt lymphomas contain mutations within the c-myc locus, predominantly affecting the transactivation domain [18-20].

We compared the transrepression of the adML promoter by MycB2 with that of wild-type Myc [12]. We found that MycB2 was a stronger repressor of the adML promoter than wild-type Myc in transient transfections. To determine if this more potent repressor activity correlated with transformation, rat fibroblasts that overexpressed either Myc or MycB2 were plated in soft agar and the ability of these cells to form colonies in soft agar, a measure of cell transformation, was assessed. MycB2 overexpressing cells formed more and larger colonies than wild-type Myc, suggesting that the more potent repressor activity of this mutant conferred enhanced transforming potential.

Having determined that a Burkitt lymphoma-derived Myc mutant with enhanced repressive and transforming properties exists, we then focused on the biologic properties of a previously described synthetic mutant which also contains a mutation within the transrepression domain [21]. This mutant, called MycW136E, contains a point mutation at position 136 in mouse Myc (correlates with 135 in human). Compared to the wild-type Myc transactivation domain, the MycW136E transactivation domain when fused to the yeast Gal4 DNA binding domain more potently transactivates Gal4 reporter plasmid [21]. Intriguingly, despite its enhanced transactivation ability, MycW136E could not transform rat embryo fibroblasts in the Ras cotransformation assay. In transient transfection experiments we found that MycW136E was significantly weaker than wild-type Myc in its ability to repress the adenoviral major late promoter. Thus it appears that MycW136E cannot transform because it has lost its ability to repress. Rat fibroblasts overexpressing MycW136E could not form colonies in soft agar as could stable cells overexpressing wild-type Myc.

The Inr-dependent mechanism of c-Myc transrepression is probably only one of several that exist. c-Myc could indirectly downregulate expression of genes by altering the activity of other transcription factors. At least two examples of this indirect suppression by Myc have been described. The suppressed expression of collagen genes in 3T3-L1 cells by c-Myc appears to occur through alterations in phosphorylation and hence activity of NF-1 isoforms, the primary regulators of collagen gene expression [22]. Both c-Myc and N-Myc suppress expression of MHC class I [10, 23]. N-Myc downregulates the p50 subunit of NFkB resulting in the down-regulation of MHC class I [24].

The function of c-Myc is extremely complex and appears to have many facets. c-Myc transactivation of genes involved in cell growth such as ornithine decarboxylase and cdc25A undoubtedly contribute to the transformed phenotype, as overexpression of these genes is sufficient for cell transformation. c-Myc transrepression is emerging as another mechanism by which c-Myc transforms cells. As Inr elements are found principally in genes highly expressed in differentiated cells, it seems plausible that down-regulation of such genes may be important for cell transformation to occur. Despite this interesting theory, it has yet to be shown that down-regulation of any of the genes in Table 1 is necessary or sufficient for the Myc transformed phenotype.

References

1.Tikhonenko, A., D. Black, and M. Linial. 1996. In press.

2.Inghirami, G., F. Grignani, L. Sternas, L. Lombardi, D. M. Knowles, and R. Dalla-Favera. 1990. Down-regulation of LFA-1 adhesion receptors by c-myc oncogene in human B lymphoblastoid cells. *Science* 250:682-686.

3.Akeson, R., and R. Bernards. 1990. N-myc down regulates neural cell adhesion molecule expression in rat neuroblastoma. *Mol Cell Biol* 10:2012-2016.

4.Yang, B.-S., T. J. Geddes, R. J. Pogulis, B. de Crombrugghe, and S. O. Freytag. 1991. Transcriptional suppression of cellular gene expression by c-Myc. *Mol Cell Biol* 11:2291-2295.

5.Antonsen, P., M. Pray, A. Jacobsson, and G. Xanthopoulos. 1995. Myc inhibits CCAAT/enhancer-binding protein alph-gene expression in HIB-1B hibernoma cells through interactions with the core promoter region. *Eur J Biochem* 232:397-403.

6.Christy, R., K. Kastner, D. Geiman, and M. Lane. 1991. CCAATT/enhancer binding protein gene promoter: binding of nuclear factors during differentiation of 3T3-L1 preadipocytes. *Proc Natl Acad Sci USA* 88:2593-2597.

7.Suen, T.-C., and M.-C. Hung. 1991. c-myc reverses neu-induced transformation morphology by transcriptional repression. *Mol Cell Biol* 11:354-362.

8.Kaddurah-Daouk, R., J. M. Greene, A. S. Baldwin Jr., and R. E. Kingston. 1987. Activation and repression of mammalian gene expression by the c-myc protein. *Genes Dev* 1:347-357.

9.Ziff, E. B., and R. M. Evans. 1978. *Cell* 14:1463-1475.

10.Versteeg, R., I. Noordermeer, M. Kruse-Wolters, D. Ruiter, and P. Schrier. 1988. c-*myc* down-regulates class I HLA expression in human melanomas. *EMBO J* 7:1023-1029.

11.Van Antwerp, M. E., D. G. Chen, C. Chang, and E. V. Prochownik. 1992. A point mutation in the MyoD basic domain imparts c-Myc-like properties. *Proc Natl Acad Sci USA* 89:9010-9014.

12.Lee, L. A., C. Dolde, J. Barrett, C. S. Wu, and C. V. Dang. 1996. A link between c-Myc-mediated transcriptional repression and neoplastic transformation. *J Clin Invest* 97:1687-1695.

13.Roy, A. L., C. Carruthers, T. Gutjahr, and R. G. Roeder. 1993. Direct role for Myc in transcription initiation mediated by interactions with TFII-I. *Nature* 365:359-361.

14.Hernandez, N. 1993. TBP, a universal eukaryotic transcription factor? *Genes Dev* 7:1291-1308.

15.Smale, S. T., and D. Baltimore. 1989. The "initiator" as a transcription control element. *Cell* 57:103-113.

16.Li, L.-H., C. Nerlov, G. Prendergast, D. MacGregor, and E. B. Ziff. 1994. c-Myc represses transcription in vivo by a novel mechanism dependent on the initiator element and Myc box II. *EMBO J* 13:4070-4079.

17.Mai, S., and I.-L. Mårtensson. 1995. The c-myc protein represses λ5 and TdT initiators. *Nuc Acids Res* 23:1-9.

18.Yano, T., C. Sander, H. Clark, M. Dolezal, E. Jaffe, and M. Raffeld. 1993. Clustered mutations in the second exon of the MYC gene in sporadic Burkitt's lymphoma. *Oncogene* 8:2741-2748.

19.Raffeld, M., T. Yano, A. T. Hoang, B. Lewis, H. M. Clark, T. Otsuki, and C. V. Dang. 1995. Clustered Mutations in the transcriptional activation domain of Myc in 8q24 translocated lymphomas and their functional consequences. *Curr Top Microbiol Immunol. 194:265-72.*

20.Clark, H. M., T. Yano, T. Otsuki, E. S. Jaffe, D. Shibata, and M. Raffeld. 1994. Mutations in the coding region of c-MYC in AIDS-associated and other aggressive lymphomas. *Cancer Res* 54:3383-3386.

21.Brough, D., T. Hofmann, K. Ellwood, R. Townley, and M. Cole. 1995. An essential domain of the c-Myc protein interacts with a nuclear factor that is also required for E1A-mediated transformation. *Mol Cell Biol* 15:1536-1544.

22.Yang, B., J. Gilbert, and S. Freytag. 1993. Overexpression of myc suppresses CCAAT transcription factor/nuclear factor 1-dependent promoters in vivo.*Mol Cell Biol* 13:3093-3102.

23.Lenardo, M., A. Rustgi, A. Schievella, and R. Bernards. 1989. Suppression of MHC class 1 gene expression by N-myc through enhancer inactivation. *EMBO J* 8:3351-3355.
24.van't Veer, L., R. Beijersbergen, and R. Bernards. 1993. N-myc suppresses major histocompatibility complex Class I gene expression through down-regulation of the p50 subunit of NF-kB. *EMBO J* 12:195-200.

Association of Myc with the Zinc-finger Protein Miz-1 Defines a Novel Pathway for Gene Regulation by Myc

A. SCHNEIDER, K. PEUKERT[1], M. EILERS and F. HÄNEL[1]
Zentrum für Molekulare Biologie Heidelberg (ZMBH), Im Neuenheimer Feld 282, 69120 Heidelberg, Germany
[1] Hans-Knöll-Institut für Naturstoff-Forschung, Department of Cell and Molecular Biology, Beutenbergstraße 11, 07745 Jena, Germany

SUMMARY

The Myc protein activates transcription as part of a complex with its partner protein, Max. Myc-transformed cells are also characterised by the loss of expression of a number of genes and this repressive effect of Myc on gene expression may not be mediated by the Myc/Max complex. We recently isolated by two-hybrid cloning a novel zinc-finger protein that associates with the carboxy-terminus of Myc. We have termed this protein Miz-1 (Myc-interacting zinc finger protein). Some of the properties of Miz-1 suggest that it may be involved in gene repression by Myc *in vivo*.

INTRODUCTION

Myc proteins have emerged as central regulators of mammalian cell proliferation and of cell death, apoptosis (for review, see Henriksson and Lüscher, 1996). Cells transformed by Myc are characterised by multiple changes in gene expression and phenotype. One pathway by which Myc exerts its biological effects has been clearly defined: Myc associates with the partner protein, Max, binds to specific sequence on DNA and activates transcription of a number of genes which carry this sequence within their regulatory elements (for review, see Bernards, 1995). Association with Max is necessary not only for transcriptional activation, but also for activation of cell proliferation, apoptosis and cell transformation by Myc (Amati et al., 1993; Amati et al., 1993).

Cells transformed by Myc are also characterised by the loss of expression of genes. Indeed, by now quite a large and diverse number of genes have been described that are repressed by Myc *in vivo*. They fall into three large groups:

- *c-myc* itself (Penn et al., 1990)
- genes encoding cell surface proteins like integrins (Flickinger et al., 1994; Inghirami et al., 1990) and collagens (Yang et al., 1991).
- cell cycle regulators like cyclin D1 (Marhin et al., 1996) and c/EBP (Freytag and Geddes, 1992).

Taken together, the identity of these genes suggest that gene repression by Myc may contribute significantly to the phenotype of transformed cells; in a few instances, this has been demonstrated directly. For example, loss of the LFA-1 protein upon expression of Myc has direct functional consequences for the adhesive properties of B-cells in culture (Paganin et al., 1994).The mechanism(s) by which Myc exerts this negative effect on gene expression have not been clearly defined yet. However, there are several indications that they may not simply occur as an indirect consequence of the transformed state. First, sequences that determine the extent of repression by Myc have been identified in several promoters; these sequences lie close to the start site of transcription ("initiator elements") and are distinct from the E-box elements which are bound by Myc/Max complexes (Li et al., 1994). Second, repression of the endogenous *c-myc* gene is a rapid process and does not lag behind the acquisition of a transformed phenotype (L.Penn, personal communication). Third, mutants of Myc have been identified that are capable of repression, but not transcriptional activation and vice versa (Philipp et al., 1994).

The data suggest that partner proteins of Myc other than Max may exist which mediate gene repression by Myc. Two candidate proteins have been identified, YY-1 (Shrivastava et al., 1993) and TFII-I (Roy et al., 1993), both of which can associate with start sites of transcription. Our own analysis (Philipp et al., 1994) had suggested that for repression of cyclin D1 by Myc, interactions with the helix-loop-helix domain of Myc, but not with the leucine zipper of Myc were critical. This prompted us to search for novel proteins that interacted with the HLH domain of Myc. In this report, we describe the characterisation of one such protein, which we have termed Miz-1, for Myc interacting zinc finger protein.

RESULTS

Miz-1 was isolated in a two-hybrid screen using a GAL-Myc (355-439) chimeric protein as a bait to screen a HeLa-cDNA library. A single clone was recovered and further characterised. Figure 1 summarises the interaction data obtained and gives a schematic representation of the clone we have isolated.

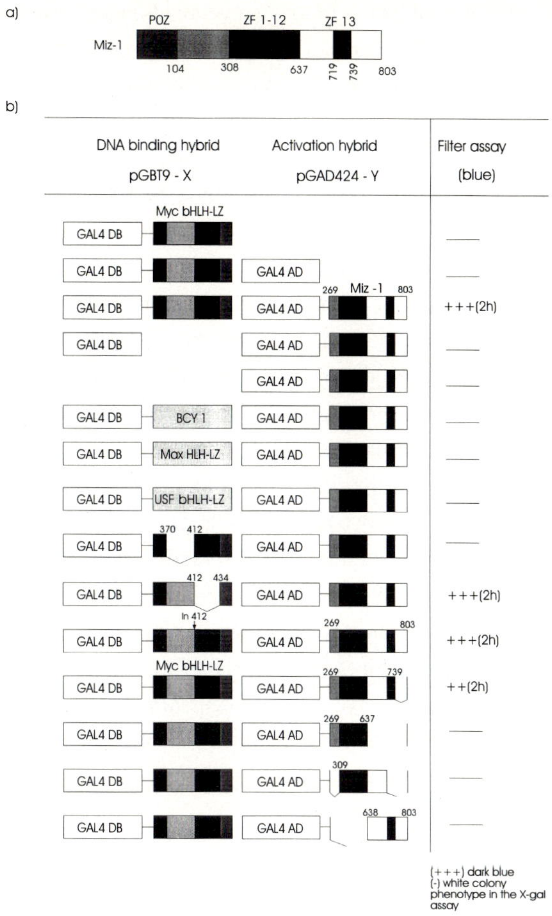

Figure 1: Structural features of Miz-1 (panel A) and summary of two hybrid data obtained in yeast (panel B).

Miz-1 is an zinc finger protein with thirteen zinc fingers; twelve of them are clustered in the carboxy-terminal half of the protein, the last one follows with a spacer of 40 amino acids. Closely homologous cDNAs have been isolated from mouse and chicken and are ubiquitously expressed in mouse (Schulz et al., 1995). At its amino-terminus, Miz-1 carries a POZ/BTB-domain: this is a protein/protein interaction domain found both in other zinc finger proteins and in otherwise unrelated cytosolic proteins (e.g.Bardwell and Treisman, 1994). Interaction with Myc occurs a region encompassing the zinc finger region; at its carboxy-terminus, deletion mutants of Miz-1 define a region predicted to form a coiled-coil structure reminiscent of an HLH motif as critical for interaction, while the structure at the amino-terminal border of the interaction domain is not obvious. Miz-1 interacts with the helix-loop-helix, but not the leucine zipper domain of Myc. This interaction is specific for Myc, as neither USF nor Max interact with Miz-1 (Figure 1). Miz-1 and Myc interact *in vitro* and co-immunoprecipitate *in vivo* after transient expression of both proteins in HeLa cells (not shown). While *in vitro* data point to the possibility that a ternary Myc/Miz-1/Max complex may exist, Max and Miz-1 appear to compete for binding to Myc *in vivo* (see below).

Miz-1 binds DNA in a zinc-dependent manner; specific binding of Miz-1 to the start sites of the Adenovirus Major Late, the polyoma late and the cyclin D1 promoter has been detected. On both the Adenovirus Major Late Promoter and the cyclin D1 promoter, Miz-1 acts as a transcriptional activator (see Figure 2). This is somewhat surprising as many POZ-domain proteins appear to repress, rather than activate transcription and the POZ-domain has been defined as a transcriptional repression domain (Albagli et al., 1996; Dhordain et al., 1995). However, it may be related to the finding that the POZ-domain of Miz-1, in contrast to that of other members of the family, does not mediate homo-dimerization (K. Peukert, unpublished observation). Also, Miz-1 carries a domain strikingly reminiscent of acidic activation domains (amino acids 208-270).
Transactivation by Miz-1 is inhibited by Myc (see Figure 2); for inhibition, the integrity of the carboxy-terminal domain of Myc is both necessary and sufficient (Figure 2), suggesting that inhibition is mediated by direct complex formation between Myc and Miz-1.

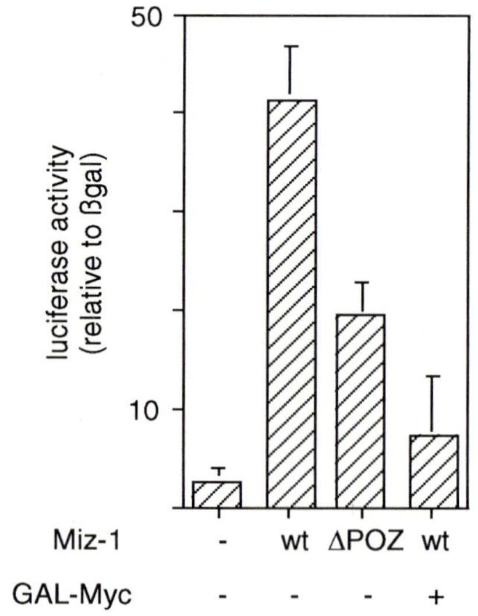

Figure 2: Transactivation of the AdML promoter by Miz-1 is inhibited by Myc.

These observations also show that inhibition of Miz-1 transactivation by Myc is also not due to transcriptional squelching by the potent transactivation domain of Myc. Whether Myc directly inhibits DNA binding by Miz-1 has not been determined.

Any proposed mechanism in which Myc inhibits gene expression by complexing another transcriptional activator *in vivo* must explain how such a mechanism can be efficient given the vanishing amounts of Myc protein present even in a transformed cell. One way this could happen would be if Myc limited the amount of functional Miz-1 protein in the cell nucleus. Inspection of the Miz-1 primary sequence suggested one potential mechanism how this might be achieved: we detected only a single very weak homology to a consensus nuclear import signal (amino acids 381-383). Indeed, fusion of amino acids 376-389 to green fluorescent protein (GFP) failed to stimulate nuclear import of GFP (A.S., unpublished), suggesting that a nuclear import signal may altogether be absent from Miz-1. Consistent with this notion, most cells ectopically expressing Miz-1 after transient transfection showed only a weak nuclear fluorescence and much of the protein was localised in the cytosol; in the cytosol, Miz-1 associated with microtubuli (see below). The same was observed in cells co-expressing Miz-1 and an allele of Myc that does not interact with Miz-1 (MycΔHLH, see Figure 3). Within the nucleus, Miz-1 showed a homogeneous distribution excluding the nucleoli.

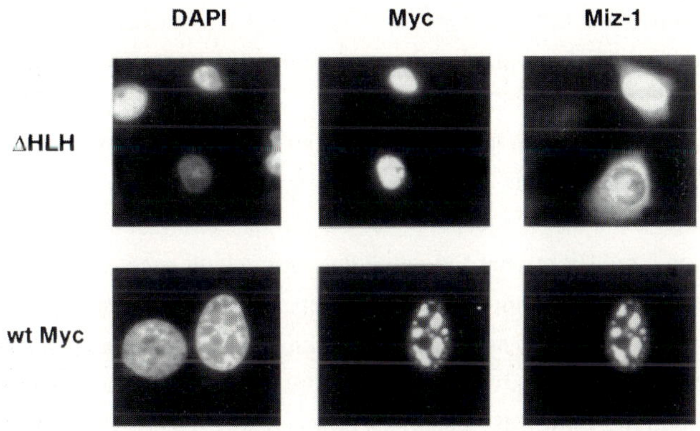

Figure 3: Intracellular distribution of Myc, MycΔHLH and Miz-1. Shown are photomicrographs from transiently transfected HeLa cells stained with monoclonal (9E10) anti-Myc and polyclonal anti-Miz-1 antibodies. The magnification of the lower panels is two-fold higher than for the upper panels.

Upon co-expression of Myc, however, essentially all of Miz-1 was localised in the cell nucleus (see Figure 3). Thus, Myc stimulates nuclear import of Miz-1. Indeed, Miz-1 may depend on Myc for its import, as expression of Max seemed to further increase the number of cells showing an exclusive cytosolic staining (not shown). Within the nucleus, distribution of Miz-1 and Myc was no longer homogeneous; rather, both proteins co-aggregate in a number of discrete foci. A similar "speckled" intranuclear distribution has previously been reported for Myc and for other POZ-domain proteins: most likely, these foci represent non functional protean aggregates (e.g. Spector et al., 1987). We concluded that the amount of Miz-1 present in the cell nucleus may be limited by Myc as Miz-1 depends on Myc for its nuclear import.

Association with Miz-1 was required, but not sufficient for Myc to stimulate nuclear import of Miz-1; rather, amino-terminal domains of Myc were required for stimulation. Indeed, Miz-1 inhibited nuclear import of the GAL-Myc chimera used as a bait in the two hybrid assay. Under these conditions, much of GAL-Myc was retained in the cytosol and was recruited by Miz-1 to microtubuli (see cover photograph of this volume). Precisely which domains of Myc are required to stimulate nuclear import of Miz-1 remains to be determined.

DISCUSSION

We describe the identification of a novel partner protein of Myc which we have termed Miz-1. The biochemical properties of Miz-1 suggest that association of Myc with Miz-1 may explain some of the well documented repressive effects Myc exerts on gene expression. For example, Miz-1 interacts specifically with both the Adenovirus Major Late and the cyclin D1 promoter, two genes shown to be repressed by Myc *in vivo*. Second, transactivation by Miz-1 is blocked by complex formation with Myc; inhibition of transactivation is not due to squelching, as the carboxy-terminal domain of Myc (which does not contain a transcriptional activation domain) is both necessary and sufficient for inhibition. Finally, nuclear import of Miz-1 depends on Myc, suggesting a model in which release from Myc in the nucleus may be critical for transactivation by Miz-1: in this view, the amount of Myc would be almost certainly sufficient for efficient inhibition of Miz-1 function. In this view, Miz-1 acts as a downstream effector of Myc.

However, our data are also compatible with a function of Miz-1 upstream of Myc, e.g. in regulating nuclear import of Myc. Myc protein accumulates in the cytosol of differentiating neuronal (Wakamatsu et al., 1993)and myeloid cells (Craig et al., 1993) and has been found to associate with microtubuli in HL-60 and HeLa cells (Alexandrova et al., 1995): thus, the Myc/Miz-1 complex may also regulate nuclear import of Miz-1 and/or stabilise an inactive conformation of Myc. In this view, Miz-1 may also act as an upstream regulator for Myc function.

At present, we can only speculate as to what the biological function of Miz-1 might be. One potential clue to its function comes from its chromosomal localisation at 1p36.1-1p36.2 in a region which is frequently mutated in human neoplasias. In neuroblastoma,

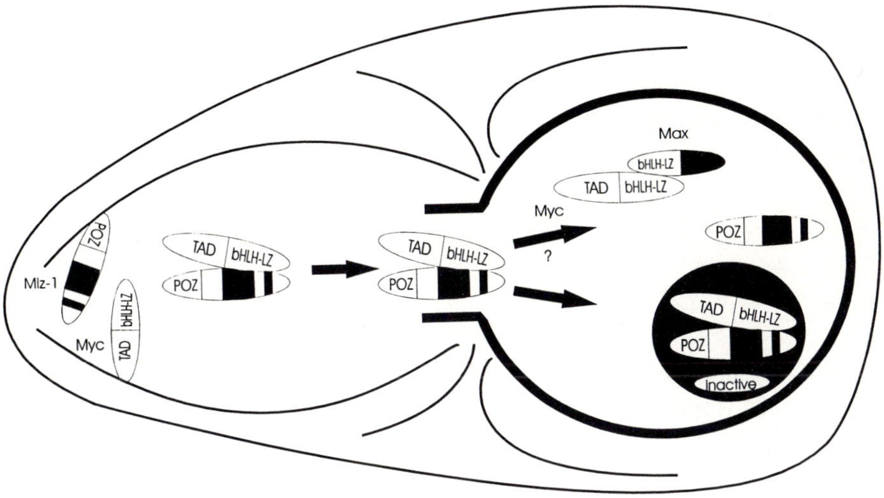

Figure 4: Model describing our findings.

this region appear two harbour two distinct tumour suppressor loci, one of which is associated with amplification of N-Myc (Schwab et al., 1996). The homologous region in mouse carries one locus that determines the susceptibility of different strains of mice to pristane-induced plasmacytomas (B.Mock, personal communication). Thus, Miz-1 may be a negative regulator of cell proliferation or tumorigenesis and its function may be ablated by Myc.

Clearly, the critical issue which remains to be resolved is whether gene repression by Myc represents a malfunction that occurs specifically in transformed cells or whether it is a physiologically important function of Myc in the decision between proliferation and differentiation. The identification of Miz-1 could potentially help to address this issue.

ACKNOWLEDGEMENTS

We would like to thank Gordon Carmichael for sharing results prior to publication and Ilona Hallwax, Claudia Franke, Vera Hanemann and Grit Mrotzek for excellent technical assistance, Eckhard Birch-Hirschfeld and Rainer Frank for oligonucleotide synthesis and Hans Krügel and Berta Reiner for assistance with computer analysis. Work in our laboratories is supported by the DFG and the BMBF.

REFERENCES

Albagli, O., Dhordain, P., Bernardin, F., Quief, S., Kerkaert, J. P., and Leprince, D. (1996). Multiple domains participate in distance-independent LAZ3/BCL6-mediated transcriptional repression. Biochem Biophys Res Commun *220*, 911-915.

Alexandrova, N., Niklinski, J., Bliskovsky, V., Otterson, G. A., Blake, M., Kaye, F. J., and Zajac Kaye, M. (1995). The N-terminal domain of c-Myc associates with alpha-tubulin and microtubules in vivo and in vitro. Mol. Cell. Biol. *15*, 5188-5195.

Amati, B., Brooks, M. W., Levy, N., Littlewood, T. D., Evan, G. I., and Land, H. (1993). Oncogenic activity of the c-Myc protein requires dimerization with Max. Cell *72*, 233-245.

Amati, B., Littlewood, T. D., Evan, G. I., and Land, H. (1993). The c-Myc protein induces cell cycle progression and apoptosis through dimerization with Max. EMBO J. *13*, 5083-5087.

Bardwell, V. J., and Treisman, R. (1994). The POZ domain: A conserved protein-protein interaction motif. Genes Dev. *8*, 1664-1677.

Bernards, R. (1995). Transcriptional regulation. Flipping the Myc switch. Curr. Biol. *5*, 859-561.

Craig, R. W., Buchan, H. L., Civin, C. I., and Kastan, M. B. (1993). Altered cytoplasmic/nuclear distribution of the c-myc protein in differentiating ML-1 human myeloid leukemia cells. Cell Growth Differ *4*, 349-357.

Dhordain, P., Albagli, O., Ansieau, S., Koken, M. H. M., Deweindt, C., Quief, S., Lantoine, D., Leutz, A., Kerckaert, J.-P., and Leprince, D. (1995). The BTB/POZ domain targets the LAZ3/BCL6 oncoprotein to nuclear dots and mediated homomerisation *in vivo*. Oncogene *11*, 2689-2697.

Flickinger, K. S., Judware, R., Lechner, R., Carter, W. G., and Culp, L. A. (1994). Integrin expression in human neuroblastoma cells with or without N-myc amplification and in ectopic/orthotopic nude mouse tumors. Exp Cell Res *213*, 156-163.

Freytag, S. O., and Geddes, T. J. (1992). Reciprocal regulation of adipogenesis by Myc and C/EBPα. Science *256*, 379-382.

Henriksson, M., and Lüscher, B. (1996). Proteins of the Myc network: Essential regulators of cell growth and differentiation. Cancer Research *68*, 109-182.

Inghirami, G., Grignani, F., Sternas, L., Lombardi, L., Knowles, D. M., and Dalla Favera, R. (1990). Down-regulation of LFA-1 adhesion receptors by C-myc oncogene in human B lymphoblastoid cells. Science *250*, 682-686.

Li, L., Nerlov, C., Prendergast, G., MacGregor, D., and Ziff, E. B. (1994). c-Myc represses transcription *in vivo* by a novel mechanism dependent on the initiator element and Myc box II. EMBO J. *13*, 4070-4079.

Marhin, W. W., Hei, Y.-J., Chen, S., Jiang, Z., Gallie, B., Phillips, R. A., and Penn, L. Z. (1996). Loss of Rb and Myc activation co-operate to suppress cyclin D1 and contribute to transformation. Oncogene *12*, 43-55.

Paganin, C., Bianchi, G., Lombardi, L., Dalla Favera, R., Mantovani, A., and Allavena, P. (1994). Role of leukocyte function-associated antigen-1 and very late antigen-4 in the adhesion and transmigration of c-myc-transfected B-lymphoblastoid cell lines across vascular endothelium. Int J Clin Lab Res *24*, 29-32.

Penn, L. J. Z., Brooks, M. W., Laufer, E. M., and Land, H. (1990). Negative autoregulation of c-myc transcription. EMBO J. *9*, 113-121.

Philipp, A., Schneider, A., Väsrik, I., Finke, K., Xiong, Y., Beach, D., Alitalo, K., and Eilers, M. (1994). Repression of Cyclin D1: a Novel Function of MYC. Mol. Cell. Biol. *14*, 4032-4043.

Roy, A. L., Carruthers, C., Gutjahr, T., and Roeder, R. G. (1993). Direct role for Myc in transcription initiation mediated by interactions with TFII-I. Nature *365*, 359-361.

Schulz, T. C., Hopwood, B., Rathjen, P. D., and Wells, J. R. E. (1995). An unusual arrangement of 13 zinc fingers in the vertebrate gene *Z13*. Biochem. J. *311*, 219-224.

Schwab, M., Praml, C., and Amler, L. C. (1996). Genomic instability in 1p and human malignancies. Genes Chromosom Cancer *16*, 211-229.

Shrivastava, A., Saleque, S., Kalpana, G. V., Artandi, S., Goff, S. P., and Calame, K. (1993). Inhibition of transcriptional regulator Yin-Yang-1 by association with c-Myc. Science *262*, 1889-1891.

Spector, D. L., Watt, R. A., and Sullivan, N. F. (1987). The v- and c-myc oncogene proteins colocalize in situ with small nuclear ribonucleoprotein particles. Oncogene *1*, 5-12.

Wakamatsu, Y., Watanabe, Y., Shimono, A., and Kondoh, H. (1993). Transition of localization of the N-Myc protein from nucleus to cytoplasm in differentiating neurons. Neuron *10*, 1-9.

Yang, B. S., Geddes, T. J., Pogulis, R. J., de Crombrugghe, B., and Freytag, S. O. (1991). Transcriptional suppression of cellular gene expression by c-Myc. Mol. Cell Biol. *11*, 2291-2295.

C-Myc Protein Interactions: Max, Mad, Mxil

Regulated Expression and Function of the c-Myc Antagonist, Mad1, During a Molecular Switch from Proliferation to Differentiation

C. M. Cultraro[1], T. Bino[1] and S. Segal[1,2*]

[1] NCI-Navy Medical Oncology Branch, National Cancer Institute, NIH, and [2] Uniformed Services, University of Health Sciences, Bethesda, MD 20889-5105, USA

Introduction

Myc, Max, Mad, Mxi1 and mSin3 comprise a transcription factor superfamily in which the central protein is Max. All family members (except mSin3) must dimerize with Max through their respective helix loop helix (HLH) and leucine zipper (LZ) domains to cooperatively bind DNA in a sequence specific manner (reviewed in [15]). In contrast to the transactivating property of Myc/Max heterodimers [1, 18, 21], Max heterodimerization with Mad or Mxi1, followed by the tethering of mSin3, to target genes results in suppression of transcription [3, 33]. Although Mad/Max heterodimers have been shown to antagonize Myc function in transformation and the mechanism(s) involved require multiple protein-protein and protein-DNA interactions [4, 20, 23, 33], how Mad functions in differentiation is unknown.

c-*myc* and *mad* family genes are regulated in a reciprocal fashion during cell growth and differentiation. While c-*myc* is up-regulated in proliferating cells and down-regulated during differentiation (reviewed in [26]), expression of *mad* is barely detectable in proliferating cells and highly induced during differentiation [2, 9, 11, 16, 24, 25, 37]. In murine erythroleukemia (MEL) cells induced to differentiate with N'N'-hexamethylene bisacetamide (HMBA) G_1 arrest is thought to occur through a cascade of events leading to sequestration of the transcription factor E2F and the subsequent down-regulation of proteins involved in cell cycle progression, such as DNA polymerase α, dihydrofolate reductase, thymidylate synthase, c-*myc* and c-*myb* [27]. In contrast, overexpression of exogenous c-Myc is believed to block inducer-mediated differentiation by precluding G_0/G_1 arrest [13, 14, 17, 31], and ectopic expression of Mad1 arrests cells in G_1 [5, 32]. Therefore, increased expression of Mad may provide a mechanism of exit from the cell cycle during differentiation. The reciprocal expression of these two genes taken together with the inverse manner in which they influence cell cycle progression, suggest that Myc and Mad each play an important, yet distinct, role in the switch from proliferation to differentiation.

In this study we sought to investigate the mechanism by which Mad functions during a molecular switch from proliferation to differentiation. MEL cells were transfected with an inducible Mad expression vector, and the effect of the transfected gene on the growth and differentiation properties of the transfectants was examined. In general, the cells were growth retarded and exhibited a low level of spontaneous differentiation. However, over time cells expressing *mad* were lost from the pool. In order to more precisely study the mechanism by which Mad functions in these cells, we modified our transfection strategy. To overcome growth inhibition imposed by ectopically expressed Mad, we cotransfected the cells with a constitutive c-*myc* gene. Whereas cells grown in HMBA in the absence of zinc fail to differentiate, addition of zinc up-regulates Mad expression by several fold, and differentiation proceeds normally. Furthermore, we mapped the motifs required for Mad to function in the switch and show that the Sin-binding, basic region and leucine zipper motifs are essential. These results suggest that Mad functions by an active repression mechanism to antagonize the growth-promoting function(s) of Myc and bring about a transition from cellular proliferation to differentiation.

Results and Discussion

Reciprocal regulation of c-Myc and Mad1 in differentiating MEL cells
MEL cells can be induced to differentiate in vitro by treatment with a variety of chemical reagents [28]. In most hematopoietic cells this process is accompanied by a characteristic down-regulation of c-Myc expression [19, 22, 29, 30, 35], and up-regulation of Mad and Mxi1 [2, 9, 11, 16, 24, 25, 37]. Furthermore, this reciprocal regulation of Myc and Mad expression is accompanied by a switch in the composition of Max heterocomplexes from growth-promoting Myc-Max to growth-inhibitory Mad-Max [2]. Therefore, it appears that both the up-regulation of Mad and down-regulation of Myc are necessary for cellular differentiation.

To characterize the regulation of Myc and Mad in differentiating MEL cells, C19 cells were treated with HMBA for up to three days and expression of the respective mRNAs and proteins examined. Three *mad* mRNA species (5.7, 3.2 and 2.1 Kb) are detected (Fig. 1). Levels of the 5.7 and 3.2 Kb species increased in response to HMBA, while c-*myc* decreased. The contrasting expression patterns is also evident at the protein level, as seen by Western analysis. Within four hours of treatment, there is a pronounced induction of the Mad 35 KDa doublet that is paralleled by an equally dramatic decline in c-Myc expression. Furthermore, this inverse pattern of regulation continues through day three, where Myc is expressed at comparatively low levels but Mad expression is high. The ratio of Myc/Max to Mad/Max heterocomplexes in these cells is in favor of Mad/Max (data not shown). Since the two proteins are reciprocally regulated in differentiating MEL cells, we utilized this cell culture system to study their functional antagonism.

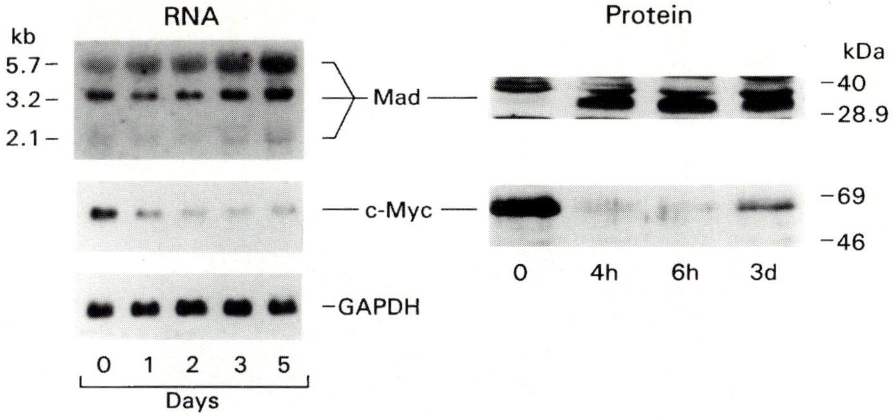

Fig. 1. c-Myc and Mad1 expression in differentiating MEL cells. C19 cells were induced to differentiate with HMBA (final concentration 3.5 mM) and maintained in logarithmic phase by diluting daily with fresh medium. Total cytoplasmic RNA and proteins were isolated [8] at the indicated time points. RNA was analyzed on Northern blots by sequential hybridization to the following probes: murine *mad*1, murine c-*myc* and GAPDH. Proteins were analyzed on Western immunoblots with c-Myc (raised against full-length fusion protein; Upstate Biotechnology, Inc.) and Mad (C-19; Santa Cruz Biotechnology, Inc.) polyclonal antiserum. Immunoreactive bands were detected by enhanced chemiluminescence (ECL, Amersham).

Ectopic Mad expression suppresses cell growth and induces a low level of spontaneous differentiation

To determine whether ectopically expressed Mad is able to trigger the cells to enter a differentiation program, cells were transfected with either the pMTH-*neo* control or the pMTH-*mad* expression vector, with *mad* under the transcriptional control of the zinc-inducible mouse metallothionein promoter [7]. Clonogenicity of the transfectants was examined two weeks after transfection by plating cells in selective medium at a density of 10^5 cells/ml/well either in the absence or presence of zinc. A marked inhibition in cloning efficiency was detected in the pMTH-*mad* transfectants with only 11% of the wells containing viable cells. In contrast, the cloning efficiency of the pMTH-*neo* controls was 80%. In these transfectants *mad* expression is low and measurable only by RT-PCR analysis (Fig. 2).

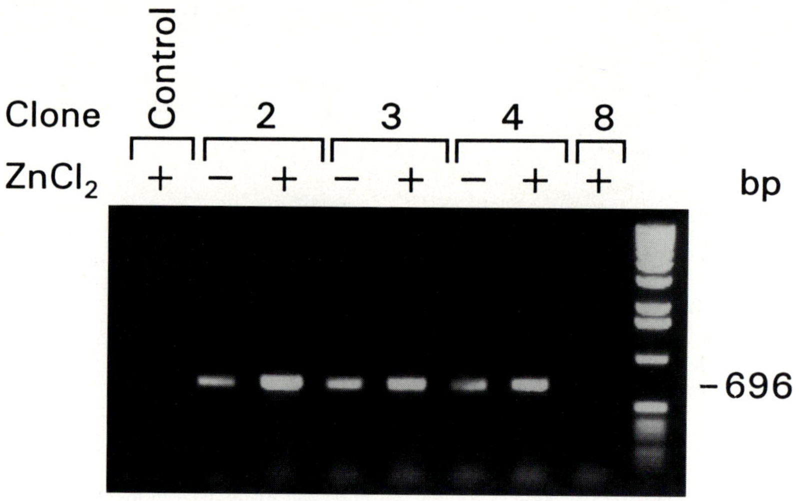

Fig. 2. Low levels of *mad* expression in transfectants. Transfectants of pMTH control and pMTH*mad*, selected in the absence of zinc, were grown in the absence (-) or presence (+) of 100 μM $ZnCl_2$ for 48 h. Total cytoplasmic RNA was isolated and analyzed by reverse transcriptase (RT)-PCR with expression vector specific primers encompassing the coding region (696 bp) of human *mad*. 1 Kb DNA molecular size marker in last lane.

We further investigated Mad-induced growth inhibition by monitoring expression in randomly selected pools of *mad*-transfected cells, grown in selective medium in the absence of zinc, 20, 50 and 80 days post-transfection. Aliquots of cells were removed at the indicated time points and grown for 48 h in the absence or presence of zinc. RNA was extracted and analyzed by RT-PCR (Fig. 3A). Although *mad* expression is detected as early as 20 days post-transfection, these levels gradually decline over time such that by 80 days, even after zinc-induction, *mad* expression is undetectable. Thus, all attempts to establish stable clones overexpressing Mad failed due to rapid loss of the *mad* transgene. Similar findings were reported for other cell systems where proliferating cells either down-regulated Mad expression or lost the transgene [6, 20, 23, 32, 36]. To examine if the loss of *mad*-expressing cells is due in part to spontaneous differentiation, in parallel with the RT-PCR experiment, cell aliquots were stained with acid benzidine for detection of hemoglobin synthesis, a marker of terminal differentiation (Fig. 3B). Twenty days post-transfection, when the zinc-induced levels of *mad* are maximal, 25% of the cells differentiate in the absence of an inducing agent. However, as *mad* levels decline on day 50, so does the level of differentiation, and by 80 days post-transfection the cells are no longer differentiating and *mad* expression is undetectable.

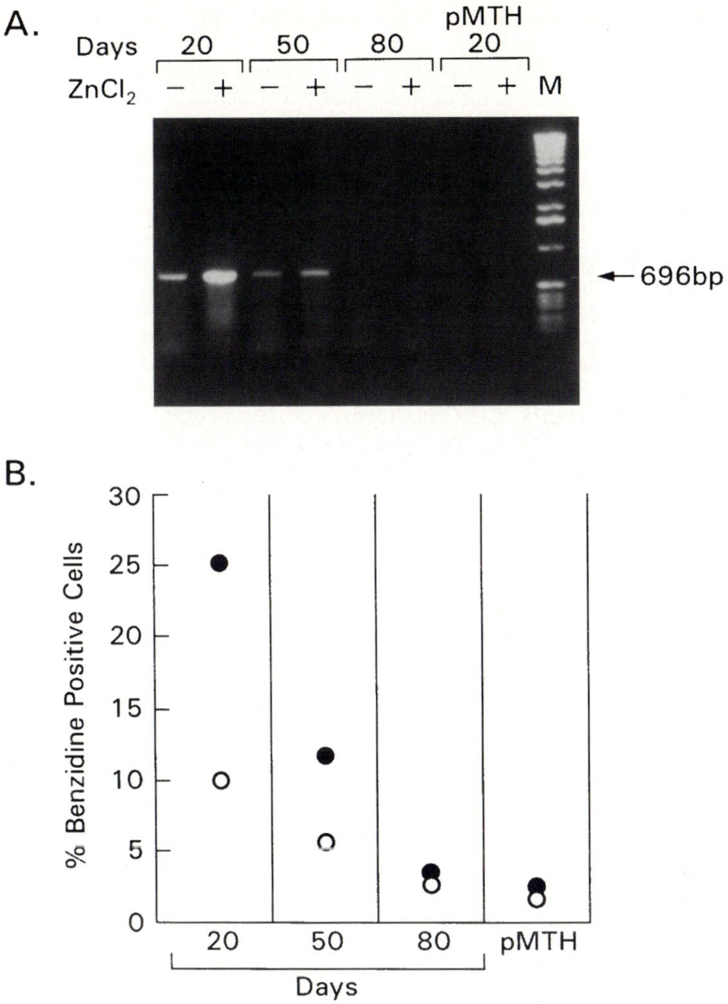

Fig. 3. Spontaneous differentiation as a result of *mad* expression in a pool of pMTH-*mad* transfected cells. Aliquots were removed from a pool of transfected cells 20, 50 and 80 days post-transfection (pMTH-neo control 20 days only). At each time point, cells were cultured in the absence (-) or presence (+) of 100 µM $ZnCl_2$. (A) Total cytoplasmic RNA was isolated and amplified by RT-PCR (see Fig. 2). M indicates 1 Kb DNA molecular size marker. (B) At each time point cells were grown for 7 days (○-without zinc; ●-with zinc) and stained with acid benzidine. Values are given as the percent of benzidine-positive cells.

Mad/Max/mSin3 interactions are essential for a switch from proliferation to differentiation

To overcome growth inhibition imposed by ectopic Mad, we exploited the ability of an overexpressed c-Myc to block inducer-mediated differentiation and cotransfected cells with c-*myc* ($pL^1hmcneo^r$). In the transfectants, Myc is constitutively expressed and overcomes growth inhibition induced by low basal levels of Mad. However, zinc-induction results in increased expression of Mad, while the level of overexpressed Myc remains unchanged. In this manner we developed a cell culture system in which a switch from proliferation to differentiation can be modulated. Furthermore, to map the motifs essential for Mad to function in this switch, we constructed a series of mutants each functionally lacking a specific interaction motif (adapted from [20]). SID(PP)Mad contains two proline substitutions in the amino terminal Sin-interaction domain which interrupt the helical structure. Thus, this mutated protein is unable to bind mSin3, but retains the ability to dimerize with Max and bind DNA [3]. ΔBRMad (basic region), ΔLZMad and ΔCTMad (carboxy terminus) are deletion mutants. ΔBRMad forms a trimeric complex with mSin3 and Max, but is unable to bind DNA. ΔLZMad lacks the ability to dimerize with Max and bind DNA, but retains the ability to bind mSin3 [3]. ΔCTMad lacks amino acids 155-221 downstream of the LZ, but retains the ability to bind mSin3, Max and DNA [4, 20]. DNA fragments encoding these mutant proteins were cloned into pMTH-*neo*. For each set of cotransfections, 30 stable clones were selected, and examined for c-*myc* and *mad* expression on Northern blots. On the average, 50% of the clones selected expressed both c-*myc* and *mad* (data not shown). For comparative analysis, one representative clone was selected from each cotransfection (Fig. 4). Each one expresses similar levels of *mad*, and comparable levels of *myc*. Included as controls are MTH-1 and Clone 56 (overexpresses c-Myc and is differentiation-blocked [10]). Although the SID(PP)Mad mutant expresses lower levels of c-Myc in comparison to the other clones, such levels are still sufficient to block differentiation. Protein levels in ΔCTMad were evaluated by using a different antibody, since the one used in general to detect Mad is against a peptide corresponding to the region deleted in this mutant.

To determine whether a switch from proliferation to differentiation can be induced in the cotransfectants such that high levels of Mad can antagonize the function of Myc and reverse a block, we examined the differentiation properties associated with the different clones. HMBA induction in the absence of zinc fails to induce differentiation in all clones tested, except the MTH-1 control. However, addition of zinc to the induction medium reverses the block only in the Myc/wild-type Mad cotransfectant. SID(PP), ΔBR and ΔLZ Mad cotransfectants behave more like Clone 56 and remain blocked (data not shown). Although Myc/ΔCTMad cotransfectants were selected, their instability prevented the characterization of their growth and differentiation properties. Taken together, these results suggest that induced levels of transfected wild-type Mad are able to overcome constitutive levels of c-Myc and reverse a block to differentiation. Furthermore, this function of Mad requires the presence of an intact SID, BR and LZ interaction domain.

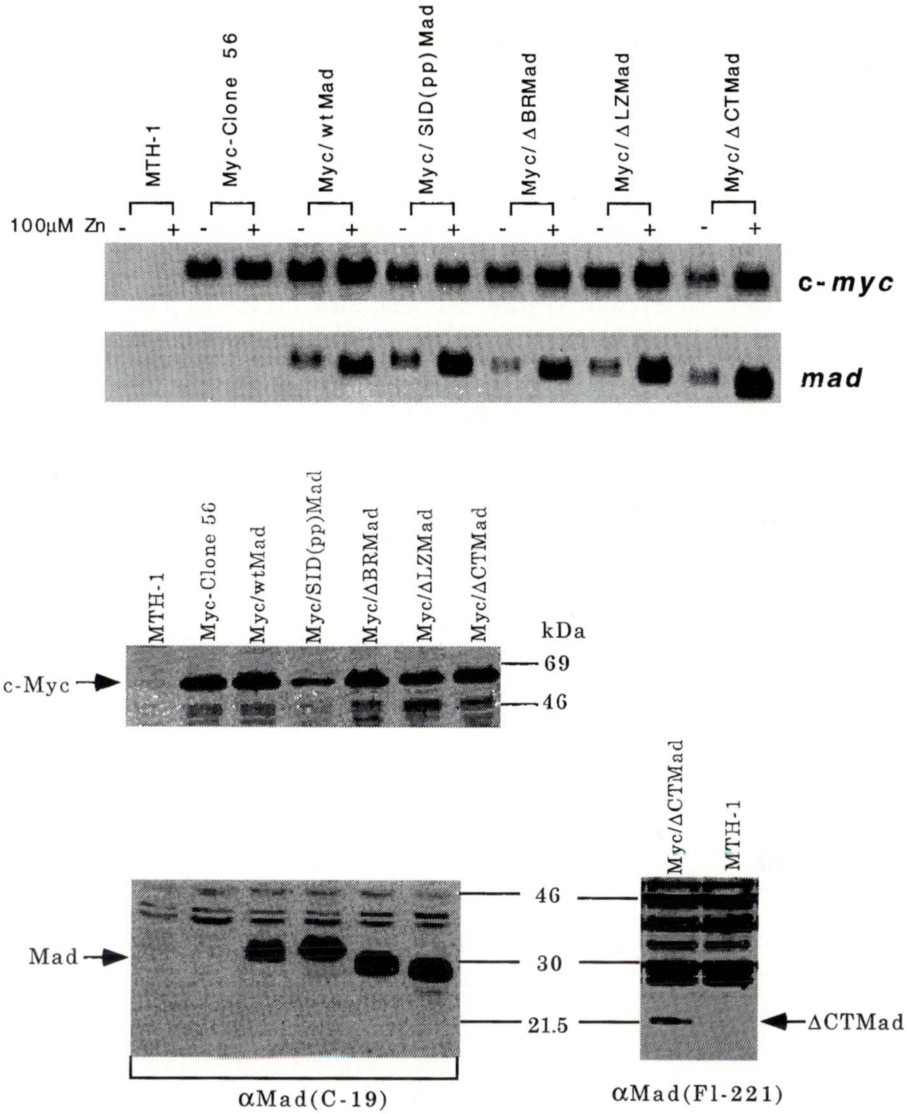

Fig. 4. c-Myc and Mad1 expression in cotransfectants. Individual clones including Clone 56 and MTH-1 were grown in the absence or presence of zinc for 48 h. Total cytoplasmic RNA and proteins (+ zinc only) were isolated. RNA was analyzed on Northern blots by first hybridizing to a human c-*myc* followed by a human *mad*1 probe. Proteins were analyzed on Western immunoblots with c-Myc (9E10; Oncogene Science) monoclonal antibodies (upper panel), Mad (C-19) polyclonal antiserum (lower panel-left) and Mad (Fl-221; Santa Cruz Biotechnology, Inc.) polyclonal antiserum (lower panel-right) (see Fig. 1).

If indeed, levels of Mad are limiting in such differentiation-blocked cells (Clone 56), one would predict that increased expression of Mad should sway the balance from Myc/Max to Mad/Max heterodimers and reverse the differentiation-block. In fact, up-regulation of a zinc-inducible Mad in cells with a Myc-imposed block restored the differentiation response. In the context of the mechanism by which these proteins exert opposing effects on cell cycle progression, it appears that the ability of Mad to arrest cells in G_1[5, 32] essentially overcomes the ability of Myc to prevent cell cycle arrest. We further substantiate this theory by mapping the interaction domains required for Mad to function in this capacity. That is, we demonstrate that mutated Mad proteins lacking cell cycle inhibitory activity [SID(PP) and ΔLZ] [32] are also defective in restoring the differentiation response. Taken together, these results suggest that Mad, Max and mSin3 must interact to form a functional complex which inhibits cell proliferation and promotes differentiation. This is in agreement with the inability of overexpressed wild-type Max to reverse a Myc-block to differentiation by simply competing with Myc for DNA-binding sites (unpublished data). In contrast, unlike the active repression imposed by Mad-Max-mSin3, a dominant-negative mutant of Max (bm-Max) reverses a Myc-imposed block to differentiation by sequestering Myc [8].

Since Mad expression is tightly associated with the transition from proliferation to differentiation, it has been proposed that Mad loss may be associated with the lack of normal differentiation ability and with tumorigenesis [16]. Moreover, it has been suggested that Mad may function as a tumor suppressor [5, 12, 34]. Our results support these hypotheses and further demonstrate that in addition to the up-regulation of Mad, the level of expression with respect to Myc is also important. The ability of Mad to antagonize Myc by restoring a switch from proliferation to differentiation in MEL cells, suggests a similar strategy may be therapeutically useful in reversing a Myc-derived malignant phenotype.

References

1. Amin C, Wagner AJ, Hay N (1993) Sequence-specific transcriptional activation by Myc and repression by Max. Mol. Cell. Biol. 13:383-390
2. Ayer DE, Eisenman RN (1993) A switch from Myc:Max to Mad:Max heterocomplexes accompanies monocyte/macrophage differentiation. Genes Dev. 7:2110-2119
3. Ayer DE, Lawrence QA, Eisenman RN (1995) Mad-Max transcriptional repression is mediated by ternary complex formation with mammalian homologs of yeast repressor Sin3. Cell 80:767-776
4. Cerni C, Bousset K, Seelos C, Burkhardt H, Henriksson M, Luscher B (1995) Differential effects by Mad and Max on transformation by cellular and viral oncoproteins. Oncogene 11:587-596
5. Chen J, Willingham T, Margraf LR, Schreiber-Agus N, DePinho RA, Nisen PD (1995) Effects of the MYC ongcogene antagonist, MAD, on proliferation, cell cycling and the malignant phenotype of human brain tumor cells. Nature Medicine 1:638-643
6. Chin L, Schreiber-Agus N, Pellicer I, Chen K, Lee H, Dudast M, Cordon-Cardo C, DePinho RA (1995) Contrasting roles for Myc and Mad proteins in cellular growth and differentiation. Proc. Natl. Acad. Sci. USA 92:8488-8492
7. Cogliati T, Dunn BK, Bar-Ner M, Cultraro CM, Segal S (1993) Transfected wild-type and mutant *max* regulate cell growth and differentiation of murine erythroleukemia cells. Oncogene 8:1263-1268
8. Cultraro CM, Cogliati C, Hearing LE, Segal S (1996) Basic mutant Max reverses a c-Myc block to differentiation. Onc. Rpts. 3:141-146

9. Delgado MD, Lerga A, Canelles M, Gomez-Casares MT, Leon J (1995) Differential regulation of Max and role of c-Myc during erythroid and myelomonocytic differentiation of K562 cells. Oncogene 10:1659-1665
10. Dmitrovsky E, Kuehl WM, Hollis GF, Kirsch IR, Bender TP, Segal S (1986) Expression of a transfected human c-*myc* oncogene inhibits differentiation of a mouse erythroleukaemia cell line. Nature 322:748-750
11. Dunn BK, Cogliati T, Cultraro CM, Bar-Ner M, Segal S (1994) Regulation of murine Max (Myn) parallels the regulation of c-Myc in differentiating murine erythroleukemia cells. Cell Growth Differ. 5:847-854
12. Edelhoff S, Ayer DE, Zervos AS, Steingrimsson E, Jenkins NA, Copeland NG, Eisenman RN, Brent R, Disteche CM (1994) Mapping of two genes encoding members of a distinct subfamily of MAX interacting proteins: MAD to human chromosome 2 and mouse chromosome 6, and MXI1 to human chromosome 10 and mouse chromosome 19. Oncogene 9:665-668
13. Einat M, Resnitzky D, Kimchi A (1985) Close link between reduction of c-*myc* expression by interferon and G_0/G_1 arrest. Nature 313:597-600
14. Freytag SO (1988) Enforced expression of the c-*myc* oncogene inhibits cell differentiation by precluding entry into a distinct predifferentiation state in G_0/G_1. Mol. Cell. Biol. 8:1614-1624
15. Henriksson M, Luscher G (1996) Proteins of the Myc network: essential regulators of cell growth and differentiation. Cancer Res. 68:110-182
16. Hurlin PJ, Foley KP, Ayer DE, Eisenman RN, Hanahan D, Arbeit JM (1995) Regulation of Myc and Mad during epidermal differentiation and HPV-associated tumorigenesis. Oncogene 11:2487-2501
17. Kaczmarek L, Hyland JK, Watt R, Rosenberg M, Baserga R (1985) Microinjected c-*myc* as a competence factor. Science 228:1313-1315
18. Kato GJ, Barrett J, Villa-Garcia M, Dang CV (1990) An amino-terminal c-Myc domain required for neoplastic transformation activates transcription. Mol. Cell. Biol. 10:5914-5920
19. Klinken PS, Holmes KL, Morse HC, Thorgeirsson SS (1988) Transcriptional and post-transcriptional regulation of c-*myc* and p53 during proliferation and differentiation of murine erythroleukemia cells treated with DFMO and DMSO. Exp. Cell. Res. 178:185-198
20. Koskinen PJ, Ayer DE, Eisenman RN (1995) Repression of Myc-Ras cotransformation by Mad is mediated by multiple protein-protein interactions. Cell Growth Differ. 6:623-629
21. Kretzner L, Blackwood EM, Eisenman RN (1992) Myc and Max proteins possess distinct transcriptional activities. Nature 359:426-429
22. Lachman HM, Skoultchi AI (1984) Expression of c-*myc* changes during differentiation of mouse erythroleukemia cells. Nature 310:592-594
23. Lahoz EG, Xu L, Schreiber-Agus N, DePinho RA (1994) Supression of Myc, but not E1a, transformation activity by Max-associated proteins, Mad and Mxi1. Proc. Natl. Acad. Sci. USA 91:5503-5507
24. Larsson L, Pettersson M, Oberg F, Nilsson K, Luscher B (1994) Expression of *mad*, *mxi*1, *max* and c-*myc* during induced differentiation of hematopoietic cells: opposite regulation of *mad* and c-*myc*. Oncogene 9:1247-1252
25. Lymboussaki A, Kaipainen A, Hatva E, Vastrik I, Jeskanen L, Jalkanen M, Werner S, Stenback R, Alitalo R (1996) Expression of Mad, an antagonist of Myc oncoprotein function, in differentiating keratinocytes during tumorigenesis of the skin. British J. Cancer 73:1347-1355
26. Marcu KB, Bossone SA, Patel AJ (1992) *myc* function and regulation. Annu. Rev. Biochem. 61:809-860
27. Marks PA, Richon VM, Kiyokawa J, Rifkind RA (1994) Inducing differentiation of transformed cells with hybrid polar compounds: A cell cycle-dependent process. Proc. Natl. Acad. Sci. USA 91:10251-10254
28. Marks PA, Rifkind RA (1978) Erythroleukemic differentiation. Annu. Rev. Biochem. 47:419-448
29. Mechti N, Piechaxzyk M, Blanchard J, Marty L, Bonnieu A, Jeanteur P, Lebleu B (1986) Transcriptional and post-transcriptional regulation of c-*myc* expression during differentiation of murine erythroleukemia Friend cells. Nucleic Acids Res. 14:9653-9666

30. Nepveu A, Marcu KB, Skoultchi AI, Lachman HM (1987) Contributions of transcriptional and post-transcriptional mechanisms to the regulation of c-*myc* expression in mouse erythroleukemia cells. Genes Dev. 1:938-945
31. Prochownik EV, Kukowska J, Rodgers C (1988) c-*myc* antisense transcripts accelerate differentiation and inhibit G_1 progression in murine erythroleukemia cells. Mol. Cell. Biol. 8:3683-3695
32. Roussel MF, Ashmun RA, Sherr CJ, Eisenman RN, Ayer DE (1996) Inhibition of cell proliferation by the Mad1 transcriptional repressor. Mol. Cell. Biol. 16:2796-2801
33. Schreiber-Agus N, Chin L, Chen K, Torres R, Rao G, Guida P, Skoultchi AI, DePinho RA (1995) An amino-terminal domain of Mxi1 mediates Anti-Myc oncogenic activity and interacts with a homolog of the yeast transcriptional repressor Sin3. Cell 80:777-786
34. Shapiro DN, Valentine V, Eagle L, Yin X, Morris SW, Prochownik EV (1994) Assignment of the human MAD and MXI1 genes to chromosomes 2p12-p13 and 10q24-25. Genomics 23:282-285
35. Spotts GD, Hann SR (1990) Enhanced translation and increased turnover of c-*myc* proteins occur during differentiation of murine erythroleukemia cells. Mol. Cell. Biol. 10:3952-3964
36. Vastrik I, Kaipainen A, Penttila T, Lymboussakis A, Alitalo R, Parvinen M, Alitalo K (1995) Expression of the *mad* gene during cell differentiation in vivo and its inhibition of cell growth in vitro. J. Cell Biol. 128:1197-1208
37. Zervos AS, Gyuris J, Brent R (1993) Mxi1, a protein that specifically interacts with Max to bind Myc-Max recognition sites. Cell 72:223-232

A Biochemical and Biological Analysis of Myc Superfamily Interactions

N. Schreiber-Agus[1], L. Alland[1], R. Muhle[1], J. Goltz[2], K. Chen[1], L. Stevens[3], D. Stein[2] and R. A. DePinho[1]

[1] Dept. of Microbiology and Immunology, Albert Einstein College of Medicine, Bronx, NY, USA

[2] Dept. of Molecular Genetics, Albert Einstein College of Medicine, Bronx, NY, USA

[3] Dept. of Developmental and Molecular Biology, Albert Einstein College of Medicine, Bronx, NY, USA

Introduction

Members of the myc family of nuclear proto-oncogenes (c-, N- and L-myc) play central roles in the control of normal growth and development and in genetic pathways linked to cellular transformation and apoptotic cell death (for reviews see [19, 40]). Accumulating structural, biochemical, and genetic evidence affords the view that the function of Myc family oncoproteins in these diverse processes relates in part to their roles as sequence-specific transcription factors (for reviews see [31, 58]). Myc family proteins possess a multi-functional amino-terminal domain with transactivation potential [32], a region rich in basic amino acid residues responsible for sequence-specific DNA binding activity to the E-box consensus CACGTG [8], and a carboxy-terminal α-helical domain required for dimerization with another basic region helix-loop-helix/leucine zipper (bHLH/LZ) protein, Max [9, 43]. Many of the biochemical and biological activities of Myc appear to be highly dependent upon its association with Max [1, 2, 9, 35, 43). In addition to its key role as an obligate partner in transactivation-competent Myc/Max complexes, Max may also repress Myc-responsive genes through the formation of transactivation-inert complexes that are capable of binding the Myc/Max recognition sequence [5, 10, 33, 35, 39, 41, 44, 65]. These complexes include Max/Max homodimers, and the heterodimers Mad/Max [5, 29] and Mxi1/Max [65]. The biochemical properties of the highly homologous Mad and Mxi1 have led to a model for their regulation of Myc activity in which these proteins compete with Myc for binding both to Max and to common target sequences [5, 29, 65].

Much of our understanding of the biological actions of vertebrate Myc family proteins has come from analysis of their oncogenic actions and developmental properties. With respect to oncogenic activity, all three Myc family genes can cooperate with a mutant H-*RAS* gene to transform early-passage rat embryo fibroblasts (REFs) [37] and can generate tumors when over-expressed in transgenic mice (for review see [40]). A role for the Myc family in normal development is supported by its dynamic pattern of stage- and cell type-specific expression (for review see [16]) and by the mid-gestational lethality associated with N- and c-myc loss-of-function in the mouse [11, 15, 49, 54; H.W. Lee and R.A. DePinho, unpublished observations). These insights on Myc function in cancer and development have been complemented recently by several mechanistic clues as to how Myc may effect its activities on the molecular level through transactivation of specific gene targets and interaction with associated proteins. For example, Myc's direct regulation of genes such as *ornithine decarboxylase* [7] and the phosphatase *cdc25A* [21] suggests a role in DNA synthesis and in G1 progression, respectively. Additionally, Myc has been shown to associate with the Rb-related protein, p107 [23], the RNA polymerase II-associated TBP [26], and the general transcription factor, YY1 [53], interactions consistent with a role in growth control and transcriptional regulation.

Preliminary analyses of members of the Mxi/Mad family in normal development and neoplastic growth have supported their roles as antagonists of Myc and putative tumor suppressors. In particular, during the approach of many cell lineages to the terminally-differentiated state, mxi and mad mRNA and protein levels increase, while those of c-myc decrease [4, 5, 13, 28, 29, 38, 45, 50, 59, 65, 66]. Overexpression of mxi1 and mad can antagonize myc activity in cellular transformation assays [34, 36, 50]. In addition, introduction of mad system into established human tumor cell lines resulted in a marked decrease in their rate of proliferation and S-phase entry [12, 46, 47] and profoundly inhibited their ability to form tumors in vivo [12]. Finally, the chromosomal loci to which mad and mxi1 genes map have been implicated in the genesis of several human cancers [18, 64; M.F. Seldin and R.A. DePinho, unpublished results].

Despite all of the aforementioned advances in the elucidation of Myc superfamily (i.e. c-, N- and L-Myc, Max, Mxi, Mad 1, 3, 4) function on the molecular level, a number of important issues have yet to be addressed. These include (I) the placement of Myc in a pathway downstream of mitogenic and differentiative signals, (ii) the elucidation of the biological relevance of Myc-responsive gene targets and interactions with associated proteins and (iii) the determination of the precise molecular mechanism of Myc's actions and Mxi/Mad's antagonism. Data from our laboratory that yield insight into these matters were presented at the meeting on c-Myc in B-cell Neoplasia and are described in this article.

Molecular Aspects of Mxi-Mediated Suppression

The Mouse Mxi-SR amino-terminal repression domain

Preliminary studies using the human forms of mad and mxi indicated that these could dramatically suppress the oncogenic activity of myc/RAS, but not E1a/RAS in the rat embryo fibroblast cooperation assay [36]. In the course of investigating the basis for this anti-oncogenic activity of Mxi, we identified two distinct mouse mxi transcripts that encode proteins with dramatically different abilities to repress myc-induced transformation [51]. These were designated Mxi-SR and Mxi-WR, for strong repressor and weak repressor, respectively, of Myc cotransformation activity (see below). The organization of mouse genomic sequences encoding the 5' regions of the mxi-SR and mxi-WR cDNAs is consistent with the existence of a single mxi1 gene capable of producing the two mRNAs through alternative RNA processing.

While mxi-SR and mxi-WR ORFs encode identical bHLH/LZ and carboxy-terminal regions, alternative utilization of 5' sequences extends the mxi1-SR ORF an additional 36 amino acids beyond the mxi1-WR ORF. This extension is highly conserved throughout vertebrate evolution of the Mxi protein [50, 65], is homologous to an analogously positioned domain in Mad 1, 3 and 4 [5, 29] and is predicted to be strongly α-helical (Fig. 1). It has been subsequently termed the SID for Sin3 interacting domain (see below).

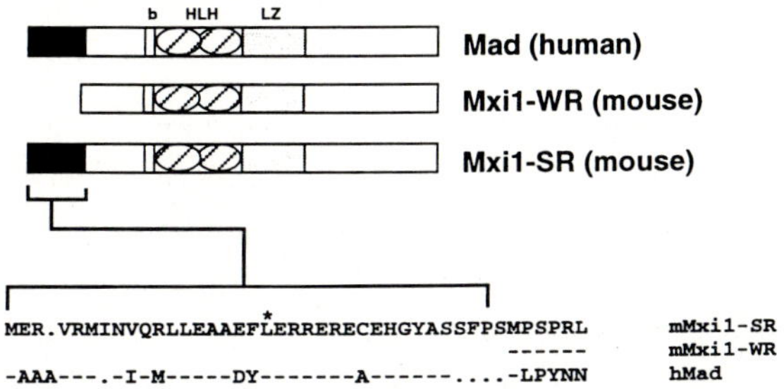

Fig. 1. Schematic maps of mouse Mxi-SR, mouse Mxi-WR, human Mxi and human Mad proteins are shown, with landmark regions indicated (blackened box, repressive region; b, basic region; HLH, helix-loop-helix; LZ, leucine zipper). Amino acid sequences were aligned using the Genetics Computer Group Sequence Analysis Software Package [17] with dashes representing residues identical to the mouse Mxi1-SR residues and dots in the sequence representing gaps that were introduced to maximize homology. Shown here is an alignment of the domains that confer repressive activity upon mouse Mxi-SR and human Mxi with a similarly positioned region in the human Mad amino terminus. This "repression domain" is absent from the weakly repressive Mxi-WR. The α-helical nature of the repression domain, as assessed by the PredictProtein algorithm (EMBL), results from the amphipathicity of these residues. The leucine residue (L19) that was converted to a proline to make Mxi-SR-pro (see below) is marked by an asterisk.

In REF cotransformation assays, the amino terminal region of Mxi-SR was shown to be essential for full anti-Myc activity [51]. In particular, Mxi-SR, Mxi-WR, and various mutant forms of Mxi-SR were tested for inhibitory potential, where inhibition was assessed by comparing the number of transformed foci generated in cotransfections containing mouse c-myc and activated Ha-ras in the presence or absence of these Mxi forms (Fig. 2). As tabulated in Fig. 2B, a significant reduction in the number of foci generated was observed when mouse mxi-SR was added to the c-myc/ras cotransfections; this level of suppression was comparable to that reported previously for the human mxi1 gene [36]. In contrast, addition of a similarly-designed expression construct encoding mouse Mxi-WR resulted in only a modest repression of c-Myc cotransformation activity. Two mutant constructs, namely mmxi-Δrep (deleted in-frame for most of the putative "repression domain" of mxi1-SR) and Mxi-SR-Pro (bearing a Pro for Leu substitution at position 19 of the repressive domain of Mxi-SR [see Fig. 1]) were found to possess weak repressive potential similar to that of Mxi-WR and markedly reduced from that of Mxi-SR (Fig. 2B, experiments 2, 3, 4 and 5). Since proline residues are known to cause disruption of α-helical structures, this loss-of-function suggests that α-helicity may be integral to amino-terminal functions. In subsequent experiments, the repression domain (or SID) was shown to be modular in nature in that it could be fused to Max [51] or to the E-box binding protein TFEB [25] and confer anti-Myc repressive potential.

A.

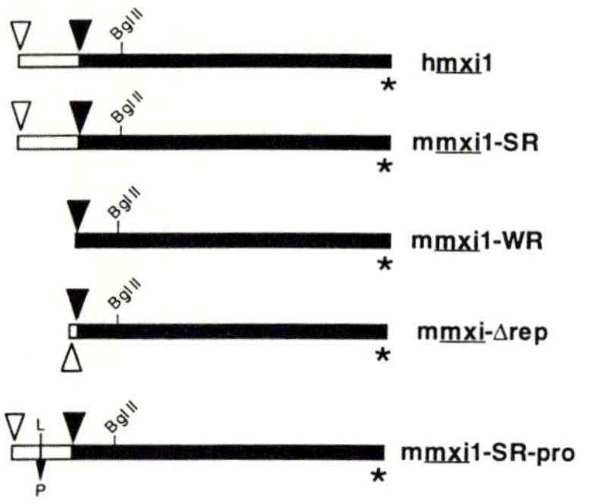

B.

DNA transfected with c-*myc* + *ras*	Total # of foci/ 6 plates				
	Exp. 1	Exp. 2	Exp. 3	Exp. 4	Exp. 5
empty vector	232	337	651	595	277
hmxi1	48	ND	ND	201	102
mmxi1-SR	38	39	142	127	36
mmxi1-WR	138	88	ND	467	255
mmxi1-Δrep	ND	141	ND	452	240
mmxi1-SR-pro	ND	ND	356	388	142

Fig 2. Structure-function analysis of various mxi1 clones as assessed by anti-Myc activity in the REF assay. (A) Inserts used to generate the various mxi expression constructs utilized in panel B are shown schematically. Initiator codon of Mxi-SR is marked by an open inverted triangle, while that of Mxi-WR is marked by a closed inverted triangle. Terminator codons are marked by asterisks. (B) Early passage cultures of REFs were cotransfected by the calcium phosphate precipitation method as previously described [41]. Each primary plate was transfected with 2 μg of the mouse c-myc expression construct, 2 μg of H-ras^{Val-12}, 2 μg of the appropriate mxi expression construct (or empty vector) as indicated in the transfected DNA column, and 30 μg of genomic carrier DNA. The total number of foci on 6 plates (derived from 2 transfected plates that were split 1 to 3) was counted approximately ten days post transfection in five separate experiments. Exp., experiment; ND, not determined.

Interaction of the SID with a Mammalian Homolog of Yeast Sin3.

The predicted α-helical configuration of the repressive domain of Mxi (and Mad) proteins raised the possibility that the molecular mechanisms governing its biological activities may be executed through protein-protein interactions. To identify proteins that associate with these repression domains, a modified version of the yeast two-hybrid method [20, 61] was employed using the amino-terminal region of human Mad [5] fused in-frame to LexA as a bait. Nucleic acid sequence analysis of an interacting clone, identified in a mouse T-cell lymphoma cDNA library subcloned in the GAL4 transactivation domain (TAD)-containing pACT vector, revealed that it was capable of encoding a mammalian protein possessing 49% similarity (33% identity) to the yeast transcriptional repressor Sin3 [42, 55, 56, 60, 62, 63]. The region of homology between mouse Sin3 (mSin3) and yeast Sin3 (ySin3) corresponded to the region surrounding the second of four paired amphipathic helices (PAH) found in the yeast protein [62]. Coimmunoprecipitations of epitope-tagged proteins in mammalian cells demonstrated (I) a specific interaction between Mxi-SR and Sin3PAH2 (i.e. the region of interaction identified in two hybrid screens) (ii) lack of interaction between Max and Sin3PAH2, and (iii) the formation of a ternary complex in vivo between Mxi-SR, Sin3 and Max [51]. A similar ternary interaction was described for Mad, Max and Sin3, and mutations that disrupted the Mad-Sin3 association were also shown to block Mad transcriptional repression [6].

Our observations with respect to the requirement of the amino-terminal extension for full suppression (Fig. 2B) and to the formation of an Mxi/Sin3/Max ternary complex in vivo prompted us to revise the prevailing view of how Myc activity is regulated by Mxi1 or Mad (for review see [3]). In the then current model, regulation of Myc-responsive genes was thought to involve Mxi's titration of a limited intracellular pool of Max and occupation (as an Mxi/Max heterodimer) of consensus recognition sequences in promoters of commonly regulated genes. Once bound, the transactivation-incompetent Mxi/Max heterodimer could serve to deny access to the active Myc/Max complex [4, 5, 36, 65; for review see 3). The observation that Mxi-WR possessed only modest repressive potential (despite having the identical bHLH/LZ region as Mxi-SR and thus able to complex with Max and bind consensus sites) argues against the simple view that Mxi regulates Myc activity in such a passive manner. Rather, since the ability of a given Mxi1 complex to fully antagonize Myc function requires activities encoded within the amino-terminal region, Mxi-SR [51] (and Mad [6]) appears to play a more active role in negative regulation. This regulation is achieved through the recruitment, by the ternary complex, of specific proteins that together mediate transcriptional repression of Myc-responsive gene targets.

Mammalian Sin3: Interaction with Mxi and Other Nuclear Proteins

Subsequent analysis of the mammalian homologue of yeast Sin3 at the level of Southern blot revealed the presence of two sin3-related loci in the mouse and human genomes; these loci were termed sin3a and sin3b, the latter of which encoded the yeast two hybrid isolate identified in our repression-domain screens [6, 45, 51]. Initial studies with the Sin3A form showed that it was capable of interacting in vivo with Mxi-SR as had been shown for the PAH2 region of Sin3B, and that it colocalized with Mxi-SR to the nucleus where the two proteins are purported to act. High endogenous mSin3 levels in REFs precluded the analysis of the effects of exogenously-added mSin3 upon Mxi-mediated repression [45], and prompted the development of a REF-based assay that employed fusion constructs of full length mouse Sin3A placed in-frame with the Mxi-SR ORF just downstream to the SID.

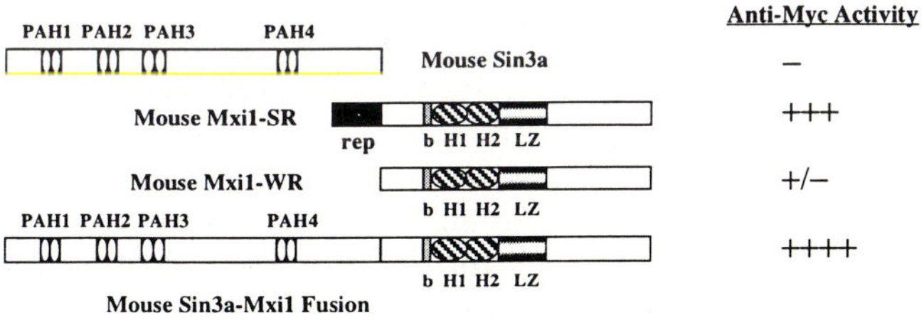

Fig. 3. mSin3A mediates the anti-Myc activity of Mxi-SR in the REF cotransformation assay. Schematic diagram of the inserts that were used to generate expression constructs that were used in the REF assay are shown. The mouse Sin3a-Mxi fusion construct was generated by fusing the entire ORF of mSin3A in frame with a PCR-generated fragment of Mxi-SR that was deleted for most of the amino-terminal repression domain. Early passage cultures of REFs were cotransfected by the calcium phosphate precipitation method as previously described [41]. The effects of addition of the various constructs to myc/ras cotransfections are shown qualitatively on the right.

As presented in Fig. 3 above, although in trans mSin3A does not augment the suppressive activity of Mxi-SR in the Myc/RAS cotransformation assay (presumably because of the abundant and ubiquitous expression of sin3 in many tissues and cell types including REFs [6, 24, 45]), it could do so effectively when fused in cis to a repression domain-lacking form of Mxi-SR. This observation strongly implies that the amino-terminal repression domain of Mxi-SR functions as a key mediator of Mxi suppression, primarily if not exclusively through recruitment of Sin3.

The above findings were recently shown to hold true for the Sin3B form as well (L. Alland and R.A. DePinho, in preparation), and further evidence for the functional linkage between Mxi and Sin3B was derived from genetic mapping studies demonstrating concordance in tumor types associated with cytogenetic lesions in the loci to where these two genes map [45, 51]. As an aside, the mouse sin3b gene was shown to give rise to two alternative transcripts that encode distinct proteins with identical amino-termini--a 3.2 kb mSin3b cDNA that encodes a 952 amino acid protein designated $mSin3b_{LF}$, and a ~1.8 kb cDNA predicted to encode a protein of 293 amino acids designated $mSin3b_{SF}$. As suggested by the terminology, the $mSin3B_{LF}$ (LF for long form) comprises all four PAH domains (as does mSin3A), while the $mSin3B_{SF}$ (SF for short form) contains PAHs 1 and 2 only (L. Alland and R.A. DePinho, in preparation).

Based on their marked conservation to ySin3, the PAH motifs are likely to be involved in protein-protein interactions that would place Sin3 (itself a non-DNA binding protein) in a promoter context where it could repress transcription. While the PAH2 motif had been previously shown to engage in an essential interaction with DNA binding proteins of the Mxi/Mad family (see above), the remainder of the PAHs could foster association with co-repressors that operate through one or more mechanisms. Postulated mechanisms include recruitment of accessory repressor proteins, modification of the activity of transcriptional activators or components of the basic transcriptional machinery, and/or induction of the repressed heterochromatic state in surrounding chromatin [45, 51; for review see 14].

Along these lines, yeast two-hybrid interaction screens have led recently to the determination that the PAH1 motif of mSin3 associates with N-CoR (L. Alland and R.A. DePinho, in preparation), a previously identified co-repressor that mediates transcription silencing by the thyroid-hormone and retinoic-acid nuclear receptors [27]. Putative functional importance of this interaction was supported by reporter assays that revealed that it appeared necessary for Sin3B-mediated active transcriptional repression (L. Alland and R.A. DePinho, in preparation). Nevertheless, results from REF-based assays similar to the ones described above (Fig. 3) but employing Sin3B PAH1-2 only fused to Mxi argued against a role for this region in the suppression of Myc-induced transformation. In contrast, utilization of fusion constructs containing Sin3 sequences carboxy-terminal to PAH2 (present only in mSin3bLF and mSin3a) showed that they were absolutely essential and possibly sufficient to suppress neoplastic growth. This study in mammalian cells, along with structure-function analyses performed in yeast [30, 63] strongly suggested that the PAH3 and PAH4 regions may play a critical role. Genetic studies performed in yeast implicating a tight functional relationship between Sin3 and Rpd3p (yeast homologue of the mammalian histone deacetylase, HD-1) [57] may provide some clues as to the mediators of Sin3 carboxy-terminal region function.

Taken together, our findings suggest that the N-CoR interaction is essential for the potent repression of basal and Myc-induced transcriptional activation, while other interactions may be more relevant for the ability of Mxi/Sin3 to antagonize the oncogenic actions of Myc in vivo (see model in Fig. 4). The existence of two distinct forms of the Sin3B protein suggests that an additional level of Mxi-mediated regulation could take place at the level of recruiting different combinations of co-repressors molecules. In the case of $mSin3_{SF}$, the sole recruitment of N-CoR could provide a more readily reversible level of regulation operating primarily at the level of modulating RNA polymerase II activity. In contrast, the ability of $mSin3_{LF}$ to associate with N-CoR as well as to effect repression through its carboxy-terminal domain may provide a more effective multi-level means of gene repression as one might need in settings such as terminal differentiation or the suppression of neoplastic growth.

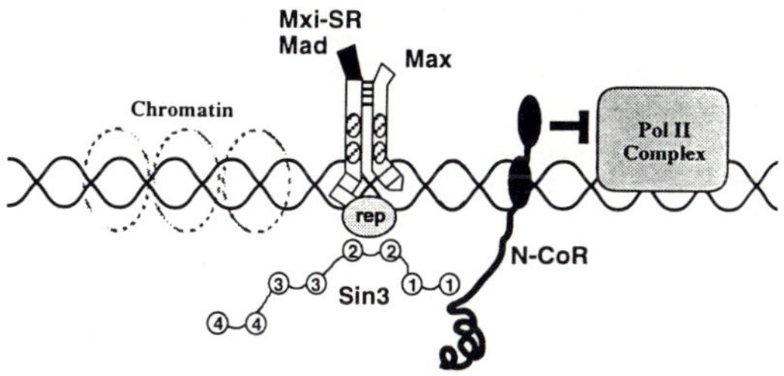

Fig. 4. Model for repression by the Mxi/mSin3 complex through interaction with co-repressors like N-CoR.

Future Prospects

As mentioned in the introduction above, a prime objective of Myc biologists is the establishment of a clear genetic link between the Myc superfamily and specific physiological pathways of growth, differentiation and death through the identification of additional associated proteins and gene targets. Among the attempts to accomplish this have been those that have characterized of Myc superfamily homologues in organisms that are more amenable to genetic analysis and experimental manipulation. Recently, our previous observation that the DNA binding/dimerization region of Max is absolutely conserved throughout vertebrate evolution [50] provided the basis for a yeast two hybrid interaction screen that led to the isolation of the *Drosophila* Myc (dMyc1) protein [52; also see 22]. Structural conservation in regions of known functional significance is consistent with the ability of dMyc1 to interact with vertebrate Max, to transactivate gene expression in yeast cells, and to cooperate with activated H-*RAS* to effect the malignant transformation of primary mammalian cells. In addition, the ability of P-element mediated ectopic expression of *dmyc1* to reverse a subset of the phenotypic alterations associated with the *diminutive* (*dm*) mutation suggests that *dm* may correspond to *dmyc1*. This finding, along with the localization of *dmyc1* expression to zones of high proliferative activity in the embryo, implicate dMyc1 as an integral regulator of *Drosophila* growth and development [52]. In the immediate future, dMyc1 will allow for the genetic analysis of functional interactions among conserved members of the Myc superfamily. In addition, the cloning of *dmyc* will enable the determination of the cell biological basis for the *diminutive* mutation that was first described sixty years ago. Ultimately, the power of the *Drosophila* model system [48] will permit one to place the dMyc network into pathways that likely lie at a nexus where mitogenic and differentiative signals are integrated in the execution of a normal growth and developmental program.

References

1. Amati B, Littlewood TD, Evan GI, Land H (1993a) The c-Myc protein induces cell cycle progression and apoptosis through dimerization with Max. EMBO J. 12: 5083-5087
2. Amati B, Brooks MW, Levy M, Littlewood TD, Evan GI, Land, H (1993b) Oncogenic activity of the c-Myc protein requires dimerization with Max. Cell 72:233-245
3. Amati B, Land H (1994) Myc-Max-Mad: a transcription factor network controlling cell cycle progression, differentiation and death. Curr. Opin. Genet. Dev. 4:102-108
4. Ayer DE, Eisenman RN (1993) A switch from Myc:Max to Mad:Max heterocomplexes accompanies monocyte/macrophage differentiation. Genes Dev. 7:2110-2119
5. Ayer DE, Kretzner L, Eisenman RN (1993) Mad: a heterodimeric partner for Max that antagonizes Myc transcriptional activity. Cell 72:211-222
6. Ayer DE, Lawrence QA, Eisenman RN (1995) The amino-terminus of Mad mediates ternary complex formation with mammalian homologs of the yeast repressor Sin3 and is required for Mad:Max transcriptional repression. Cell 80:767-776
7. Bello-Fernandez C, Packham G, Cleveland JL (1993) The ornithine decarboxylase gene is a transcriptional target of c-Myc. Proc. Nat'l Acad. Sci. USA 90:7804-7808
8. Blackwell TK, Kretzner L, Blackwood EM, Eisenman RN, Weintraub H (1990) Sequence-specific DNA binding by the c-myc protein. Science 250:1149-1151
9. Blackwood EM, Eisenman RN (1991) Max: A helix-loop-helix zipper protein that forms a sequence-specific DNA binding complex with Myc. Science 251:1211-1217
10. Blackwood EM, Luscher B, Eisenman RN (1992) Myc and Max associate in vivo. Genes Dev. 6:71-80
11. Charron J, Malynn B, Fisher P, Stewart V, Jeannotte L, Goff SP, Robertson L, Alt FW (1992) Embryonic lethality in mice homozygous for a targeted disruption of the N-myc gene. Genes Dev. 6:2248-2257
12. Chen J, Willingham T, Margraf LF, Schreiber-Agus N, DePinho RA, Nisen PD (1995) Effects of the Myc oncogene antagonist, MAD, on proliferation, cell cycling and the malignant phenotype of human brain tumor cells. Nature Med. 1:638-643
13. Chin L, Schreiber-Agus N, Pellicer I, Chen K, Lee HW, Dudast M, Cordon-Cardo C, DePinho RA (1995) Contrasting roles for Myc and Mad proteins in cellular growth and differentiation. Proc. Natl. Acad. Sci. USA 92:8488-8492
14. Cowell IG (1994) Repression versus activation in the control of gene transcription. Trends Biochem. Sci. 19:38-42
15. Davis AC, Wims M, Spotts GD, Hann S, Bradley A (1993) A null c-myc mutation causes lethality before 10.5 days of gestation in homozygotes and reduced fertility in heterozygous female mice. Genes Dev. 7:671-682
16. DePinho RA, Schreiber-Agus N, Alt FW (1991) myc family oncogenes in the development of normal and neoplastic cells. Adv. Cancer Res. 57:1-46
17. Devereux J, Haeberli P, Smithies O (1984) A comprhensive set of sequence analysis programs for the VAX. Nucleic Acids Res. 12:387-395
18. Edelhoff S, Ayer DE, Zervos AS, Steingrimsson E, Jenkins NA, Copeland NG, Eisenman RN, Brent R, Disteche CM (1994) Mapping of two genes encoding members of a distinct subfamily of MAX interacting proteins: MAD to human chromosome 2 and mouse chromosome 6, and MXI1 to human chromosome 10 and mouse chromosome 19. Oncogene 9:665-668
19. Evan, GI, Littlewood TD (1993) The role of c-myc in cell growth. Current Biol. 3:44-49

20. Fields S, Song O (1989) A novel genetic system to detect protein-protein interactions. Nature 340:245-246
21. Galaktionov K, Chen X, Beach D (1996) Cdc25 cell cycle phosphatase as a target of c-myc. Nature 382:511-517
22. Gallant P, Shiio Y, Cheng PF, Parkhurst SM, Eisenman RN (1996) Myc and Max Homologs in Drosophila. Science 274:1523-1527
23. Gu W, Bhatia K, Magrath, IT, Dang CV, Dalla-Favera R (1994) Binding and suppression of the Myc transcriptional activation domain by p107. Science 264:251-254
24. Halleck MS, Pownall S, Harder KW, Duncan AM, Jirik FR, Schlegel RA (1995) A widely distributed putative mammalian transcriptional regulator containing multiple paired amphipathic helices, with similarity to yeast SIN3. Genomics 26:403-406
25. Harper SE, Qiu Y, Sharp PA (1996) Sin3 corepressor function in Myc-induced transcription and transformation. Proc. Natl. Acad. Sci. USA 93:8536-8540
26. Hateboer G, Timmers HT, Rustgi AK, Billaud M, van't Veer LJ, Bernards R (1993) TATA-binding protein and the retinoblastoma gene product bind to overlapping epitpoes on c-Myc and adenovirus E1A protein. Proc. Natl. Acad. Sci. U.S.A. 90:8489-8493
27. Horlein AJ, Naar AM, Heinze T, Torchia J, Gloss B, Korokawa R, Ryan A, Kamei Y, Soderstrom M, Glass CK, Rosenfeld MG (1995) Ligand-independent repression by the thyroid hormone receptor mediated by a nuclear co-repressor. Nature 377:397-404
28. Hurlin PJ, Foley KP, Ayer DE, Eisenman RN, Hanahan D, Arbeit JM (1995) Regulation of Myc and Mad during epidermal differentiaion and HPV-associated tumorigenesis. Oncogene 11:2487-2501
29. Hurlin PJ, Queva C, Koskinen PJ, Steingrimsson E, Ayer DE, Copeland NG, Jenkins NA, Eisenman RN (1996) Mad3 and Mad4: novel Max-interacting transcriptional repressors that suppress c-myc dependent transformation and are expressed during neural and epidermal differentiation. EMBO J. 14:5646-5659
30. Kasten MM, Ayer DE, Stillman DJ (1996) SIN3-dependent transcriptional repression by interaction with the Mad1 DNA-binding protein. Mol. Cell. Biol. 16:4215-4221.
31. Kato GJ, Dang CV (1992) Function of the c-Myc oncoprotein. FASEB 6:3065-3072
32. Kato GJ, Barret J, Villa-Garcia M, Dang CV (1990) An amino-terminal c-Myc domain required for neoplastic transformation activates transcription. Mol. Cell. Biol. 10:5914-5920
33. Kato GJ, Lee WMF, Chen L, Dang CV (1992) Max: functional domains and interaction with c-Myc. Genes Dev. 6:81-92
34. Koskinen PJ, Ayer DE, Eisenman RN (1995) Repression of Myc-Ras cotransformation by Mad is mediated by multiple protein-protein interactions. Cell Growth Diff. 6:623-629
35. Kretzner L, Blackwood EM, Eisenman RN (1992) Myc and Max proteins possess distinct transcriptional activities. Nature (London) 359:426-429
36. Lahoz EG, Xu L, Schreiber-Agus N, DePinho RA (1994) Suppression of Myc, but not E1a, transformation activity by Max-associated proteins, Mad and Mxi1. Proc. Natl. Acad. Sci. USA 91:5503-5507
37. Land H, Parada LF, Weinberg RA (1983) Tumorigenic conversion of primary embryo fibroblasts requires at least two cooperating oncogenes. Nature (London) 304:596-602
38. Larsson LG, Pettersson M, Oberg F, Nilsson K, Luscher B (1994) Expression of mad, mxi1, max and c-myc during induced differentiation of hematopoietic cells: opposite regulation of mad and myc. Oncogene 9:1247-1252
39. Makela TP, Koskinen PJ, Vastrik I, Alitalo K (1992) Alternative forms of Max as enhancers or suppressors of Myc-Ras cotransformation. Science 256:373-376
40. Morgenbesser SD, DePinho RA (1994) Use of transgenic mice to study *myc* family gene function in normal mammalian development and in cancer. Seminars in Cancer Biol. 5:21-36
41. Mukherjee B, Morgenbesser SD, DePinho RA (1992) Myc-family oncoproteins function through a common pathway to transform normal cells in culture: cross interference by Max and trans-acting dominant mutants. Genes Dev. 6:1480-1492
42. Nasmyth K, Stillman D, Kipling D (1987) Both positive and negative regulators of HO transcription are required for mother-cell-specific mating-type switching in yeast. Cell 48:579-587
43. Prendergast GC, Lawe D, Ziff EB (1991) Association of Myn, the murine homolog of Max, with c-Myc stimulates methylation-sensitive DNA Binding and Ras cotransformation. Cell 65:395-407

44. Prendergast GC, Hopewell R, Gorham BJ, Ziff EB (1992) Biphasic effect of Max on Myc cotransformation activity and dependence on amino- and carboxy-terminal Max functions. Genes Dev. 6:2429-2439
45. Rao G, Alland L, Guida P, Schreiber-Agus N, Chen K, Chin L, Rochelle JM, Seldin MF, Skoultchi AS, DePinho RA (1996) Mouse Sin3A interacts with and can functionally substitute for the amino-terminal repression domain of the Myc antagonist Mxi. Oncogene 12:1165-1172
46. Roussel MF, Ashmun RA, Sherr CJ, Eisenman RN, Ayer DE (1996) Inhibition of cell proliferation by the Mad1 transcriptional repressor. Mol. Cell Biol. 16:2796-2801
47. Roy B, Reisman, D (1995) Inducible expression of Mad accelerates growth arrest of serum deprived human glioblastoma cells. Cell Biol. Intl. 19:307-313.
48. Rubin GM, (1988) Drosophila melanogaster as an experimental organism. Science 243:1453-1459
49. Sawai SA, Shimono K, Yakamatsu Y, Palmes C, Hanaoka K, Kondoh H (1993) Defects of embryonic organogenesis resulting from targetd disruption of the N-myc gene in the mouse. Development 117:1445-1455
50. Schreiber-Agus N, Chin L, Chen K, Torres R, Thomson C, Sacchettini JC, DePinho RA (1994) Evolutionary relationships and functional conservation among vertebrate Max-associated proteins: the zebra fish homolog of Mxi1. Oncogene 9:3167-3177
51. Schreiber-Agus N, Chin L, Chen K, Torres R, Rao G, Guida P, Skoultchi AI, DePinho RA (1995) An amino-terminal domain of Mxi1 mediates anti-Myc oncogenic activity and interacts with a homolog of the yeast transcriptional repressor SIN3. Cell 80:777-786
52. Schreiber-Agus N, Stein D, Chen K, Goltz JS, Stevens L, DePinho RA (1997)Drosophila Myc is oncogenic in mammalian cells and plays a role in the *diminutive* phenotype. Proc. Natl. Acad. Sci., U.S.A., in press
53. Shrivastava A, Saleque S, Kalpana GV, Artandi S, Goff SP, Calame K (1993) Inhibition of transcriptional regulator Yin-Yang-1 by association with c-Myc. Science 262:1889-1892
54. Stanton BR, Perkins A, Tessarollo L, Sassoon D, Parada L (1992) Loss of N-myc function results in embryonic lethality and failure of the epithelial component of the embryo to develop. Genes Dev. 6:2235-2247
55. Sternberg PW, Stern MJ, Clark I, Herskowitz I (1987) Activation of the yeast HO gene by release from multiple negative controls. Cell 48:567-577
56. Strich R, Slater MR, Esposito RE (1989) Identification of negative regulatory genes that govern the expression of early meiotic genes in yeast. Proc. Natl. Acad. Sci. U.S.A. 86:10018-10022
57. Taunton J, Hassig CA, Schreiber SL (1996) A mammalian histone deacetylase related to the yeast transcriptional regulator Rpd3p. Science 272:408-411
58. Torres R, Schreiber-Agus N, Morgenbesser SD, DePinho RA (1992) Myc and Max: a putative transcriptional complex in search of a cellular target. Curr. Opin. Cell Biol. 4:468-474
59. Vastrik I, Kaipainen A, Penttila TL, Lymboussakis A, Alitalo R, Parvinen M, Alitalo K (1995) Expression of the mad gene during cell differentiation in vivo and its inhibition of cell growth in vitro. J. Cell Biol. 128:1197-1208
60. Vidal M, Strich R, Esposito RE, Gaber RF (1991) RPD1 (SIN3/UME4) is required for maximal activation and repression of diverse yeast genes. Mol. Cell. Biol. 11:6306-6316
61. Vojtek AB, Hollenberg SM, Cooper JA (1993) Mammalian Ras interacts directly with the serine/threonine kinase Raf. Cell 74:205-214
62. Wang H, Clark I, Nicholson PR, Herskowitz I, Stillman DJ (1990) The Saccharomyces cerevisiae SIN3 gene, a negative regulator of HO, contains four paired amphipathic helix motifs. Mol. Cell. Biol. 10:5927-5936
63. Wang H, Stillman DJ (1993) Transcriptional repression in Saccharomyces cerevisiae by a SIN3-LexA fusion protein. Mol. Cell. Biol. 13:1805-1814
64. Wechsler DS, Hawkins AL, Li X, Jabs EW, Griffin CA, Dang CV (1994) Localization of the human Mxi1 transcription factor gene (MXI1) to chromosome 10q24-q25. Genomics 21:669-672
65. Zervos AS, Gyuris J, Brent R (1993) Mxi1, a protein that specifically interacts with Max to bind Myc-Max recognition sites. Cell 72:223-232
66. Zimmerman KA, Yancopoulos GD, Collum RG, Smith RK, Kohl NE, Denis KA, Nau MM, Witte ON, Toran-Allerand D, Gee CE, Minna JD, Alt FW (1986) Differential expression of *myc* family genes during murine development. Nature (London) 319:780-783

Design of Dominant Negatives to bHLHZip Proteins that Inhibit DNA Binding

D. Krylov[1], D. R. Echlin[2], E. J. Taparowsky[2] and C. Vinson[1]

[1] Building 37, Room 4D06, Laboratory of Biochemistry, National Cancer Institute, National Institutes of Health Bethesda, Maryland 20892, USA, Tel: (301) 496-8753, Fax: (301) 402-3095, E mail: Vinsonc@dc37a.nci.nih.gov

[2] Department of Biological Sciences, Purdue University, West Lafayette, Indiana, 47907, USA

Introduction

The Myc oncogene is a transcription factor that heterodimerizes with a partner protein termed Max to bind sequence-specific DNA (Blackwood and Eisenman, 1991). Both Myc and Max are members of the basic-helix-loop-helix/leucine zipper (bHLHZip) family of transcription factors (Murre, et al., 1989). The Myc/Max heterodimer binds the DNA sequence CACGTG, termed the Myc E box, and activates transcription from these sites (Blackwood, et al., 1992; Henriksson and Luscher, 1996). Provocatively, several other bHLHZip proteins, including the two USF family members and the four TFE family members, also bind and can transactivate E box DNA sequences (Desbrarats, et al., 1996). These proteins however have not been implicated in oncogenesis suggesting a more subtle mechanism exists to discriminate between the promoters relevant to cellular transformation by Myc. An unresolved question is if there is competition between different bHLHZip proteins for binding to the same cis element, with some bHLHZip proteins acting as repressors while others can act as activators, depending on the exact context of the promoter. An alternative possibility is that the subtle difference in DNA binding which can be observed between different proteins reflects the preference of proteins to bind to different, though related, cis elements in vivo. In mammalian cells, the primary bHLHZip protein that binds to E box DNA is USF. The possibility exists that in vivo Myc activity is regulated by the binding of USF to the same cis elements where it acts as a transcriptional repressor. To help unravel these possibilities, we are developing dominant-negatives (D-N) (Herskowitz, 1987) to bHLHZip family members that inhibit DNA binding in an equimolar competition. Such reagents will help determine if there is a competition between different bHLHZip proteins in vivo for the same DNA sequences.

Previously, we developed D-N to bZIP family members that inhibited DNA binding in an equimolar competition (Krylov, et al., 1995). This was accomplished by replacing the basic region critical for DNA binding with an acidic amphipathic region. The amphipathic acidic extension formed a coiled coil structure with the wild type basic region. This interaction stabilized the heterodimer 2.5 to 5 kcal/mol, depending on the particular example. We are presently are applying a similar logic to the development of D-N to bHLHZip proteins. We are able to purify the Myc and Max bHLHZip domain and determine their dimerization constants using thermal denaturation monitored by circular dichroism spectroscopy. Using this system, we are designing new proteins that dimerize preferentially with Myc better than Max.

Results and Discussion

DNA binding stabilizes the Max homodimer

The three-dimensional structure of the bHLHZip domain of Max bound to DNA reveals a dimeric parallel four-helix bundle (Ferre-D'Amare, et al., 1993). The helical nature of the dimerization domain allows us to determine the stability of different bHLHZip dimers by thermal denaturation monitored by circular dichroism spectroscopy. A fortunate property of the bHLHZip domain is that it does not aggregate when denatured and readily refolds. The monomers are not helical and the dimers are helical. This allows for biophysical characterization using circular dichroism (CD) thermal denaturation which monitors the presence of α-helical structure. We have expressed different bHLHZip domains in E coli, purified them as described earlier (Krylov, et al., 1995) and determined their CD spectra and thermal stability. The development of D-N that can inhibit DNA binding in an equimolar competition is complicated by the stabilizing effects of DNA binding. In the absence of DNA, the DNA binding or basic region is not helical. Upon DNA binding, helix 1 extends N-terminally into the basic region creating a long α-helix (Anthony-Cahill, et al., 1992) which stabilizes the dimer (data not shown). Therefore, D-N which inhibit DNA binding must demonstrate an ability to interact with Myc better that the Myc/Max heterodimer bound to DNA.

Figure 1 presents a schematic of the amino acid sequence organization of the four proteins described in this report. These include the Myc bHLHZip domain (Myc), the Max bHLHZip domain (Max bHLHZip), the Max HLHZip domain with the DNA binding

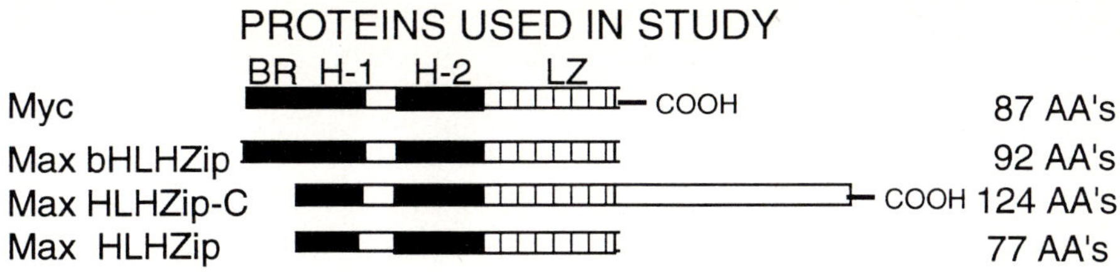

Fig. 1 Schematic of the four proteins used in this study. The BR (basic region) H-1 (Helix 1), H-2 (helix 2), and LZ (leucine zipper) are indicated. If the protein proceeds to its natural C-terminus, this is indicated by a COOH. The Myc sample is 87 amino acids long (starting at amino acid 439) and contains only the bHLHZip domain. The human Max construct (Max bHLHZip) is 92 amino acids long and starts at amino acid 21. Max HLHZip-C has 15 amino acids deleted from the basic region but does include the C-terminal 47 amino acids which contains the nuclear localization sequence. Max HLHZip is 77 amino acids long and contains only the HLHZip domain. All of the proteins contain a 13 amino acid N-terminal sequence as a cloning linker which has been described elsewhere (Krylov, et al., 1994).

sequence deleted (Max HLHZip), and the Max HLHZip domain with the basic region deleted but including the C-terminal 47 amino acids which has been shown to contain a nuclear localization sequence (Makela, et al., 1992) (Max HLHZip-C). Figure 2 presents three CD spectra from 200 nm to 250 nm of Max bHLHZip in the absence and presence of DNA. The first spectra is of Max, whose X-ray structure has been determined. The ellipticity minima at 208 nm and 222 nm indicate that Max is predominately α-helical. The second spectra is of a double stranded 28 bp DNA oligonucleotide containing a Myc E box. There is little signal at these wavelengths. The third spectra is of an equimolar mixture of double stranded DNA and dimeric Max. An increase in ellipticity at 208 and 222 nm is observed indicating that there is more α-helical structure with the addition of DNA which we interpret to represent the basic region becoming helical upon DNA binding. This increase in α-helical structure which is observed following DNA binding also stabilizes the structure. This stabilization is what complicates the design of D-N to bHLHZip proteins.

The deletion of the Max basic region.

We were interested in inhibiting Myc/Max DNA binding by building a construct that heterodimerizes with Myc with a stronger affinity than the myc/Max heterodimer bound to DNA. In an

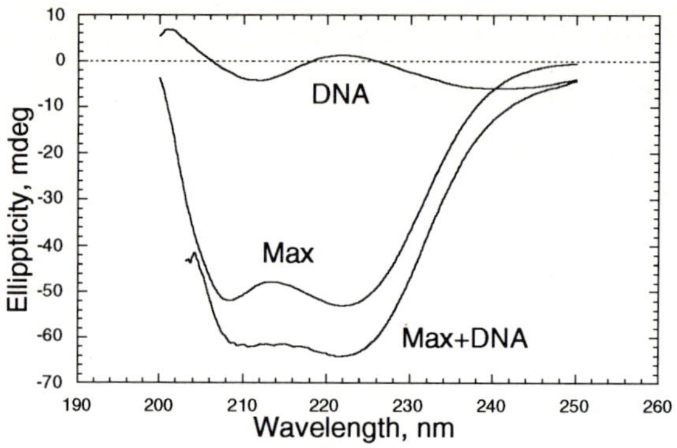

Fig. 2. Circular dichroism spectra of Max with and without DNA. The spectra from 200 nm to 250 nm of Max, a 28 bp double stranded DNA oligonucleotide containing a Myc E box, and a mixture of Max + DNA. The increase in ellipticity in the mixture is suggestive of additional α-helical structure for the Max dimer.

equimolar competition, such a reagent would inhibit myc/max DNA binding. Several groups have built D-Ns of Max by mutating the basic region (Billaud, et al., 1993; Cogliati, et al., 1993). We have determined the thermal stability of such D-Ns to determine if they inhibit binding of Myc/Max to a consensus DNA oligonucleotide in an equimolar competition.

Figure 3 presents five circular dichroism (CD) spectra from 200 to 250 nm. The samples are 1) the 87 amino acid Myc bHLHZip domain (Myc), 2) the 92 amino acid Max bHLHZip domain , 3) a mixture of Myc + Max, 4) a mixture of Myc + Max without the basic region but containing the C-terminal 47 amino acids, and 5) a mixture of Myc + Max without the basic region and missing 47 amino acids of the C-terminus. Myc alone very little α-helical structure which is not unexpected as Myc alone is unable to bind efficiently to DNA. The Max spectra, as seen in Figure 2, shows a clear minimum at 208 and 222 nm indicative of an α-helical structure. The mixture of Myc and Max shows more helicity than the sum of the two individual spectra, suggesting that Myc forms heterodimers with Max and adopts an α-helical conformation. The mixture of Myc + Max without the Max basic region shows slightly less ellipticity to Myc + Max with the basic region suggesting that the basic region of Max supports α-helix formation. The mixture of Myc + Max with the C-terminal 47 amino acids shows no significant change in ellipticity suggesting that the C-terminus is not helical.

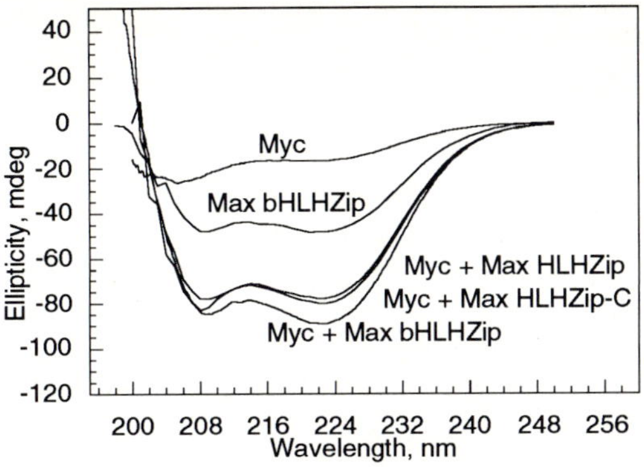

Fig. 3. Circular dichroism spectra of Myc + Max. The spectra of Myc, Max, Myc + Max, and Myc with two possible D-N are shown from 200 nm to 250 nm. There is 4 μM monomer of each protein in the sample. The minima at 208 and 222 nm are indicate the presence of α-helices. See text for details.

The thermal denaturation profiles of six HLHZip samples are shown in Figure 4. Max shows a clear transition with a dimerization constant $K_d(37)$ of $6x10^{-6}$. The two Max samples deleted for the basic region show a similar thermal denaturation profile as Max. This indicates that the basic region does not contribute to the stability of the complex. This is in contrast to bZIP proteins where the C/EBP basic region has been shown to be repulsive by 0.6 kcal/mol (Krylov, et al., 1995). The absolute ellipticity is less suggesting that the basic region deletion disrupts the ability of the basic region-helix 1 α-helix to form. The mixture of Myc with all three Max proteins shows both an increase in ellipticity and an increase in thermal stability. The Myc + Max mixture has a dimerization constant $K_d(37)$ of $3x10^{-8}$. The mixture of Myc + Max without the basic region (Max HLHZip-C) shows a similar thermal denaturation profile suggesting that the Max basic region does not affect the stability of the Max interaction with Myc. The mixture of Myc + Max with a deleted basic region and C-terminus (Max HLHZip) showed similar ellipticity and stability properties to HLHZip-C indicates that the C-terminal of Max does not interact with Myc.

Presently, we are appending onto the N-terminal of the Max HLHZip dimerization domain different acidic extensions (Krylov, et al., 1995) to stabilize the interaction of Max with Myc and thus inhibit the ability of Myc + Max to bind to DNA. Our initial results appear promising. These new reagents should be more effective in vivo at inhibiting the oncogenic properties of Myc.

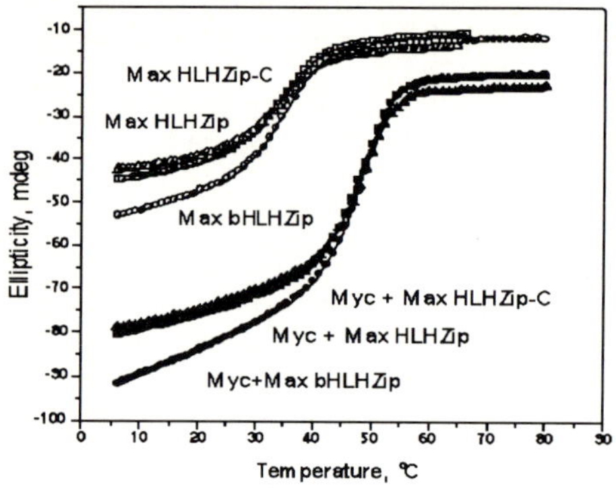

Fig. 4. Circular dichroism (CD) thermal denaturations for six samples: three homodimers (open shapes) of the Max bHLHZip domain (circles), the Max HLHZip domain (squares), and the Max HLHZip-C domain (triangles); three heterodimers (closed shapes) formed from an equimolar mixture of Myc + the three Max proteins described above.

protein	homodimer				heterodimer with Myc			
	T_m	ΔH	ΔG	k_d	T_m	ΔH	ΔG	k_d
Max bHLHZip	36.2	-92	-7.5	6e-6	48.6	-95	-10.7	3e-8
Max HLHZip	34.6	-77	-7.0	1e-5	48.0	-101	-10.8	3e-8
Max HLHZip-C	34.2	-80	-7.0	1e-5	48.4	-104	-11.0	2e-8

Table 1. Thermal stability of D-Ns with Myc. Thermal stability of potential D-Ns, either alone or mixed with Myc, was determined by CD spectroscopy. The Table presents the designation of the protein sample the melting temperature (T_m,°C); Gibbs free energy, ΔG(37 °C); and the dissociation constant at 37°C (k_d), k_d. The Table contains values for three potential D-Ns, either as homodimers or as an equimolar mixture with Myc. If the mixture has a higher melting temperature than either homodimer alone, we infer that the sample is composed of heterodimers.

Myc + Max DNA binding

Gel shift assays were performed to establish if deletion of the Max basic region inhibits Myc/Max binding to a Myc E box site. The top panel of Figure 5 shows a titration of Myc/Max binding indicating that binding is on the order of 10^{-9} M. The bottom panel of Figure 5 shows a competition between Myc + Max binding to DNA and increasing amounts of Max with the basic region deleted (Max HLHZip) to determine if Max HLHZip can inhibit Myc + Max DNA binding. Thermal denaturation studies indicate that the Max HLHZip

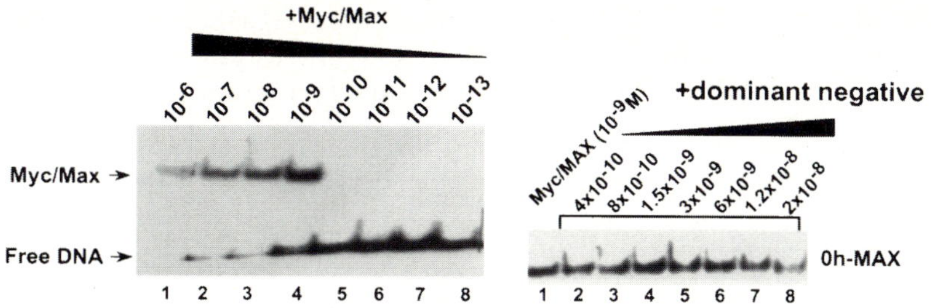

Fig. 5. Myc + Max binding to a 28 bp double stranded DNA oligonucleotide containing a Myc E box. The top panel presents the DNA properties of a equimolar mixture of the bHLHZip domains of Myc and Max. 100 pM of radiolabeled DNA is shifted with the indicated amount of Myc + Max. DNA binding appears to be $1x0^{-9}$ M. The bottom panel shows the results of competition reactions using increasing amounts of the Max HLHZip domain. An inhibition of Myc + Max is only beginning to be seen at a 20-fold molar excess.

protein heterodimerizes with Myc as well as Max bHLHZip. Only at a 20-fold molar excess does Max HLHZip begin to compete for Myc/Max DNA binding. The ineffectualness of Max HLHZip on inhibiting Myc + Max DNA binding reflects the stabilizing influence of DNA binding on the Myc/Max heterodimer. We are presently using this thermal denaturation assay to develop proteins that interact more stability with the Myc bHLHZip domain. we are presently appending onto the N-terminus of the HLHZip domain of Max different acidic extension as we have done with the bZIP family of DNA binding proteins (Krylov, et al., 1995).

Inhibition of cellular transformation

The ability of these different D-Ns to inhibit cellular transformation was tested using a Ras + Myc cotransformation assay in C3H10T1/2 cells (Table 2) (Taparowsky, et al., 1987). Ras alone is able to generate a modest level of focus formation in this cell line. The cotranfection of Ras + Myc triples the number of foci observed in the transformation assay as has been reported earlier (Henriksson and Luscher, 1996). Max proteins, deleted for the DNA binding region, are more effective D-Ns to Ras + Myc mediated transformation than Max itself. The C-terminal 47 amino acids of Max, although it does not effect the interaction of Max + Myc (see figure 4), does increase the potency of the D-N, presumably since the inclusion of the C-terminus allows effective transport of the D-N Max to the nucleus. Experiments underway in the lab but not reported here suggest that the potency of the Max D-Ns can be increased by appending an acidic extension on to the Max HLHZip domain and thus stabilizing the Myc/Max heterodimer (Krylov, et al., 1995). These D-Ns should inhibit Myc mediated transformation better than the reagents reported here.

Groups	number of foci per experiment			relative focus formation
Ras	580	855	1730	0.39
Ras + Myc	1915	2180	3670	1.00
Ras + Myc + Max HLHZip	1820	1635	2600	0.80
Ras + Myc + Max HLHZip-C	925	1350	2150	0.56

Table 2. Transformation of C3H10T1/2 cells. C3H10T1/2 cells were transfected with expression vectors for the activated human H-ras oncogene (Ras) and the viral myc oncogene (Myc) as described previously (Taparowsky, et al., 1987). A 3-fold molar excess of the Max HLHZip of Max HLHZip-C constructs was added to asses the effect of overexpression of these D-Ns on transformation in this model system. Relative focus formation is calculated using the average number of foci from three independent transfection experiments and is expressed as a percent of focus formation by Ras + Myc which is set at 1.00.

Acknowledgments

We thank Ron DePinho for the Myc DNA construct, and G. Prendergast for the bHLHZip Max DNA construct.

References

Anthony-Cahill, S., Benfield, P., Fairman, R., Wasserman, Z., Brenner, S., Stafford, W., Altenbach, C., Hubbell, W., and DeGrado, W. (1992) Molecular characterization of helix-loop-helix peptides. Science 255, 979-983

Billaud, M., Isselbacher, K., and Bernards, R. (1993) A dominant-negative mutant of Max that inhibits sequence-specific DNA binding of Myc proteins. PNAS 90, 2739-2743

Blackwood, E., and Eisenman, R. (1991) Max: A helix-loop-helix zipper protein that forms a sequence-specific DNA-binding complex with Myc. Science 251, 1221-1227

Blackwood, E., Kretzner, L., and Eisenman, R. (1992) Myc and Max function as a nucleoprotein complex. Current Opinion in Genetics and Development 227-235

Cogliati, T., Dunn, B., Bar-Ner, M., Cultraro, C., and Segal, S. (1993) Transfected wild-type and mutant max regulate cell growth and differentiation of murine erthroleukemia cells. Oncogene 8, 1263-1268

Desbrarats, L., Gaubatz, S., and Eilers, M. (1996) Discrimination between different E-Box-binding proteins at an endogenous target gene of c-myc. Genes and Development 10, 447-460

Ferre-D'Amare, A., Prendergast, G., Ziff, E., and Burley, S. (1993) Recognition by Max of its cognate DNA through a dimeric b/HLH/Z domain. Nature 363, 38-44

Henriksson, M., and Luscher, B. (1996) Proteins of the Myc network: essential regulators of cell growth and differentiation. Adv. Cancer Res. 68, 109-182

Herskowitz, I. (1987) Functional inactivation of genes by dominant negative mutations. Nature 329, 219-222

Krylov, D., Mikhailenko, I., and Vinson, C. (1994) A thermodynamic scale for leucine zipper stability and dimerization specificity: e and g interhelical interactions. EMBO 13, 1849-1861

Krylov, D., Olive, M., and Vinson, C. (1995) Extending dimerization interfaces: the bZIP basic region can form a coiled coil. EMBO

Makela, T., Koskinen, P., Vastrik, I., and Alitalo, K. (1992) Alternative forms of Max as enhancers or suppressers of Myc-ras cotransformation. Science 256, 373-377

Murre, C., McCaw, P., and Baltimore, D. (1989) A new DNA binding and dimerization motif in immunoglobulin enhancer binding, daughterless, MyoD, and myc proteins. Cell 56, 777-783

Taparowsky, E., Heaney, M., and Parsons, T. (1987) oncogene-mediated multistep transformation of C3H10T1/2 cells. Cancer Research 47, 4125-4129

Myc Targets

Myc Target Genes in Neoplastic Tranformation

H. Shim, B. C. Lewis, C. Dolde, Q. Li, C.-S. Wu, Y. S. Chun and C. V. Dang
Department of Medicine, The Johns Hopkins University School of Medicine, Baltimore, MD, USA

Deregulated expression of the c-*myc* oncogene as a consequence of specific genetic alterations is sine-qua-non for certain B-cell neoplasms. Dissection of the c-Myc protein over the last decade reveals a structural organization that is characteristic of a transcription factor. c-Myc function is regulated by a complicated network of proteins that developed through millions of years of evolution and is likely to include a large repertoire of interacting proteins. Yet, the mechanism by which c-Myc or its retroviral counterpart v-Myc transforms cells is only beginning to emerge. Clues to the molecular basis of c-Myc mediated cellular transformation are being revealed by studies that identify target genes and events linking the deregulated expression of Myc and transformed phenotypes.

What is a Myc target gene?

In the broadest sense, any gene that c-Myc transactivates may be considered a target. This definition does not distinguish, however, between direct and indirect targets and does not address the relevance of the targets to Myc-mediated phenotypes. A direct target gene may be defined as those genes whose expression is altered as a consequence of a direct interaction of the c-Myc protein with the gene regulatory *cis*-acting DNA elements or with the *trans*acting factors that bind these *cis* elements. Thus, the induction of an artificially construed promoter-reporter plasmid is insufficient to establish the identity of a target gene. Regulation of the endogenous cellular target gene expression by c-Myc as demonstrated by nuclear run-on studies is also required to authenticate a target gene. Conversely, the absence of transactivation of artificial promoter-reporter constructs by c-Myc should not be sufficient to exclude a target gene that may require chromosomal context as well as other *trans*acting factors to be transactivated. To date, the only system that is able to test the direct effect of Myc is the Myc-estrogen receptor (Myc-ER) fusion protein system initially developed by Eilers and Bishop (see below). In this system, the Myc-ER fusion is tethered to chaperone proteins in the absence of estrogenic ligands. The fusion protein is activated by binding to ligand, released from chaperone proteins and enter the nucleus to activate Myc target genes as a complex with Max. Thus, simultaneous exposure of cells expressing the fusion Myc-ER protein to estrogens and cycloheximide would directly activate gene transcription in the absence of new protein synthesis. This system, therefore, allow an experimental approach to determine the direct effect of Myc on target genes.

It stands to reason that the time course of induction of a direct target gene follows the expression of Myc within several hours. This reasoning may unnecessarily exclude the possibility of genes whose expression depends on the presence of c-Myc protein but whose expression is delayed and requires another transacting factor that appears late after the induction of Myc expression. Indirect target genes of c-Myc may be considered as those whose expressions require new protein synthesis after induction of Myc activity and whose expressions are directly connected to c-Myc mediated phenotypes such as cellular proliferation, transformation or apoptosis. Although the search for target genes usually implies identification of the direct ones, the uncovering of indirect targets may provide the much needed clues to link deregulated c-Myc expression to neoplastic transformation.

The lack of a clear set of criteria to identify relevant target genes stems in part from difficulties with providing evidence that a putative target gene is biologically relevant. This difficulty is further confounded by the fact that target genes may be necessary but not sufficient for Myc-associated phenotypes (Figure 1). In such case, antisense experiments appear to be a reasonable approach to establish the necessity of a specific target gene for a Myc-associated phenotype. The difficult with this experimental approach, however, is when a target gene (for example a cyclin gene) is one whose disruption leads to dramatic cellular changes. Considering these caveats, we will review putative c-Myc target genes and use the above definitions to guide our discussion.

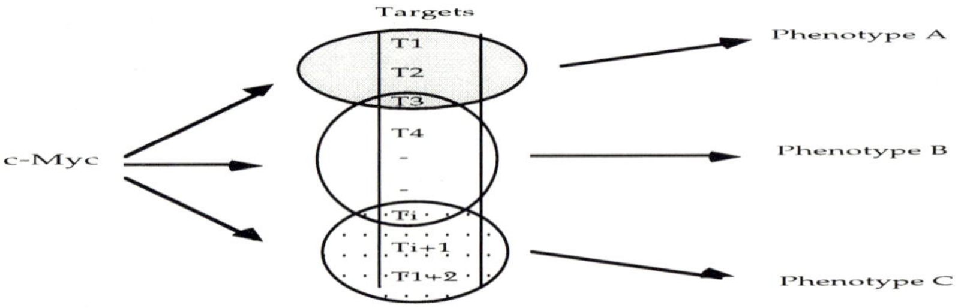

Figure 1. Hypothetical scheme of Myc target genes and their participation in c-*myc* induced phenotypes. The scheme depicts subsets of Myc targets, which may be overlapping with other subsets and are shown to be necessary for specific phenotypes.

Identifying Target Genes Through Differential Cloning

Using differential cloning, the Cole group reported that plasminogen activator inhibitor-1 (PAI-1) gene expression is augmented by c-Myc [1, 2]. Their studies suggest that c-Myc alters the levels of PAI-1 mRNA at the post-trancriptional level. A recent report also suggests that Myc plays a role in post-transcriptional regulation of ribosomal RNA levels; whether this is a direct effect of c-Myc was not addressed [3]. Although PAI-1 may be a target of c-Myc (the PAI-1 gene promoter contains several E-boxes), it is not clear what the role of PAI-1 is in the biology of c-Myc. TGFβ1 induces PAI-1 in cultured fibroblasts. The TGFβ1 responsive element was mapped to a sequence located about 550 bp upstream of the human gene start site [4]. It is composed of overlapping sites for CCAAT-binding protein (NF-1/CTF1) and the E-box sequence CACGTG. The upstream stimulatory factor or USF was found to bind the E-box as determined by supershift experiment with an anti-USF antibody. c-Myc does not appear to participate in this pathway.

The Freytag group demonstrated through differential cloning that collagen gene expression (types α1(I), α2(I), and α3(VI)) is down-regulated in fibroblasts over-expressing c-Myc [5, 6]. This group went on further to demonstrate that c-Myc suppresses promoters driven by NF-1 DNA binding sites [6]. In addition, the form of transcriptional factor NF-1, which exists as a family of polypeptides, was altered by enforced c-Myc expression. In this case, the promoters of collagen genes do not appear to contain direct binding sites for c-Myc; nevertheless, c-Myc reproducibly down-regulate collagen expression in fibroblasts. Thus, it appears that collagen is an indirect target of c-Myc [6]. Cells transformed by other oncogenes, such as p53, *mos*, *ras*, *raf* or *src*, also resulted in decreased collagen gene expression [7-12]. It is intriguing to note that ectopic expression of NF-1 or increased collagen expression inhibit transformation [13-15]. Based on these observations, it may be speculated that indirect targets such as collagen genes may play a key role in Myc-associated phenotypes such as anchorage-independent growth.

Another approach to identifying c-Myc target genes is to clone cDNAs corresponding to differentially expressed mRNAs in a system in which c-Myc expression is inducible. A differentially expressed gene encoding alpha-prothymosin was identified using cells that express a Myc-estrogen receptor (ER) fusion protein [16,17]. Alpha-prothymosin protein levels have been shown to correlate with cell proliferation, although its function remains unknown [18-20]. Eilers and coworkers reported that E-boxes located in intron 1 of the alpha-prothymosin gene mediate transactivation of this gene by c-Myc [21, 22]. Subsequently, this group reported the existence of AP-2 sites overlapping E-boxes in the alpha-prothymosin gene as well as other putative c-Myc target genes [23]. AP-2 appears to suppress transcription in this context. The induction of alpha-prothymosin by c-Myc appears to be cell type specific, since c-Myc does not induce alpha-prothymosin in 3T3 fibroblasts [21, 24]. The fact that induction of alpha-prothymosin gene expression is cell specific does not exclude it as a c-Myc target. Rather, it is possible that the genetic background of a cell determines which targets are rate-limiting for cell proliferation.

Tavtigian et al. undertook a unique effort to clone cDNAs corresponding to midserum-response genes which are also upregulated in two inducible c-Myc cell lines [24]. This work showed that transcription of the lactate dehydrogenase-A and ornithine decarboxylase genes are upregulated by c-Myc. A cDNA sequence with limited homology to methylenetetrahydrofolate synthetase (clone I-8-29) sequence was also upregulated. Alpha-prothymosin was found to be upregulated only in certain cells. p53 appears to be upregulated by c-Myc but only in the zinc inducible Myc NIH3T3 cell line. Among genes that may be repressed by c-Myc, alpha-1(III) collagen was repressed in the NIH3T3 cell line but remains unchanged in the MycER Balb/c 3T3 cells after exposure to estrogen. This study underscores the difficulty in studying c-Myc target genes in only selected cell lines, since there may be cell specific effects of c-Myc.

Utilizing subtraction cloning, an embryonically expressed gene ECA39 was identified as a Myc target that appears to have a cell specific response to c-Myc [25]. In this study a cDNA library that was generated from a brain tumor caused by transgenic HTLV-1 LTR-*myc* was depleted of cDNAs found in normal brain through subtractive hybridization [26]. One clone that was highly expressed in Myc-induced brain tumors and in Myc-mediated T-lymphomas in transgenic animals was selected for further study and found to be a previously cloned cDNA termed ECA39. This gene is not overexpressed, however, in other transgenic c-Myc induced tumors such as mammary tumor or B-cell lymphomas. Thus ECA39 appears to be associated with Myc expression only in specific types of tumors derived from transgenic animals. The promoter region of ECA39 revealed a

CACGTG E-box 105 bp 3' of the transcriptional start site. Cotransfection experiments with the ECA39 promoter-reporter construct and c-Myc expression vector suggests that c-Myc is capable of activating transcription through this promoter region in an E-box dependent manner. These observations are interpreted to suggest that ECA39 is a direct target of c-Myc. The evidence presented suggest that ECA39 may be a target of c-Myc in certain tumors, but its expression is not altered in other Myc-associated tumors. The *Saccharomyces cerevisiae* homologs of ECA39 were recently found to encode proteins that are involved in the transport of neutral amino acids [27-29]. Whether the mammalian ECA39 protein also functions in transporting amino acids and how ECA 39 links Myc to neoplastic transformation remains to be established.

In our own studies, we identified a set of c-Myc responsive genes in the Rat1a fibroblast, which can be transformed to grow in soft agar by overexpression of c-Myc alone. These genes were identified by the application of cDNA Representational Difference Analysis (cDNA RDA) to cDNAs isolated from non-adherent Rat1a and Rat1a-myc cells, Rat1a cells stably transfected to express human c-Myc [30,31]. We hypothesized that genes differentially expressed between Rat1a and Rat1a-myc cells under non-adherent conditions contribute to the anchorage independent growth phenotype of Rat1a-myc cells and do not simply reflect differences between growth arrested cells and proliferating cells. The collection of genes identified includes previously described targets of *c-myc* including ODC, as well as several novel genes and known genes not previously linked to c-Myc. We have fully characterized lactate dehydrogenase-A as a direct target of c-Myc.

The characteristic ability of cancer cells to produce excess lactic acid aerobically was recognized by Warburg about seventy years ago, although the molecular mechanisms underlying the Warburg effect have been elusive [32]. The lactate dehydrogenase-A (*LDH-A*) gene, whose product converts pyruvate to lactic acid participates in normal anaerobic glycolysis and is frequently increased in human cancers, was identified as a c-Myc responsive gene. The Myc-estrogen receptor fusion protein was able to activate the transcription of LDH-A in the presence of cycloheximide indicating that LDH-A is a direct Myc target. Moreover, the elevation of LDH-A mRNA in Rat1a-Myc cells is largely due to transcription as determined by nuclear run-on studies. Stably transfected Rat1a fibroblasts that overexpress *LDH-A* alone or those transformed by c-Myc overproduce lactate in excess of that produced by the control Rat1a cells, suggesting that overexpression of LDH-A is sufficient to induce the Warburg effect. Lowering LDH-A expression by antisense technology reduces soft agar clonogenicity of c-Myc-transformed Rat1a fibroblasts, c-Myc-transformed human lymphoblastoid and Burkitt's lymphoma cells suggesting that LDH-A overexpression is required for c-Myc-mediated transformation. To assess whether deregulated *LDH-A* expression alters cell cycle regulation by nutrients, we determined the effects of glucose withdrawal on cell growth and survival. Glucose deprivation or treatment with the glucose antimetabolite, 2-deoxyglucose, causes non-transformed cells to arrest in the G_1 phase of the cell cycle, whereas c-Myc transformed fibroblasts, lymphoblastoid or lung carcinoma cells undergo extensive apoptosis that is blocked by Bcl-2. Overexpression of LDH-A alone in Rat1a fibroblasts is sufficient to induce apoptosis with glucose deprivation, but not with serum withdrawal, suggesting that LDH-A mediates the apoptotic effect of c-Myc when glycolysis is blocked. Our studies have linked c-Myc to the induction of *LDH-A* whose expression is sufficient for the Warburg effect and sensitizes cells to a unique apoptotic pathway induced by glucose deprivation.

Cell proliferation and candidate Myc target genes

Candidates have been tested as Myc target genes based on the biology of c-Myc and the candidate genes. The ornithine decarboxylase (ODC) gene represents such a target, whose expression was noted to correlate with the level of c-Myc expression [33]. In addition, ODC has been known to be a key enzyme in the synthesis of polyamines which are required for cell proliferation. In fact, deregulated expression of ODC appears to contribute to neoplastic transformation [34] and an inhibitor of ODC, difluoromehylornithine (DFMO), inhibits cell growth in vitro and has been used as an anti-neoplastic agent in clinical trial [34]. ODC has now been shown to be a target for c-Myc in several independent studies [35-37]. Specifically, the time course of ODC is compatible with it being a Myc target. The ODC upstream (-491 bp to -474 bp in the human ODC promoter) sequence contains an E-box that has been implicated in Myc regulation [36,38]. In other studies, however, two E-boxes in intron 1 have been shown to respond to c-Myc [35]. The occurence of intronic E-boxes in both prothymosin and ODC genes and an E-box element downstream of the start site of ECA39 suggest that the position of E-boxes may be important for c-Myc mediated transactivation. Work by the Cleveland group, however, failed to demonstrate significant differences in transactivation when the E-box elements were moved to various positions relative to the transcriptional start site [39].

Studies of gene promoters have also led to the recognition of the Myc/Max binding site or E-box (CACGTG) in a variety of genes. It should be noted that this E-box could be bound by USF, TFE-3 or TFE-B in addition to c-Myc [40-42]. So its existence in promoter regions should include the possibility that USF, TFE-3 or TFE-B act as the transactivator. In fact, it is as yet unclear what the role of the ubiquitous USF is in the regulation of these so-called Myc E-boxes. Notwithstanding these concerns, several promoters have been proposed to be c-Myc targets based on the presence of E-boxes amidst other *cis* elements in these promoters. The promoters of genes for dihydrofolate reductase (*dhfr*) and carbamoyl-phosphate synthase (*cad*) both contain E2F as well as the Myc E-box sequences [43, 44]. Both genes are proposed to be c-Myc target genes based on the time course of expression of these genes relative to c-*myc* expression, although *dhfr* expression may be dependent on E2F and is not inhibited by dominant negative c-*myc* alleles [44]. In the case of *dhfr*, electrophoretic mobility shift assays with the putative Myc binding sequence revealed bands that were supershifted with anti-c-Myc antibodies. Whereas *dhfr* is required for cellular metabolism and proliferation, its role in c-Myc mediated neoplastic transformation remains to be studied.

A novel view of c-Myc function emerges from its connection with the expression of cyclins, CDKs and CDK inhibitors, all key regulators of the cell cycle. Overexpression of c-Myc has been known to shorten the G1 phase of the cell cycle of fibroblasts [45] and induction of its activity is tightly associated with entry into S-phase [22, 23]. Removal of a copy of c-*myc* through homologous recombination results in Rat1 fibroblasts that have a delayed entry into S-phase and a prolonged G1 phase [46-48]. These observations suggest a connection between c-Myc and the cell cycle machinery.

A link between deregulated c-Myc expression in BALB/c 3T3 fibroblasts and increased cyclin A and E mRNA levels was first demonstrated by Jansen-Durr et al. [49]. Estrogen activated MycER suppresses the expression of cyclin D1 very early in the cell cycle whereas it induces the expression of cyclins A and E [50]. Another study contrasts with that of Jansen-Durr et al.; cyclin D1 expression was shown to be induced in the activated MycER system [51]. Cyclin D1 protein level was found to be elevated, although its mRNA level remained essentially unchanged, in yet another MycER system [52]. It is postulated in this study that cyclin D1 protein level was augmented by elevated levels of the translational initiation factor eIF4E (see below). The conflicting data regarding the potential regulation of cyclin D1 by c-Myc is presently not fully resolved; however, the use of estradiol versus hydrotamoxifen (an estrogen analog) to activate the Myc-ER fusion protein may contribute to different reported results.

The correlation of c-Myc expression with elevated cyclin A expression has been independently observed in several studies [48.49,51,53]. Using heterozygous *myc* cells derived by homologous recombination, it was observed that reduced c-*myc* expression is associated with a delayed expression of cyclin E and reduced expression of cyclin A protein [48]. Overexpression of c-Myc correlated with an increase in cyclin D protein level, early expression of cyclin E and an increase in cyclin A protein protein level. Cdk2 protein levels were unaltered by changes in c-*myc* expression. The effect of c-Myc on cyclin D expression is at present unclear, since the results of different studies are conflicting. The observation that c-Myc expression correlates with that of cyclin A has been independently verified by all independent studies published to date. The available sequence of the cyclin A promoter (>3kb) does not contain a concensus c-Myc E-box [54,55]. More recently, the critical element in the cyclin A promoter that regulates its expression appears to be a binding site for ATF/CREB [56-58]. The time course of induction of cyclin A following c-Myc expression suggests that this induction is indirect. Activation of cyclin E, however appears to be required for subsequent increases in cyclin A expression. Induction of cyclin A and E expression may in part explain a number of c-Myc-related phenotypes. Overexpression of cyclin E shortens G1 by inducing early entry into S phase. Cyclin A expression was observed to be anchorage-dependent in a variety of different fibroblast cell lines [59-60].

The effect of c-Myc on CDKs is unclear. In one study, c-Myc cooperates with *RAS* to induce the *CDC2* promoter which does not contain a concensus Myc E-box [63]. This promoter, however, contains an NRF1 site (CGCATT) which is similar but not identical to a non-canonical Myc binding site, CGCATG, identified by *in vitro* studies. In an independent study induction of c-Myc expression was shown to elevated *CDC2* gene expression [64]. Thus, this intriguing observation needs additional verification specifically with regard to regulation of cellular *CDC2* gene expression by c-Myc.

A recently published study provides compelling arguments for *cdc25A* as a target of c-Myc [65]. CDC25A is a phosphatase that activates cyclin dependent CDK2 and CDK4 kinases through removal of specific phosphate residues. Its overexpression has been shown to transform cells in cooperation with activated Ras. The study by Galaktionov shows that *cdc25A* gene expression is induced by c-Myc directly. The *cdc25A* gene contains three intronic E-boxes that are activatable in transient transfection experiments. Furthermore, overexpression of *cdc25A* is shown to induce serum-deprivation-dependent apoptosis suggesting that this target gene may underlie Myc-induced apoptosis upon serum withdrawal. Taken together, the *cdc25A* gene may be a critical link between c-Myc and the cell cycle. How *cdc25A* may account for the pleiotropic effects of c-Myc remains to be established, however.

Transient transfection experiments indicate that c-Myc expression vectors transactivate the tumor suppressor p53 promoter-reporter constructs, which contain an E-box resembling a Myc binding site [66,67]. It is notable that this promoter is also transactivated by USF in transient transfection experiments. In fact, nuclear extracts demonstrated the binding of USF to this E-box, and a Myc-related shifted band was not demonstrated. Although alterations of endogenous p53 levels as a consequence of deregulated c-Myc was not studied, it is intriguing that lymphoma cell lines with high c-Myc expression tend to also have elevated p53 levels [67]. This latter observation is a correlation, which inherently does not reveal any mechanistic link between Myc and p53, and may simple reflect a function interaction between these proteins or the pathways they elicit. Thus, additional evidence using inducible Myc systems to demonstrate alterations of endogenous p53 levels by c-Myc appear necessary to further establish this connection.

c-Myc stimulates the expression of the eukaryotic translational elongation factor 2α (eIF-2α) through an NRF1 site (CGCATG), which is identical to a non-canonical Myc binding site [68,69]. eIF4E is also elevated by c-Myc through E-boxes [70]. eIF-4E in turn appears to increase the translational of cyclin D1 mRNA resulting in elevated cyclin D1 protein level. It is intriguing to note that eIF-2α appears to possess neoplastic transforming activity and eIF-4E overexpression rescues cells from c-Myc induced apoptosis. The ability of eIF-4E to inhibit apoptosis is not intuitive as overexpression of c-Myc induces eIF-4E expression and predisposes cells to apoptosis. NRF1 (nuclear respiratory factor) was identified as a factor that binds CGCATG which is found in a number of genes encoding the respiratory chain proteins [70-72]. It may be surmised that c-Myc and NRF1 share common binding sites, but c-Myc only augments the expression of NRF1 target genes under proliferative conditions. NRF1 may serve as a constitutive positive signal in the expression of these genes.

In summary, the studies from various laboratories reviewed here suggest that c-Myc activates genetic programs that provide the underpinnings of the effects of c-Myc on cell proliferation, differentiation and apoptotic cell death. We surmise that the oncogenic transcription factor c-Myc acts pleiotropically to transform cells by upregulating expression of components of the cell cycle machinery, stimulating the production of biosynthetic enzymes such as ornithine decarboxylase to prepare cells for S-phase entry, and activating the expression of metabolic enzymes such as LDH-A to ensure an adequate supply of energy or signals for cell proliferation.

Acknowledgments

This work was supported in part by grants from the National Institutes of Health and the Wilbur-Rogers Foundation. C.V.D. is Scholar of the Leukemia Society of America, Inc. B.C.L. is a Howard Hughes Predoctoral Fellow. H.S. is Fellow of the Lymphoma Research Foundation of America, Inc. Y.S.C. received the American Society of Hematology Summer Medical Student Scholarship. Q. L. is with the Program in Cellular and Molecular Medicine, and B.C.L. and C.D. are with the Program in Human Genetics & Molecular Biology.

References

1. Prendergast GC, Cole MD. Posttranscriptional regulation of cellular gene expression by the c-myc oncogene. Mol Cell Biol 1989; 9:124-34.
2. Prendergast GC, Diamond LE, Dahl D, Cole MD. The c-myc-regulated gene mrl encodes plasminogen activator inhibitor 1. Mol Cell Biol 1990; 10:1265-9.

3. Gibson AW, Ye R, Johnston RN, Browder LW. A possible role for c-Myc oncoproteins in post-transcriptional regulation of ribosomal RNA. Oncogene 1992; 7:2363-7.
4. Riccio A, Pedone PV, Lund LR, Olesen T, Olsen HS, Andreasen PA. Transforming growth factor beta 1-responsive element: closely associated binding sites for USF and CCAAT-binding transcription factor-nuclear factor I in the type 1 plasminogen activator inhibitor gene. Mol Cell Biol 1992; 12:1846-55.
5. Yang BS, Geddes TJ, Pogulis RJ, de Crombrugghe B, Freytag SO. Transcriptional suppression of cellular gene expression by c-Myc. Mol Cell Biol 1991; 11:2291-5.
6. Yang BS, Gilbert JD, Freytag SO. Overexpression of Myc suppresses CCAAT transcription factor/nuclear factor 1-dependent promoters in vivo. Mol Cell Biol 1993; 13:3093-102.
7. Schmidt A, Setoyama C, de Crombrugghe B. Regulation of a collagen gene promoter by the product of viral mos oncogene. Nature 1985; 314:286-9.
8. Slack JL, Parker MI, Robinson VR, Bornstein P. Regulation of collagen I gene expression by ras. Mol Cell Biol 1992; 12:4714-23.
9. Setoyama C, Liau G, de Crombrugghe B. Pleiotropic mutants of NIH 3T3 cells with altered regulation in the expression of both type I collagen and fibronectin. Cell 1985; 41:201-9.
10. Eizenberg O, Oren M. Reduced levels of alpha 1 (I) collagen mRNA in cells immortalized by mutant p53 or transformed by ras. Biochim Biophys Acta 1991; 1129:34-42.
11. Frankfort BJ, Gelman IH. Identification of novel cellular genes transcriptionally suppressed by v-src. Biochem Biophys Res Commun 1995; 206:916-26.
12. Hampton LL, Worland PJ, Yu B, Thorgeirsson SS, Huggett AC. Expression of growth-related genes during tumor progression in v-raf-transformed rat liver epithelial cells. Cancer Res 1990; 50:7460-7.
13. Schuur ER, Kruse U, Iacovoni JS, Vogt PK. Nuclear factor 1 interferes with transformation by nuclear oncogenes. Cell Growth Diff 1995; 6:219-227.
14. Lim A, Greenspan DS, Smith BD. Expression of alpha 2 type I collagen in W8 cells increases cell adhesion and decreases colony formation in soft agar. Matrix Biol 1994; 14:21-30.
15. Wiseman RW, Montgomery JC, Hosoi J, et al. Identification of genes associated with tumor suppression in Syrian hamster embryo cells. Environ Health Perspect 1991; 93:105-9.
16. Eilers M, Picard D, Yamamoto KR, Bishop JM. Chimaeras of myc oncoprotein and steroid receptors cause hormone-dependent transformation of cells. Nature 1989; 340:66-8.
17. Eilers M, Schirm S, Bishop JM. The MYC protein activates transcription of the alpha-prothymosin gene. EMBO J 1991; 10:133-41.
18. Eschenfeldt WH, Berger SL. The human prothymosin alpha gene is polymorphic and induced upon growth stimulation: evidence using a cloned cDNA. Proc Natl Acad Sci U S A 1986; 83:9403-7.
19. Sburlati AR, Manrow RE, Berger SL. Prothymosin alpha antisense oligomers inhibit myeloma cell division. Proc Natl Acad Sci U S A 1991; 88:253-7.
20. Manrow RE, Sburlati AR, Hanover JA, Berger SL. Nuclear targeting of prothymosin alpha. J Biol Chem 1991; 266:3916-24.
21. Gaubatz S, Meichle A, Eilers M. An E-box element localized in the first intron mediates regulation of the prothymosin alpha gene by c-myc. Mol Cell Biol 1994; 14:3853-3862.
22. Meichle A, Philipp A, Eilers M. The functions of Myc proteins. Biochim Biophys Acta 1992; 1114:129-46.
23. Gaubatz S, Imho FA, Dosch R, et al. Transcriptional activation by Myc is under negative control by the transcription factor AP-2. EMBO J 1995; 14:1508-1519.
24. Tavtigian SV, Zabludoff SD, Wold BJ. Cloning of mid-G(1) serum response genes and identification of a subset regulated by conditional myc expression. Mol Biol Cell 1994; 5:375-388.
25. Benvenisty N, Leder A, Kuo A, Leder P. An embryonically expressed gene is a target for c-Myc regulation via the c-Myc-binding sequence. Genes Dev 1992; 6:2513-2523.
26. Benvenisty N, Ornitz DM, Bennett GL, et al. Brain tumours and lymphomas in transgenic mice that carry HTLV-I LTR/c-myc and Ig/tax genes. Oncogene 1992; 7:2399-405.
27. Eden A, Simchen G, Benvenisty N. Two yeast homologs of ECA39, a target for c-Myc regulation, code for cytosolic and mitochondrial branched-chain amino acid aminotransferases. J Biol Chem 1996; 271:20242-5.
28. Schuldiner O, Eden A, Ben-Yosef T, Yanuka O, Simchen G, Benvenisty N. ECA39, a conserved gene regulated by c-Myc in mice, is involved in G1/S cell cycle regulation in yeast. Proc Natl Acad Sci U S A 1996; 93:7143-8.

29. Hutson SM, Bledsoe RK, Hall TR, Dawson PA. Cloning and expression of the mammalian cytosolic branched chain aminotransferase isoenzyme. J Biol Chem 1995; 270:30344-52.
30. Hubank M, Schatz DG. Identifying differences in mRNA expression by representational difference analysis of cDNA. Nucleic Acids Res 1994; 22:5640-8.
31. Lisitsyn N, Lisitsyn N, Wigler M. Cloning the differences between two complex genomes. Science 1993; 259:946-51.
32. Warburg O. On the origin of cancer cells. Science 1956; 123:309-314.
33. Askew DS, Ashmun RA, Simmons BC, Cleveland JL. Constitutive c-myc expression in an IL-3-dependent myeloid cell line suppresses cell cycle arrest and accelerates apoptosis. Oncogene 1991; 6:1915-22.
34. Auvinen M, Paasinen A, Andersson LC, Holtta E. Ornithine decarboxylase activity is critical for cell transformation. Nature 1992; 360:355-358.
35. Bello-Fernandez C, Packham G, Cleveland JL. The ornithine decarboxylase gene is a transcriptional target of c-Myc. Proc Natl Acad Sci USA 1993; 90:7804-7808.
36. Pena A, Reddy CD, Wu S, et al. Regulation of human ornithine decarboxylase expression by the c-Myc.Max protein complex. J Biol Chem 1993; 268:27277-85.
37. Wagner AJ, Meyers C, Laimins LA, Hay N. c-Myc induces the expression and activity of ornithine decarboxylase. Cell Growth Differ 1993; 4:879-83.
38. Pena A, Wu S, Hickok NJ, Soprano DR, Soprano KJ. Regulation of human ornithine decarboxylase expression following prolonged quiescence: role for the c-Myc/Max protein complex. J Cell Physiol 1995; 162:234-45.
39. Packham G, Bellofernandez C, Cleveland JL. Position and orientation independent transactivation by c-Myc. Cell Molec Biol Res 1994; 40:699-706, 1994.
40. Gregor PD, Sawadogo M, Roeder RG. The adenovirus major late transcription factor USF is a member of the helix-loop-helix group of regulatory proteins and binds to DNA as a dimer. Genes Dev 1990; 4:1730-1740.
41. Beckmann H, Kadesch T. The leucine zipper of TFE3 dictates helix-loop-helix dimerization specificity. Genes Dev. 1991; 5:1057-1066.
42. Fisher DE, Carr CS, Parent LA, Sharp PA. TFEB has DNA-binding and oligomerization properties of a unique helix-loop-helix/leucine-zipper family. Genes Dev 1991; 5:2342-52.
43. Mai S, Jalava A. C-myc binds to 5' flanking sequence motifs of the dihydrofolate reductase gene in cellular extracts - role in proliferation. Nuc Acids Res 1994; 22:2264-2273.
44. Miltenberger RJ, Sukow KA, Farnham PJ. An E-box-mediated increase in *cad* transcription at the G1/S-phase boundary is suppressed by inhibitory c-Myc mutants. Mol Cell Biol 1995; 15:2527-2535
45. Karn J, Watson J, Lowe A, Green S, Vedeckis W. Regulation of cell cycle duration by c-*myc* levels. Oncogene 1989; 4:773-787.
46. Prouty SM, Hanson KD, Boyle AL, et al. A cell culture model system for genetic analyses of the cell cycle by targeted homologous recombination. Oncogene 1993; 8:899-907.
47. Shichiri M, Hanson KD, Sedivy JM. Effects of c-myc expression on proliferation, quiescence, and the G0 to G1 transition in nontransformed cells. Cell Growth Differ 1993; 4:93-104.
48. Hanson KD, Shichiri M, Follansbee MR, Sedivy JM. Effects of c-myc expression on cell cycle progression. Mol Cell Biol 1994; 14:5748-5755.
49. Jansen-Durr P, Meichle A, Steiner P, et al. Differential modulation of cyclin gene expression by MYC. Proc Natl Acad Sci USA 1993; 90:3685-3689.
50. Philipp A, Schneider A, Vasrik I, et al. Repression of cyclin D1 - a novel function of myc. Mol Cell Biol 1994; 14:4032-4043.
51. Daksis JI, Lu RY, Facchini LM, Marhin WW, Penn LJ. Myc induces cyclin D1 expression in the absence of de novo protein synthesis and links mitogen-stimulated signal transduction to the cell cycle. Oncogene 1994; 9:3635-45.
52. Rosenwald IB, Lazariskaratzas A, Sonenberg N, Schmidt EV. Elevated levels of cyclin D1 protein in response to increased expression of eukaryotic initiation factor 4E. Mol Cell Biol 1993; 13:7358-7363.
53. Hoang AT, Cohen KJ, Barrett JF, Bergstrom DA, Dang CV. Participation of cyclin A in Myc-induced apoptosis. Proc Natl Acad Sci U S A 1994; 91:6875-6879.
54. Henglein B, Chenivesse X, Wang J, Eick D, Brechot C. Structure and cell cycle-regulated transcription of the human cyclin A gene. Proc Natl Acad Sci U S A 1994; 91:5490-4.

55. Yamamoto M, Yoshida M, Ono K, et al. Effect of tumor suppressors on cell cycle-regulatory genes: RB suppresses p34cdc2 expression and normal p53 suppresses cyclin A expression. Exp Cell Res 1994; 210:94-101.
56. Yoshizumi M, Hsieh CM, Zhou F, et al. The ATF site mediates downregulation of the cyclin A gene during contact inhibition in vascular endothelial cells. Mol Cell Biol 1995; 6:3266-3272.
57. Desdouets C, Matesic G, Molina CA, et al. Cell cycle regulation of cyclin A gene expression by the cyclic AMP-responsive transcription factors CREB and CREM. Mol Cell Biol 1995; 6:3301-3309.
58. Nakamura T, Okuyama S, Okamoto S, Nakajima T, Sekiya S, Oda K. Down-regulation of the cyclin A promoter in differentiating human embryonal carcinoma cells is mediated by depletion of ATF-1 and ATF-2 in the complex at the ATF/CRE site. Exp Cell Res 1995; 216:422-430.
59. Guadagno TM, Ohtsubo M, Roberts JM, Assoian RK. A link between cyclin A expression and adhesion-dependent cell cycle progression. Science 1993; 262:1572-5.
60. Guadagno TM, Assoian RK. G1/S control of anchorage-independent growth in the fibroblast cell cycle. J Cell Biol 1991; 115:1419-25.
61. Han EK, Guadagno TM, Dalton SL, Assoian RK. A cell cycle and mutational analysis of anchorage-independent growth: cell adhesion and TGF-beta 1 control G1/S transit specifically. J Cell Biol 1993; 122:461-71.
62. Barrett JF, Lewis BC, Hoang AT, Alvarez JRJ, Dang CV. Cyclin A links c-Myc to adhesion-independent cell proliferation. J Biol Chem 1995; 270:15923-15925.
63. Born TL, Frost JA, Schonthal A, Prendergast GC, Feramisco JR. C-myc cooperates with activated ras to induce the cdc2 promoter. Mol Cell Biol 1994; 14:5710-5718.
64. Kim YH, Buchholz MA, Chrest FJ, Nordin AA. Up-regulation of c-myc induces the gene expression of the murine homologues of p34(cdc2) and cyclin-dependent kinase-2 in T lymphocytes. J Immunol 1994; 152:4328-4335.
65. Galaktionov K, Chen X, Beach D. Cdc25 cell-cycle phosphatase as a target of c-myc. Nature 1996; 382:511-7.
66. Reisman D, Elkind N, Roy B, Beamon J, Rotter V. c-Myc trans-activate the p53 promoter through a required downstream CACGTG motif. Cell Growth Diff 1993; 4:57-65.
67. Roy B, Beamon J, Balint E, Reisman D. Transactivation of the human p53 tumor suppressor gene by c-Myc/Max contributes to elevated mutant p53 expression in some tumors. Mol Cell Biol 1994; 14:7805-15.
68. Rosenwald IB, Rhoads DB, Callanan LD, Isselbacher KJ, Schmidt EV. Increased expression of eukaryotic translation initiation factors eIF-4E and eIF-2 alpha in response to growth induction by c-myc. Proc Natl Acad Sci U S A 1993; 90:6175-8.
69. Blackwell TK, Huang J, Ma A, et al. Binding of myc proteins to canonical and noncanonical DNA sequences. Mol Cell Biol 1993; 13:5216-24.
70. Jones RM, Branda J, Johnston KA, et al. An essential E box in the promoter of the gene encoding the mRNA cap-binding protein (eukaryotic initiation factor 4E) is a target for activation by c-myc. Mol Cell Biol 1996; 16:4754-64.
71. Chau CM, Evans MJ, Scarpulla RC. Nuclear respiratory factor 1 activation sites in genes encoding the gamma-subunit of ATP synthase, eukaryotic initiation factor 2 alpha, and tyrosine aminotransferase. Specific interaction of purified NRF-1 with multiple target genes. J Biol Chem 1992; 267:6999-7006.
72. Virbasius CA, Virbasius JV, Scarpulla RC. NRF-1, an activator involved in nuclear-mitochondrial interactions, utilizes a new DNA-binding domain conserved in a family of developmental regulators. Genes Dev 1993; 7:2431-45.
73. Virbasius JV, Scarpulla RC. Activation of the human mitochondrial transcription factor A gene by nuclear respiratory factors: a potential regulatory link between nuclear and mitochondrial gene expression in organelle biogenesis. Proc Natl Acad Sci U S A 1994; 91:1309-13.

Cytokine-induced Inhibition of Myc Activity in Monocytic Cells

L.-G. Larsson[1,2], F. Bahram[1], S. Wu[1], F. Öberg[1], K. Nilsson[1] and B. Lüscher[2]

[1] Laboratory of Tumor Biology, Department of Pathology, University of Uppsala, S-75185 Uppsala, Sweden

[2] Institut für Molekularbiologie, Medizinische Hochschule Hannover, 30623 Hannover, Germany

Introduction

The c-*myc* proto-oncogene plays an important role in the regulation of cell proliferation, differentiation and apoptosis. It encodes a transcription factor of the basic region/helix-loop-helix/leucine zipper (bHLHZip) family and binds specifically to certain E-box DNA elements and activates transcription from promoters containing such elements by forming heterodimers with the bHLHZip protein Max (Blackwood et al. 1991, Prendergast et al. 1991, for review see Henriksson and Lüscher 1996). Max on the other hand was recently shown to form heterodimers with a number of other bHLHZip proteins; Mad1, Mxi1, Mad3 and Mad4, referred to as the Mad family (Ayer et al. 1993, Zervos et al. 1993, Hurlin et al. 1995a). These are, like c-Myc, dependent on Max for their activity and bind the same DNA elements as Myc:Max heterodimers. The Mad proteins seem to act as negative regulators of growth and inhibit the transactivating and transforming capacity of Myc (for review see Henriksson & Lüscher 1996). This repressive activity depends on the N-terminus of Mad which is required for interaction with mammalian homologues of the yeast repressor protein Sin3 (Ayer et al. 1995, Schreiber-Agus et al. 1995).

Myc, Max and Mad proteins thus participate in a network of protein-protein and protein-DNA interactions. An attractive hypothesis is that this network may constitute a switch for growth/growth arrest and/or growth/differentiation. According to this hypothesis the relative amounts of the positively or negatively acting components will balance the network in favor of a proliferative or anti-proliferative outcome. In accordance with this model *mad*1 and *mxi*1 are induced during *in vitro* differentiation of myeloid cells (Ayer and Eisenman 1993, Zervos et al. 1993, Larsson et al. 1994) and keratinocytes (Hurlin et al. 1995b) whereas c-*myc* is down-regulated during the same process, resulting in a shift in the ratio of Mad1:Max to c-Myc:Max heterodimers in the cell. Furthermore, studies of embryonic and adult neuronal and epithelial tissues suggest that most *mad* genes are expressed in resting, differentiated cells whereas the *myc* genes are predominantly expressed in the proliferative, undifferentiated compartments (Hurlin et al. 1995a, Västrik et al. 1995).The network is assumed to control crucial genes involved in growth, differentiation and apoptosis. Suggested target genes include α-prothymosine, ODC, cdc25a, eIF2, cad and MrDb among others (for review see Henriksson and Lüscher 1996). We have in this report continued our studies of the Myc/Max/Mad network in U-937 cells by investigating the DNA-binding activity of these proteins during induced differentiation. Our results suggest that Mad1 DNA-binding complexes are rapidly induced in response to TPA whereas c-Myc DNA-binding declines. These data thus give further support for the network model described above.

We have previously reported that constitutive expression of v-Myc blocks phorbol ester (TPA) induced differentiation of U-937 monoblasts (Larsson et al. 1988). However, interferon (IFN)–γ treatment in combination with TPA restores differentiation and growth arrest despite continuous expression of v-Myc (Öberg et al. 1991, Larsson et al. 1992). TPA+IFN–γ thus directly or indirectly interfere with the activity of v-Myc. The present investigation has addressed the question whether also other cytokines have the capacity to restore differentiation and/or growth arrest in v-Myc expressing cells. Our results suggest that other cytokines such as IL-6 and TFGβ indeed induce such activity. We have also further investigated the mechanism by with TPA+IFN–γ counteract the activity of v-Myc. This question was addressed by investigating the expression, *in vivo* interaction, DNA-binding activity, and transcriptional activity of components of the Myc/Max/Mad network during TPA+IFN–γ-induced differentiation of v-Myc expressing U-937 cells. Our results show that TPA+IFN–γ do not affect the expression or activity of Mad1. In contrast, the amount of v-Myc:Max heterodimers and the DNA-binding activity of Myc is reduced in TPA+IFN–γ-induced as compared to TPA-treated cells. Furthermore, the activity of a reporter gene under control of a promoter containing Myc/Max binding sites is inhibited by the costimulation. Taken together these results suggest that the activity of Myc is directly affected by TPA+IFN–γ treatment.

Results and Discussion

Expression and DNA-binding activity of c-Myc, Mad1 and Max during TPA-induced differentiation of U-937 cells

We and others have previously reported that the expression of *mad*1 mRNA and to a lesser extent *mxi*1 mRNA is rapidly increased whereas the expression of c-*myc* mRNA is reduced following induced differentiation of U-937 monoblasts (Ayer et al. 1993, Zervos et al. 1993, Larsson et al. 1994). The aim of the present study was to determine if these changes in mRNA expression result in similar changes in the synthesis of the corresponding proteins and if this is also reflected in changes in the amount of Myc:Max and Mad1:Max heterodimers with the capacity to bind to the Myc:Max DNA recognition sequence CACGTG.

U-937-1 cells were induced to differentiate by the addition of TPA after which the differentiation was monitored kinetically by analyzing the percentage of cells with nitroblue tetrazolium (NBT) reducing capacity. In addition, the incorporation of ^{3}H-thymidine was assayed as a measure of the proliferative activity of the cells. Fig. 1 shows that an increase in the percentage of cells reducing NBT and a reduction of thymidine incorporation was detectable by 12 hrs after induction. The maximal percentage of cells with NBT-reducing activity and the minimal level of thymidine incorporation was observed 48-72 hrs post induction.

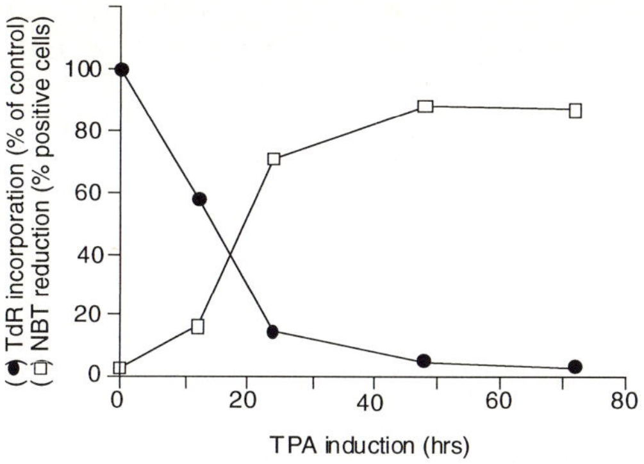

Fig. 1. TPA-induced differentiation of U-937-1 cells. Cells (10^5/ml) were stimulated by 1.6 x 10^{-7} M TPA and harvested at the indicated time points. NBT and ^{3}H-TdR incorporation assays were performed as described (Larsson et al. 1994).

Untreated and treated cells were labelled with ^{35}S-methionine and cell lysates were immunoprecipitated with Myc, Mad1 and Max antisera and analysed by SDS-PAGE. The quantification of the observed 62 kDa c-Myc, 35 kDa Mad1 and p21 and p22 kDa Max protein bands using an image analyzer is presented in Fig. 2b. As a comparison, quantification of the amount of the corresponding mRNAs, as determined by northern blot analysis (Larsson et al. 1994) is shown in Fig. 2a. The synthesis of Mad1 protein was rapidly induced following the TPA treatment and developed kinetically in a manner closely corresponding to the changes in *mad*1 mRNA expression. Both *mad*1 mRNA and protein described a biphasic pattern of expression peaking at 4 hrs and late increase starting from 24 hrs, although the expression of the two *mad*1 transcripts differed somewhat kinetically. The magnitude of the increase in Mad1 protein expression (3-4 fold) was intermediate to that of the two *mad*1 transcripts. The synthesis of c-Myc rapidly declined to 55% within an hour after TPA stimulation and thereafter continued to decrease. This reduction resembled that of c-*myc* mRNA but occurred faster at an hour of TPA stimulation. Although this might indicate a translational or post-translational regulation, we have observed slight differences in early kinetics both at the mRNA and protein levels between different experiments (data not shown). The synthesis of Max proteins was also somewhat reduced (to 70% of untreated cells by 72 hrs) starting from 12 hrs post induction. A similar reduction both kinetically and with respect to magnitude was observed at the mRNA level.

We next analysed the DNA-binding activity of c-Myc, Mad1 and Max to the CACGTG Myc:Max DNA recognition sequence. Due to the low abundance of these proteins and the presence of other proteins binding the same site, electrophoretic mobility shift assays (EMSA) have so far been unsuccessful to analyze of the DNA-binding of Myc- and Mad1-containing complexes using U-937 cell extracts. As an alternative, we have developed a solid phase DNA-binding assay based on binding of labelled oligonucleotides, containing the Myc binding site, to immunoprecipitated proteins. These immunoprecipitations are made under conditions where Myc:Max and Mad1:Max heterodimers are preserved. We have shown that this assay is very specific and sensitive (L.-G. Larsson, F. Bahram and B. Lüscher, submitted). As shown in Fig. 2c, a reduction in the DNA-binding activity of anti-Myc immunocomplexes was observed already 30 min after TPA treatment, and the binding continued to decline gradually throughout the experiment. The kinetics and magnitude of this reduction were similar to that of the synthesis of c-Myc. In contrast, a dramatic increase in the DNA-binding activity of anti-Mad1 complexes was observed, peaking 1 hr after TPA stimulation. A 3.5-6 fold increase in the level of binding as compared to untreated cells was detected at the time points thereafter. It is at present unclear whether the differences in magnitude of the Mad1 DNA-binding and Mad1 synthesis observed in these experiments represent post-translational regulation of Mad1 steady state levels, interaction with Max, or DNA-binding activity. Little variation in the DNA-binding of anti-Max immunocomplexes was observed during the experiment. In particular, no reduction in DNA-binding occurred at the later time point where the synthesis of Max was slightly reduced. The DNA-binding of Max in absolute numbers was 2-3 fold higher than that of c-Myc in untreated cells (data not shown). One should bear in mind that the DNA-binding activity of Max represent the sum of all Max-containing complexes with capacity to bind the CACGTG sequence.

We concluded from these experiments that *mad*1 mRNA and protein expression was rapidly induced in response to TPA in U-937-1 cells. The expression remained at an elevated level during the course of differentiation and described a biphasic pattern both at the mRNA and protein level. The induction of Mad1 protein synthesis resulted in an immediate formation of Mad1 complexes with DNA-binding activity. This activity remained elevated throughout the experiment and most likely represents Mad1:Max heterodimers since the Mad1 immunocomplexes contain Max (data not shown). The expression of c-*myc* mRNA and protein and the DNA-binding activity of Myc complexes declined during the same period. The DNA-binding activity of Myc and Mad1 immunocomplexes was roughly equal at late time points (data not shown). We did not have the opportunity to measure the DNA-binding of Mxi1 due to the lack of antibodies. Since the expression of *mxi*1 mRNA is quite high in these cells and increases during differentiation we would expect the combined DNA-binding of Mad1 and Mxi1 to exceed that of c-Myc at late stages of differentiation. These results would therefore support a model where c-Myc:Max DNA-binding complexes predominate in undifferentiated cells, and the sum of Mad-family:Max DNA-binding complexes predominates in differentiated cells. The kinetics of this process seems to essentially follow the expression patterns of the proteins involved although we can not exclude that other levels of regulation may occur as well. The potential role of the Mad proteins in the differentiation process, however, remains to be shown.

Fig. 2. Expression and DNA-binding activity of c-Myc, Mad1 and Max during TPA-induced differentiation of U-937-1 cells. The cells were induced as described in the legend to Fig. 1. a) Northern blot analysis. The presented data are normalised to the expression of actin. The analysis was performed as described (Larsson et al. 1994). b) Protein synthesis. The cells were labelled with ^{35}S-methionine for 40 min, lysed, immunoprecipitated with Myc, Mad1 or Max antisera and analysed on SDS-PAGE (Lüscher and Eisenman 1988). c) DNA-binding activity. The cells were lysed under low stringency conditions, immunoprecipitated with Myc, Mad1 and Max antisera, collected on protein A-Sepharose and washed (Blackwood et al. 1992). The immunoprecipitates were incubated in gelshift buffer for 25 min at 25 ^{o}C with ^{32}P-labelled CMD oligonucleotide, containing the CACGTG sequence. After washing, the amount of bound radioactivity was measured in a scintillation counter (L.-G. Larsson, F. Bahram and B. Lüscher submitted). The data are presented as percent of untreated cells (c-Myc, Max) or as fold induction (Mad1).

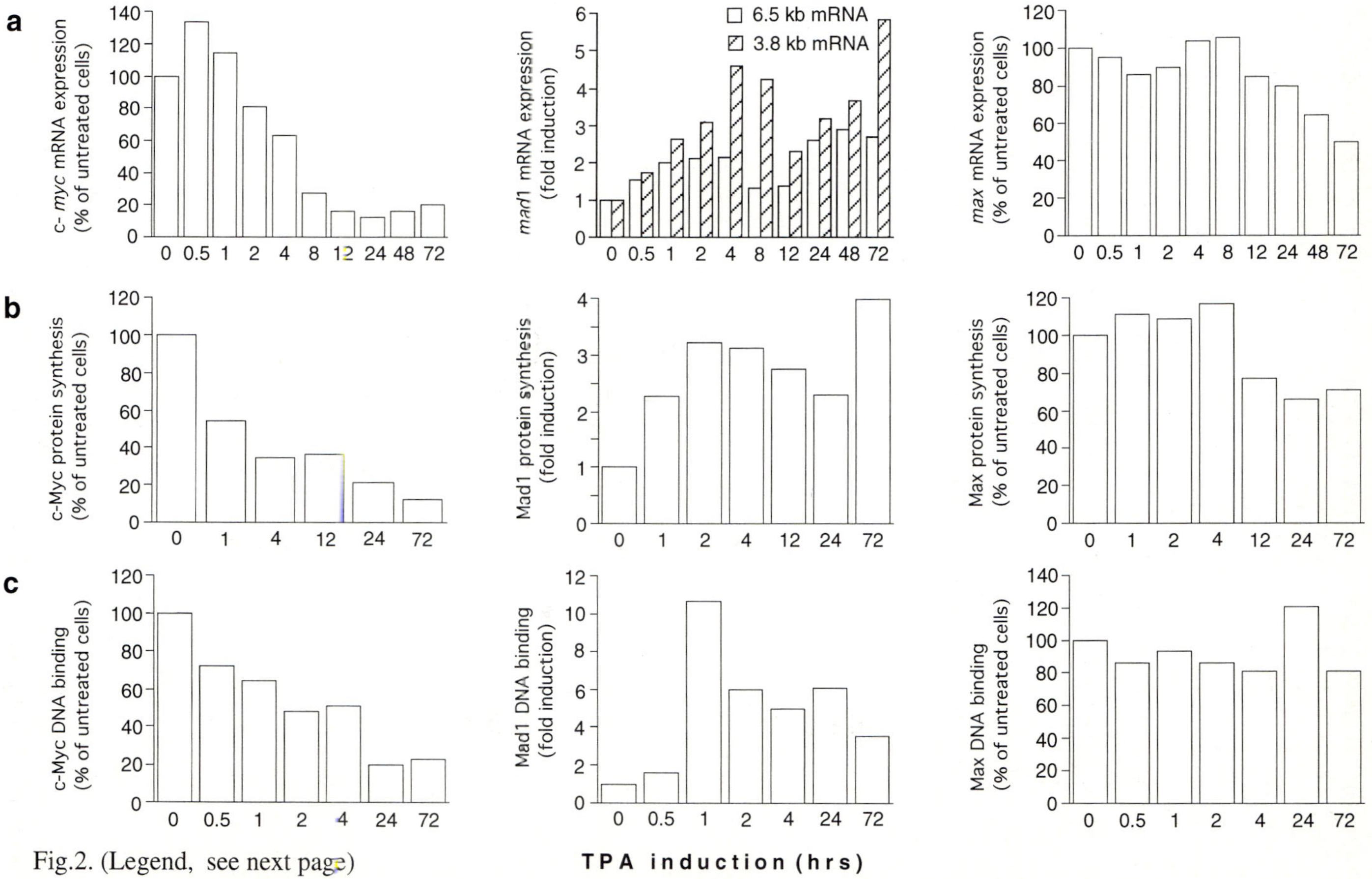

Fig.2. (Legend, see next page)

Cytokine costimulation restores TPA-induced differentiation and cell cycle arrest in v-Myc expressing U-937 cells

We have previously reported that TPA-, VitD_3- and RA-induced differentiation is inhibited in U-937 cells constitutively expressing a v-*myc* gene (Larsson et al. 1988). However, costimulation with IFN–γ, which alone is not a potent inducer of differentiation, restores differentiation and G_0/G_1 arrest induced by all three differentiation agents, despite continuous expression of v-Myc (Öberg et al. 1991, Larsson et al. 1992). Since many cytokines utilise similar signal transduction pathways, we investigated whether also other cytokines, alone or together with TPA, might have similar effects as IFN–γ.

Fig. 3a shows that the TPA-induced cell surface expression of the monocytic differentiation marker CD11c, was inhibited in U-937-myc-6 cells. These cells contain the OK10 v-*myc* gene as part of the retroviral construct MMCV-neo. In contrast, 80% of U-937-neo-6 cells, containing a similar retroviral construct lacking the v-*myc* gene, expressed CD11c after TPA stimulation. In addition, the percentage of U-937-neo-6 cells in S-phase declined (Fig. 3b) concomitantly with an increase in G_1 cells and a decrease in G_2/M cells (data not shown). No changes in the cell cycle distribution were observed in TPA-treated U-937-myc-6 cells.

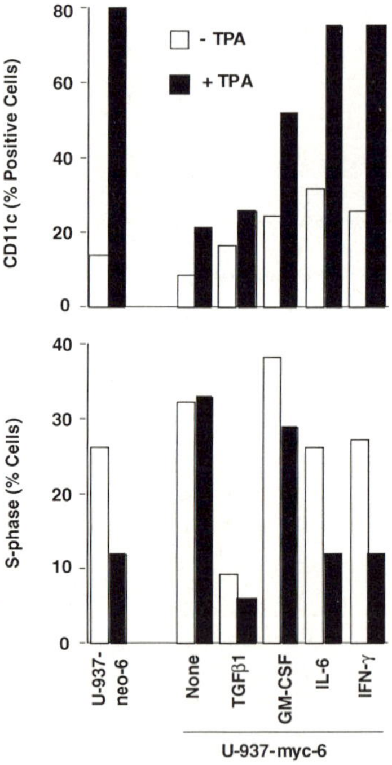

Fig. 3. Cytokine-induced differentiation and/or cell cycle arrest in v-Myc expressing U-937 cells. 1.5 x 10^5 cells/ml were stimulated with 1 ng/ml rTGFβ1, 100 ng/ml rGM-CSF, 100 U/ml rIL-6 or 100 U/ml rIFN–γ with or without $1.6x10^{-7}$ M TPA for 3 days. Viable cells were analyzed for CD11c cell surface expression and cell cycle distribution as described (Larsson et al. 1994).

In agreement with previous results (Öberg et al. 1991, Larsson et al. 1992), IFN–γ treatment of U-937-myc-6 cells in combination with TPA induced CD11c expression and reduced the percentage of cells in S phase to a similar level as in TPA-stimulated U-937-neo-6 cells. IFN–γ alone only slightly increased the expression of CD11c and had no effect on the cell cycle (Fig. 3) but induced apoptosis in a percentage of the cells (50-70 % in different experiments). The survival was higher in costimulated cells (10-30% apoptotic cells) (data not shown). Fig. 3 shows that stimulation with IL-6 in combination with TPA restored CD11c expression and reduced the percentage of S-phase cells in a manner very similar to that of IFN–γ. IL-6 alone increased the number of CD11c positive cell to 30 % but had little effect on the cell cycle. Also GM-CSF in combination with TPA partially restored CD11c expression but did not induce growth arrest. TFGβ on the other hand induced cell cycle arrest very efficiently both alone and in combination with TPA, but did not restore the expression of CD11c.

These experiments showed that other cytokines than IFN–γ, in particular IL-6 and TFGβ, restore differentiation and/or growth arrest in v-Myc expressing U-937 cells. The effects of IL-6 and GM-CSF were similar to those of IFN–γ. These cytokines had moderate effects on differentiation and cell cycle arrest alone, both in parental U-937 cells (data not shown) and U-937-myc-6 cells, but primarily seem to act by normalising the effect of TPA in the latter cells. Interestingly, IFN-γ, IL-6, and GM-CSF all utilise the JAK/STAT pathway for their signal transduction and share some of the components in this pathway (for review see Taniguchi 1995). We are at present investigating which of these induced signals are relevant for the observed anti-Myc activity. The effect of TFGβ differs from that of the other cytokines. This cytokine did not synergize with TPA and did not promote differentiation but very efficiently induced cell cycle arrest. In fact, TFGβ may even inhibit aspects of the differentiation of parental U-937 cells (data not shown). Not surprisingly, TFGβ utilises distinct signaling pathways (for review see Massague' 1996). IFN–γ alone at high concentration, like TNFα, induces apoptosis in U-937 cells. v-Myc expressing U-937 cells are, however, more sensitive to both IFN–γ- and TNFα induced apoptosis (data not shown). This resembles the enhanced TNFα-induced apoptosis observed in fibroblasts overexpressing c-Myc (Klefstrom et al. 1994). The results of these experiments are summarised in Fig. 4.

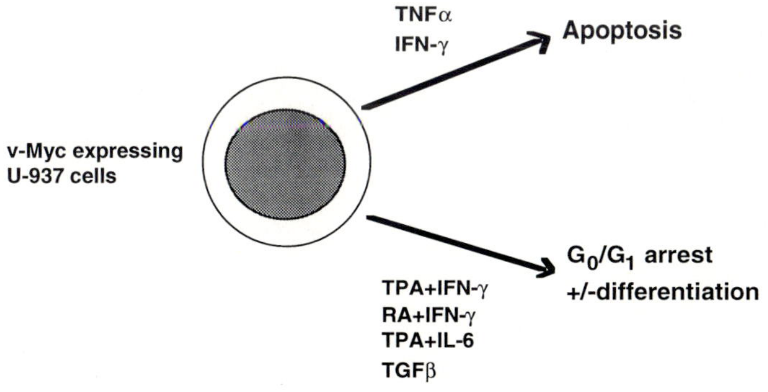

Fig. 4. Summary of effects of cytokines on differentiation, cell cycle arrest and apoptosis in v-Myc expressing U-937 cells.

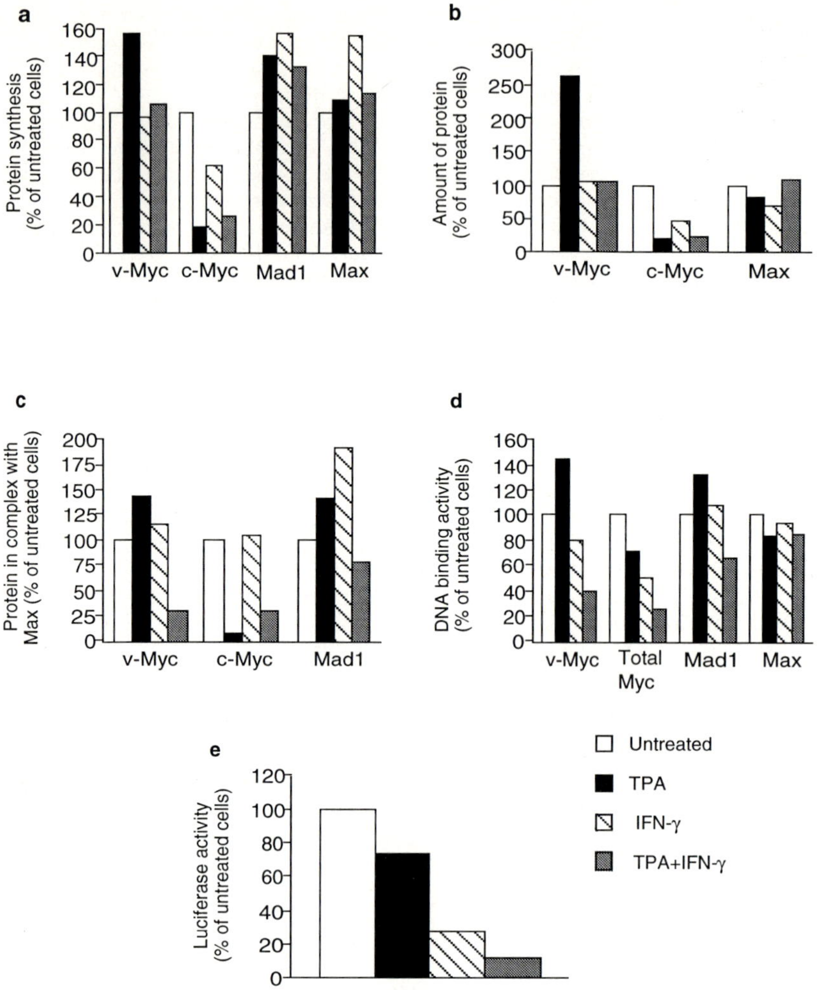

Fig. 5. TPA and IFN–γ costimulation inhibits the activity of Myc by a Mad1 independent pathway. U-937-myc-6 cells were induced by TPA, IFN–γ or TPA+IFN–γ for three days. a) Protein synthesis. Lysates from untreated and treated ^{35}S-labelled cells were immunoprecipitated and analysed on SDS-PAGE. b) Steady state level of proteins. Unlabelled cell lysates were immunoprecipitated and subjected to western blot analysis using the ECL system. c) *in vivo* interactions with Max. Unlabelled cell lysates were immunoprecipitated with Max antiserum under low stringency conditions and subjected to western blot analysis using Myc or Mad1 antisera. d) DNA- binding activity. The assay was performed as described in the legend to Fig. 2. e) Transactivation. A luciferase reporter construct containing a minimal tk-promoter driven by four copies of the Myc E box CACGTG (m4mintk-Luc) was coelectroporated with a hygromycin resistance gene into U-937-myc-6 cells, and stable transfectants were selected. One representative clone, U-937-myc-6-m112, was induced as indicated and assayed for luciferase activity. The data in a-e are presented as percent of untreated cells. The data in a-c are based on quantification using a Fuji bas image analyzer (a) or scanning of autoradiograms (b and c)

IFN–γ costimulation inhibits Myc activity in U-937 cells.

The mechanism by which IFN–γ and other cytokines restore TPA-induced differentiation in v-Myc expressing U-937 cells is unknown. One could envisage at least three different explanations for this effect: TPA+IFN–γ-induced signals may 1) directly affect the activity of Myc, 2) increase the expression or activity of members of the Mad family or other Myc antagonists, or 3) act downstream of Myc, for instance by regulating target genes of Myc. We have addressed the two first possibilities in this report by investigating the expression, *in vivo* interaction and DNA-binding activity of Myc, Mad1 and Max and the activity of a Myc-inducible reporter construct in U-937-myc-6 cells in response to TPA and IFN–γ.

Fig. 5a shows that the normal increase in Mad1 expression during TPA-induced differentiation of U-937 cells (see Fig. 2) was inhibited in v-Myc expressing cells, indicating that Mad1 is directly or indirectly regulated by Myc. Accordingly, very little increase in the amount of Mad1:Max heterodimers (Fig. 5c) or in Mad1 DNA-binding activity (Fig. 5d) occurred in response to TPA. None of these activities were restored by costimulation with IFN–γ. Moreover, no increase in *mxi*1 mRNA expression was observed (data not shown), suggesting that restoration of TPA-induced differentiation by IFN–γ is not due to activation of the Mad family.

TPA increased the expression of v-Myc (Fig. 5a and b), the amount of v-Myc:Max heterodimers (Fig. 5c) and the v-Myc DNA-binding activity (Fig. 5d), whereas the expression and activity of endogenous c-Myc declined. However, TPA+IFN–γ treatment prevented the increased expression of v-Myc, and furthermore decreased the amount of v-Myc:Max heterodimers and the DNA-binding activity of v-Myc. Accordingly, the total level of DNA-binding activity of Myc complexes (v- + c-Myc) was reduced in response to the costimulation. To measure the activity of a Myc-responsive reporter gene, the m4mintk-Luc construct, which contains four CACGTG elements upstream of a minimal tk-promoter linked to a luciferase reporter gene, was stably transfected into U-937-myc-6 cells. Selected clones containing this construct were stimulated as above and the luciferase activity was measured. IFN–γ and in particular TPA+IFN–γ treatment reduced the luciferase activity to 10-15 % of untreated cells as exemplified by clone m-112 (Fig. 5e). Similar results were obtained by transient transfections of m4mintk-Luc and a Myc-regulated α-prothymosine promoter construct (data not shown).

Taken together these results suggest that TPA+IFN–γ costimulation directly interfere with the activity of v-Myc. At least in part this seems to be due to a reduction of the amount of v-Myc:Max heterodimers and of the v-Myc-specific DNA-binding activity. In addition it is possible that the transactivation domain is negatively regulated by the two signals. Also we can not exclude that the costimulation may counteract Myc by additional indirect mechanisms, for instance by affecting the expression or activity of other Myc antagonists than Mad1 and Mxi1 or by affecting downstream targets of Myc. Experiments addressing these possibilities are presently in progress.

Acknowledgements

This work was supported by grants from the Swedish Cancer Society (to L-G.L, F.Ö. and K.N.), the Children Cancer Foundation of Sweden, the Lovisa & Thielman and Selander Foundations (to L-G.L) and the Deutsche Forschungsgemeinschaft, the Deutsche Krebshilfe and the Fonds der Chemischen Industrie (to B.L.).

References

Ayer DE, Eisenman RN (1993) A switch from Myc:Max to Mad:Max heterocomplexes accompanies monocyte/macrophage differentiation. Genes Dev 7:2110-2119.

Ayer DE, Kretzner L, Eisenman RN (1993) Mad: a heterodimeric partner for Max that antagonizes Myc transcriptional activity. Cell 72:211-222.

Ayer DE, Lawrence QA, Eisenman RN (1995) Mad-Max transcriptional repression is mediated by ternary complex formation with mammalian homologs of yeast repressor Sin3. Cell 80:767-776.

Blackwood EM, Eisenman RN (1991) Max: a helix-loop-helix zipper protein that forms a sequence-specific DNA-binding complex with Myc. Science 251:1211-1217.

Blackwood E.M, Lüscher B, Eisenman RN (1992) Myc and Max associate in vivo. Genes & Dev. 6:71-80.

Henriksson M, Luscher B (1996) Proteins of the Myc network: essential regulators of cell growth and differentiation. Adv Cancer Res 68:109-182.

Hurlin PJ, Queva C, Koskinen PJ, Steingrimsson E, Ayer DE, Copeland NG, Jenkins NA, Eisenman RN (1995a) Mad3 and Mad4: novel Max-interacting transcriptional repressors that suppress c-myc dependent transformation and are expressed during neural and epidermal differentiation. EMBO J 14:5646-5659.

Hurlin PJ, Foley KP, Ayer DE, Eisenman RN, Hanahan D, Arbeit JM (1995b) Regulation of Myc and Mad during epidermal differentiation and HPV-associated tumorigenesis. Oncogene 11:2487-2501.

Klefstrom J, Vastrik I, Saksela E, Valle J, Eilers M, Alitalo K (1994) c-Myc induces cellular susceptibility to the cytotoxic action of TNF-alpha. EMBO J 13:5442-5450.

Larsson LG, Ivhed I, Gidlund M, Pettersson U, Vennstrom B, Nilsson K (1988) Phorbol ester-induced terminal differentiation is inhibited in human U-937 monoblastic cells expressing a v-myc oncogene. Proc Natl Acad Sci U S A 85:2638-2642.

Larsson LG, Oberg F, Stockbauer P, Masucci MG, Nilsson K (1992) Suppression of basal, PMA- and IFN-alpha-, but not IFN-gamma-induced expression of HLA class I in v-myc-transformed U-937 monoblasts. Int J Cancer 52:759-765.

Larsson LG, Pettersson M, Oberg F, Nilsson K, Luscher B (1994) Expression of mad, mxi1, max and c-myc during induced differentiation of hematopoietic cells: opposite regulation of mad and c-myc. Oncogene 9:1247-1252.

Luscher B, Eisenman RN (1988) c-myc and c-myb protein degradation: effect of metabolic inhibitors and heat shock. Mol Cell Biol 8:2504-2512.

Massague', J (1996) TGFβ signalling: receptors, transducers and Mad proteins. Cell 85:947-950.

Oberg F, Larsson LG, Anton R, Nilsson K (1991) Interferon gamma abrogates the differentiation block in v-myc-expressing U-937 monoblasts. Proc Natl Acad Sci U S A 88:5567-5571.

Prendergast GC, Lawe D, Ziff EB (1991) Association of Myn, the murine homolog of max, with c-Myc stimulates methylation-sensitive DNA binding and ras cotransformation. Cell 65:395-407.

Schreiber-Agus N, Chin L, Chen K, Torres R, Rao G, Guida P, Skoultchi AI, DePinho RA (1995) An amino-terminal domain of Mxi1 mediates anti-Myc oncogenic activity and interacts with a homolog of the yeast transcriptional repressor SIN3. Cell 80:777-786.

Taniguchi T (1995) Cytokine signaling through nonreceptor protein tyrosine kinases. Science 268:251-255.

Vastrik I, Kaipainen A, Penttila TL, Lymboussakis A, Alitalo R, Parvinen M, Alitalo K (1995) Expression of the mad gene during cell differentiation in vivo and its inhibition of cell growth in vitro. J Cell Biol 128:1197-1208.

Zervos AS, Gyuris J, Brent R (1993) Mxi1, a protein that specifically interacts with Max to bind Myc-Max recognition sites. Cell 72:223-232.

c-Myc Dependent Initiation of Genomic Instability During Neoplastic Transformation

C. Taylor, A. Jalava and S. Mai
Manitoba Institute of Cell Biology and the University of Manitoba,
100 Olivia Street, Winnipeg, MB R3E 0V9, Canada

Abstract

The dihydrofolate reductase (*DHFR*) gene is a target of c-Myc in genomic instability. The induced overexpression of c-Myc in cell lines is followed by the amplification and rearrangement of the *DHFR* gene. Furthermore, the constitutive upregulation of c-Myc protein coincides with genomic instability of the *DHFR* gene in lymphoid, non-lymphoid and in tumor lines. The amplification of the *DHFR* gene is locus-specific and independent of species origins. We have now addressed the question whether inducible deregulation of c-Myc is followed by *DHFR* gene amplification *in vivo* . We show that the *DHFR* gene is a target of c-Myc-dependent neoplasia *in vivo* and propose a role for genomic instability during the initiation of neoplastic transformation.

Introduction

Gene amplification represents one feature of genomic instability in mammalian cells, although it may also occur as part of a normal developmental program in insects, amphibia, and lower organisms [1-3]. Amplified genes that are present in mammalian cells indicate that these cells have become genomically unstable, immortalized, transformed and/or tumorigenic. Therefore, the amplification of specific genes serves as prognostic marker in cancer [e.g. 4]. Gene amplification often involves the amplification of oncogenes, and it frequently is accompanied by translocations, double minutes and additional rearrangements that involve one or several distinct loci [5-9].

In mammalian cell lines and in tumors, gene amplification has been described after drug selection [10-12], during constitutive growth factor expression [13-15] or after DNA damage [16-20], and as a result of c-Myc overexpression [21, 5, 22]. Spontaneous gene amplification has also been reported [23]. With one published exception [24], gene amplification has not been observed in normal diploid mammalian cells [20, 25, 26] and therefore is associated with a transformed phenotype. Gene amplification is facilitated by the absence of the tumor suppressor protein p53 [27, 28]. Yet, gene amplification may also occur in the presence of wildtype p53 protein [29, 6] and thus may involve both p53 dependent and p53 independent pathways.

c-Myc is a key regulator of growth, proliferation, differentiation, and development. Deregulation of the c-Myc oncoprotein has been reported in apoptosis, transformation, and in malignancies of lymphoid and non-lymphoid origin [30, 31]. c-Myc plays a role in the modulation [32-38] and initiation of transcription [39-41]. It is a short-lived nuclear oncoprotein [31], which is strictly regulated during the cell cycle of normal diploid cells [31, 42, 43]. Increased half life of the protein is associated with immortalization and transformation [30, 31]. The deregulation of c-Myc is a common feature in many tumors [30, 31], where it frequently is translocated [44, 45, 7, 30, 31] and/or amplified and overexpressed [30, 31, 46, 47]. In addition, the c-myc gene is often the site of proviral insertion [30, 31]. Chromosomal aberrations involving c-myc are associated with a poor prognosis [4].

Besides its role in transcription, c-Myc promotes replication and amplification. Studies by Classon et al. [48-50] and by us [51, 52] have shown that c-Myc protein levels correlate with Simian Virus 40 (SV40) replication and binding to the SV40 replication origin. Additional evidence has been provided on c-Myc's role in DNA damage-induced protein binding to the SV40 minimal origin of replication and in SV40 gene amplification [52]. Regions of c-Myc involved in the stimulation of replication have been characterized. They include the regions of transactivation, DNA and protein interaction [50].

In addition to the amplification of SV40, c-Myc overexpression promotes gene amplification of the dihydrofolate reductase (*DHFR*) gene [21, 5, 22]. The enzyme encoded by the *DHFR* gene is a key enzyme of the folate metabolism that supplies the cell with dTTP for DNA synthesis [53]. c-Myc overexpression enhances *DHFR* gene amplification and the resistance to the drug methotrexate (MTX) [22]. Earlier, we have identified and characterized two adjacent E-box sequence motifs within the 5' flanking region of the *DHFR* gene that bind c-Myc/Max heterodimers [53]. These sites have been recently confirmed by others [54]. c-Myc/Max binding is proliferation-dependent [53]. In inducible transfectants that allow the experimental overexpression of the c-Myc oncoprotein [21], c-Myc overexpression is followed by the enhanced binding of the c-Myc/Max heterodimer to *DHFR* 5' flanking E-box motifs [21, 5]. Furthermore, the *DHFR* gene is amplified as a result of the inducible overexpression of the oncoprotein and the increase in c-Myc/Max heterodimer formation at the *DHFR* E-box sequence motifs [21, 5]. c-Myc overexpression thus affects the genomic stability of the *DHFR* locus.

The amplification of the *DHFR* gene occurs within three cell doublings and reaches levels of 1.8 to 4.2fold during this time period. The amplification is locus-specific, since other loci are unaffected irrespective of c-Myc protein levels [21, 5]. *DHFR* gene amplification as a result of c-Myc overexpression coincides with the elevated expression of the DHFR enzyme [55]. The amplification of the *DHFR* locus is transient if c-Myc overexpression is induced for a single time [5]. Constitutive c-Myc overexpression is associated with both the amplification and the rearrangement of the *DHFR* gene [5]. Moreover, the prolonged induction of c-Myc overexpression induces a significant increase in the formation of telomere-centromere-fusions and of extrachromosomal elements [7].

In conclusion, previous work performed *in vitro* has documented the non-random and locus-specific amplification of the *DHFR* gene as a result of c-Myc overexpression independent of species and cell types.

Results and Discussion

To determine whether the locus-specific amplification of the *DHFR* gene occured as a result of c-Myc overexpression *in vivo*, we have examined an animal model of c-Myc-dependent neoplasia, the mouse plasmacytoma [45]. Using plasmacytoma-susceptible Balb/c mice, we analyzed whether *DHFR* gene amplification occured during pristane-induced plasmacytomagenesis. We examined Balb/c mice that were injected i.p. with pristane [45]. Control Balb/c mice received i.p. injections of LPS (lipopolysaccharide) that elicites the transient activation of B cells concomitant with a transient upregulation of c-Myc protein levels, but does not lead to PCT genesis which requires the constitutive overexpression of c-Myc [45].

c-Myc protein levels of cells directly isolated from the peritoneal cavity [45] were analyzed by quantitative fluorescent immunohistochemistry. Pristane elicited the elevation of c-Myc protein levels (Table 1). The induction level reached 4 to 10 fold three days post pristane injection and prevailed elevated for the next four weeks. LPS induced a similar, but transient upregulation of c-Myc protein levels in B lineage cells (Table 1). Non-treated peritoneal cavity cells exhibited low c-Myc protein levels (Table 1).

We next examined whether *DHFR* gene amplification in Balb/c mice was induced as a result of the above treatments. Peritoneal cavity cells were analyzed by fluorescent *in situ* hybridization (FISH). The amplification of the *DHFR* gene was observed after a single i.p. injection of pristane (Table 1). Interestingly, LPS did not lead to the amplification of the *DHFR* gene (Table 1).

Table 1. *DHFR* gene amplification in Balb/c peritoneal cavity cells seven days after i.p. injection of pristane

Treatment	c-Myc upregulation	*DHFR* gene amplification
None	-	-(1)
LPS	+	-(1)
Pristane	+	+(2)

LPS: lipopolysaccharide; pristane: 2,6,10,14-tetramethylpentadecane; (1): background frequency of *DHFR* gene amplification: 1×10^{-5}; (2): *DHFR* gene amplification affects 40-60% of all peritoneal cavity cells within the first week after i.p. injection of pristane.

The above findings allow one to conclude that the *DHFR* gene is a molecular marker of c-Myc-dependent genomic instability *in vivo*. Moreover, these findings confirm our previous *in vitro* data on c-Myc-dependent *DHFR* gene amplification in non-lymphoid and lymphoid cell lines of mouse, hamster, rat and human [21, 5]. Interestingly, the fully developed plasmacytoma also exhibited *DHFR* gene amplification (Fig. 1).

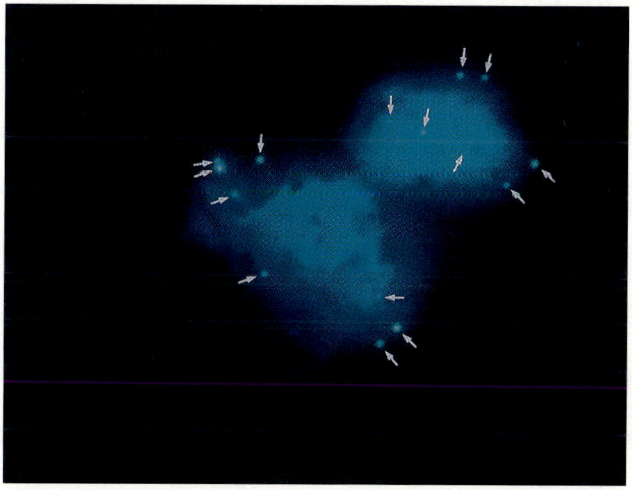

Fig. 1. *DHFR* gene amplification in fully developed plasmacytoma. Arrows point to amplified *DHFR* sequences as detected by FISH. Nuclei are counterstained with DAPI (4', 6'-diamidino-2-phenylindole).

As shown earlier, *DHFR* gene amplification and DHFR enzyme overexpression coincide [55]. It is not known whether the amplification of the *DHFR* gene is functionally important in c-Myc-induced genomic instability and neoplasia. Based on the fact that *DHFR* gene amplification occurs both early and late during pristane-induced plasmacytomagenesis in Balb/c mice, we speculate that this amplification event plays a role during the initiation of genomic instability and neoplastic transformation (Fig. 2). It has been described by others that imbalances in the nucleotide pool enhance mutation frequencies [56]. Consistent with these findings, we propose that the amplification and overexpression of DHFR enzyme, which is a key enzyme of the folate metabolism, may lead to changes in the nucleotide pool, especially in the dTTP pool, which affect both DNA synthesis and mutation frequencies. Thus *DHFR* amplification and overexpression may account in part for accelerated acquisition rates of mutations and for further genomic instability. Moreover, DNA synthesis and cellular proliferation and thus the statistically elevated probability to generate a malignant clone may be enhanced due to *DHFR* amplification and overexpression. It is noteworthy that the potential to amplify the *DHFR* gene as well as the levels of *DHFR* gene amplification correlate with the metastatic potential in a rat tumor model [57].

Fig. 2. Model : c-Myc deregulation and the initiation of genomic instability

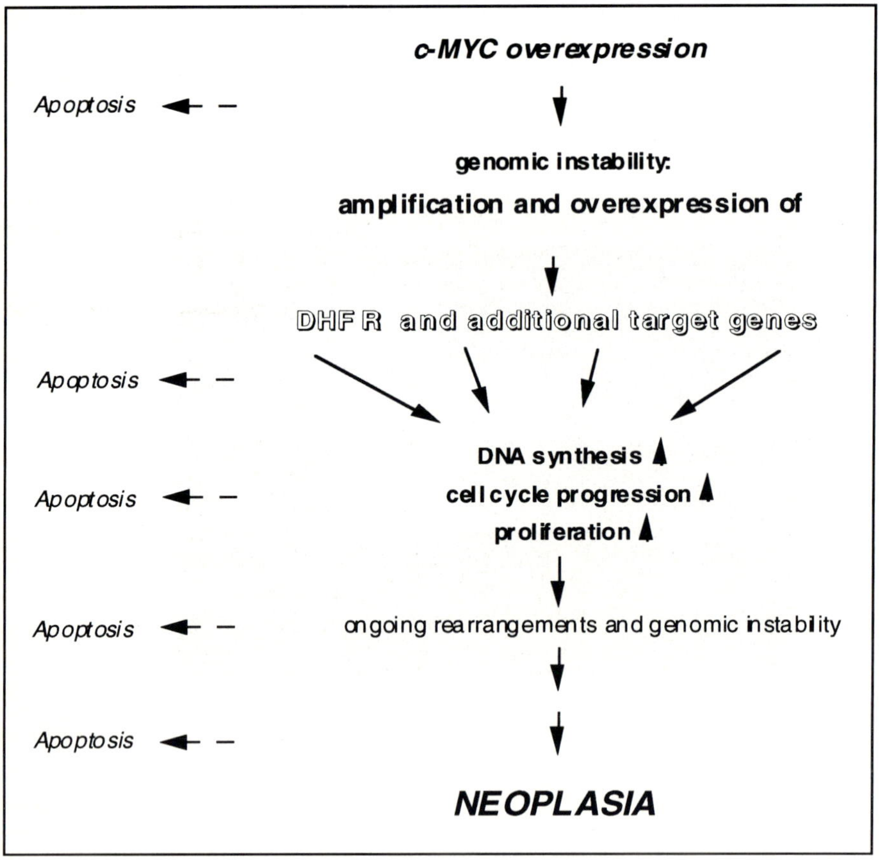

Acknowledgements

This work has been supported by grants of the National Sciences and Engineering Council (NSERC), the Thorlakson Fund and the Manitoba Cancer Treatment and Research Foundation (MTCRF) to SM and by a Manitoba Health and Research Council (MHRC) fellowship to AJ.

References

1. Santelli, R.V., Machado-Santelli, G.M., Pueyo, M.T., Navarro-Cattapan, L.D., and Lara, F.J.S. (1991). Replication and transcription in the course of DNA amplification of the C3 and C8 puffs of Rhynchosciara americana. Mech. Dev. 36: 59-66, 1991.
2. Delikadis, C. and Kafatos, F.C. (1989). Amplification enhancers and replication origins in the autosomal chorion cluster of Drosophila. The EMBO J. 8: 891-901.
3. Stark, G.R. and Wahl, G.M. (1984). Gene amplification. Ann. Rev. Biochem., 53, 447-491.
4. Yokota, Y., Tsunetsugu-Yokota, Y., Battifora, C.L., and Cline, M.J. (1986). Alterations in myc, myb, ras Ha proto-oncogenes in cancers are frequent and show clinical correlation. Science 231: 261-265.
5. Mai, S., Hanley-Hyde, J., Fluri, M. (1996). c-Myc overexpression associated DHFR gene amplification in hamster, rat, mouse and human cell lines. Oncogene 12: 277-288.
6. Mai, S., Fluri, M., Siwarski, D., Huppi, K. (1996). Genomic instability in MycER activated Rat1A-MycER cells. Chromosome Research 4: 365-372.
7. Mai, S., Hanley-Hyde, J., Coleman, A., Siwarski, D., Huppi, K. (1995). Amplified extrachromosomal elements containing c-Myc and Pvt 1 in a mouse plasmacytoma. Genome 38: 780-85.
8. Van Der Bliek, A. M., Van Der Velde-Koerts, T., Ling, V., Borst, P. (1986). Overexpression and amplification of five genes in a multidrug-resistant Chinese hamster ovary line. Mol. Cell. Biol. 6: 1671-1678.
9. Corvi, R., Amler, L. C., Savelyeva, L., Gehring, M., Schwab, M. (1994). MycN is retained in single copy at chromosome 2 band p23-23 during amplification in human neuroblastoma. Proc. Natl. Acad. Sci. (USA) 91: 5523-5527.
10. Stark, G.R. (1993). Regulation and mechanisms of mammalian gene amplification. Adv. Cancer Res. 61: 87-113.
11. Schimke, R.T., Kaufman, R.J., Alt, F.W., and Kellems, R.F. (1978). Gene amplification and drug resistance in cultured murine cells. Science 202: 1051-1055.
12. Shah, D.M., Horsch, R.B., Klee, H.J., Kishore, G.M., Winter, J.A., Tumer, N.E., Hironaka, C.M., Sanders, P.R., Gasser, C.S., Aykent, S., Siegel, N.R., Rogers, S.G., and Fraley, R.T. (1986). Engeneering herbicide tolerance in transgenic plants. Science 233: 478-481.
13. Huang, A. and Wright, J.A. (1994). Fibroblast growth factor mediated alterations in drug resistance, and evidence of gene amplification. Oncogene 9: 491-499.
14. Huang, A., Jin, H., and Wright, J.A. (1994). Aberrant expression of basic fibroblast growth factor in NIH-3T3 cells alters drug resistance and gene amplification potential. Exp. Cell Res. 213: 335-339.
15. Huang, A., Jin, H., and Wright, J.A. (1995). Drug resistance and gene amplification potential regulated by transforming growth factor-β 1 gene expression. Cancer Res. 55: 1758-1762.
16. Lavi, S. (1981). Carcinogen-mediated amplification of viral DNA sequences in simian virus 40-transformed Chinese hamster embryo cells. Proc. Natl. Acad. Sci. (USA) 78: 6144-6148.
17. Tlsty, T.D., Brown, P.E., and Schimke, R.T. (1984). UV radiation facilitates methotrexate resistance and amplification of the dihydrofolate reductase gene in cultured mouse cells. Mol. Cell.Biol. 4: 1050-1056.
18. Lücke-Huhle, C., Pech, M., and Herrlich, P. (1990). SV40 DNA amplification and reintegration in surviving hamster cells after 60 Co gamma-irradiation. Int. J. Radiat. Biol. 58: 577-588.
19. Yalkinoglu, A.Ö., Zentgraf, H., and Hübscher, U. (1991). The origin of adeno-associated virus DNA replication is a target for carcinogen-induced DNA amplification. J. Virol. 65: 3175-3184.
20. Lücke-Huhle, C. (1989). Review: gene amplification - a cellular response to genotoxic stress. Mol. Toxicol. 2: 237-253.

21. Mai, S. (1994). Overexpression of c-myc precedes amplification of the gene encoding dihydrofolate reductase. Gene 148: 253-260.
22. Denis, N., Kitzis, A., Kruh, J., Dautry, F., and Crocos, D. (1991). Stimulation of methotrexate resistance and dihydrofolate reductase gene amplification by c-myc. Oncogene 6: 1453-1457.
23. Johnston, R.N., Beverley, S.M., and Schimke, R.T. (1983). Rapid spontaneous dihydrofolate reductase gene amplification shown by fluorescence-activated cell sorting. Proc. Natl. Acad. Sci. (USA) 80: 3711-3715.
24. Prody, C.A., Dreyfus, P., Zamir, R., Zakut, H., and Soreq, H. (1989). De novo amplification within a "silent" human cholinesterase gene in a family subjected to prolonged exposure to organophosphorus insecticides. Proc. Natl. Acad. Sci. (USA) 86: 690-694.
25. Wright, J.A., Smith, H.S., Watt, F.M., Hancock, M.C., Hudson, D.L., and Stark, G.R. (1990). DNA amplification is rare in normal human cells. Proc. Natl. Acad. Sci. (USA) 87: 1791-1795.
26. Tlsty, T.D. (1990). Normal diploid cells lack a detectable frquency of gene amplification. Proc. Natl. Acad. Sci. (USA) 87: 3132-3136, 1990.
27. Yin, Y., Tainsky, M. A., Bischoff, F.Z., Strong, L. C., and Wahl, G. M. (1992). Wildtype p53 restores cell cycle control and inhibits gene amplifictaion in cells with mutant p53 alleles. Cell 70: 937-948.
28. Livingstone, L. R., White, A., Sprouse, J., Livanos, E., Jacks, T., and Tlsty, T. D. (1992). Altered cell cycle arrest and gene amplification potential accompany loss of wildtype p53. Cell 70: 923-935.
29. Zhou, P., Jiang, W., Wegorst, C. M., and Weinstein, I. B. (1996). Overexpression of cyclin D1 enhances gene amplification. Cancer Research 56:36-39.
30. Marcu, K.B., Bossone, S.A., and Patel, A.J. (1992). Myc function and regulation. Ann. Rev. Biochem. 61: 809-860.
31. Cole, M.D. (1986). The myc oncogene: its role in transformation and differentiation. Ann. Rev. Genet. 20: 361-384.
32. Benevisty, N., Leder, A., Kuo, A., and Leder, P. (1992). An embryonically expressed gene is a target for c-Myc regulation via the c-Myc binding sequence. Genes Dev. 6: 2513-2523.
33. Bello-Fernandez, C., Packham, G., and Cleveland, J.L. (1993). The ornithine decarboxylase is a transcriptional target of c-Myc. Proc. Natl. Acad. Sci. (USA) 90: 7804-7808.
34. Gaubatz, S., Meichle, A., and Eilers, M. (1994). An E-box element localized in the first intron mediates regulation of the prothymosin a gene by c-myc. Mol. Cell. Biol. 14: 3853-3862.
35. Jansen-Dürr, P., Meichle, A., Steiner, P., Pagano, M., Finke, K., Botz, J., Wessbecher, J., Draetta, G., and Eilers, M. (1993). Differential modulation of cyclin expression by MYC. Proc. Natl. Acad. Sci. (USA) 90: 3685-3689.
36. Daksis, J.I., Lu, R.Y., Facchini, L.M., Marhin, W.W., and Penn, L.J.Z. (1994). Myc induces cyclin D1 expression in the absence of de novo protein synthesis and links mitogen-stimulated signal transduction to the cell cycle. Oncogene 9: 3635-3645, 1994.
37. Philipp, A., Schneider, A., Västrik, I., Finke, K., Xiong, Y., Beach, D., Alitalo, K., and Eilers, M. (1994). Repression fo cyclin D1: a novel function of MYC. Mol. Cell. Biol. 14: 4032-4043.
38. Galaktionov, K., Chen, X., and Beach, D. (1996). Cdc25 cell-cycle phosphatase as a target of c-myc. Nature 382: 511-517.
39. Roy, A.L., Carruthers, C., Gutjahr, T., and Roeder, R.G. (1993). Direct role for Myc in transcription initiation mediated by interactions with TFII-I. Nature 365: 359-361.
40. Li, L.-h., Nerlov, C., Prendergast, G., MacGregor, D., and Ziff, E.B. (1994). c-Myc represses transcription in vivo by a novel mechanism dependent on the initiator element and Myc box II. The EMBO J. 13: 4070-4079.
41. Mai, S. and Mårtensson, I.-L. (1995). The c-myc protein represses λ5 and TdT initiators. Nucl. Ac. Res. 23: 1-9.
42. Heikkila, R., Schwab, G., Wickstrom, E., Loke, S.L., Pluznik, D.H., Watt, R., and Neckers, L.M. (1987). A c-myc antisense oligodeoxynucleotide inhibits entry into S phase but not progress from Go to G1. Nature 328: 445-449.
42. Karn, J., Watson, J.V., Lowe, A.D., Green, S.M., and Vedeckis, W. (1989). Regulation of cell cycle duration by c-myc levels. Oncogene 4: 773-787.
43. Hanson, K.D., Shichiri, M., Follansbee, M.R., and Sedivy, J.M. (1994). Effects of c-myc expression on cell cycle progression. Mol. Cell. Biol. 14: 5748-5755.
44. Stanton, L. W., Watt, R., Marcu, K. B. (1983). Translocation, breakage, and truncated transcripts of c-myc oncogene in murine plasmacytomas. Nature 303: 401-406.

45. Potter, M. and Wiener, F. (1992). Plasmacytomagenesis in mice: model of neoplastic development dependent upon chromosomal translocation. Carcinogenesis 13: 1681-1697.
46. Feo, S., Liegro, C.D., Jones, T., Read, M., and Fried, M. (1994). The DNA region around the c-myc gene and its amplification in human tumour cell lines. Oncogene 9: 955-961.
47. Alitalo, K. (1985). Amplification of cellular oncogenes in cancer cells. TIBS 10: 194-197.
48. Classon, M., Henriksson, M., Klein, G., and Hammaskjold, M.-L. (1987). Elevated c-myc expression facilitates the replication of SV40 in human lymphoid cells. Nature 330: 272-274.
49. Classon, M., Henriksson, M., Klein, G., and Hammerskjold, M.-L. (1990). The effect of c-myc protein on SV40 replication in human lymphoid cells. Oncogene 5: 1371-1376.
50. Classon, M., Wennborg, M., Klein, G., and Sümegi, J. (1993). Analysis of c-Myc domains involved in stimulating SV40 replication. Gene 133: 153-161.
51. Luecke-Huhle, C., Mai, S., Herrlich, P. (1989). UV-inducible early-domain binding factor as the limiting component of Simian Virus 40 DNA amplification in rodent cells. Mol. Cell. Biol. 9: 4812-4818.
52. Mai, S., Lücke-Huhle, C., Kaina, B., Rahmsdorf, H.J., Stein, B., Ponta, H., and Herrlich, P. (1990). Ionizing radiation induced formation of a replication origin binding complex involving the product of the cellular oncogene c-Myc. In: Ionizing Radiation Damage of DNA. Molecular Aspects. Wiley-Liss., New York, NY, 319-331.
53. Mai, S. and Jalava, A. (1994). c-Myc binds to 5' flanking sequence motifs of the dihydrofolate reductase gene in cellular extracts: role in proliferation. Nucl. Acids Res. 22: 2264-2273.
54. Wells, J., Held, P., Illenye, S., and Heintz, N.H. (1996). Protein-DNA interactions at the major and minor promoters of the divergently transcribed *dhfr* and *rep 3* genes during the Chinese hamster ovary cell cycle. Mol. Cell. Biol. 16: 634-647.
55. Luecke-Huhle, C., Mai, S., Moll, J. (1996). Correlation of gene expression and gene amplification. Proc. of the ICRR. pp. 560-564.
56. Kunz, B. A., Kohalmi, S. E., Kunkel, T. A., Mathews, C. K., Mcintosh, E. M., Reidy, J. A. (1994). Deoxyribonucleoside triphosphate levels: a critical factor in the maintenance of genetic stability. Mut. Res. 318: 1-64.
57. Luecke-Huhle, C. (1994). Permissivity for methotrexate-induced DHFR gene amplification correlates with the metastatic potential of rat adenocarcinoma cells. Carcinogenesis 15: 695-700.

C-Myc in Lymphomagenesis

The Role of c-*myc* During Normal B Cell Proliferation, and as B Cells Undergo Malignant Transformation

E. C. Snow
Department of Microbiology and Immunology, University of Kentucky Medical Center, Lexington, Kentucky 40536-0084, USA

Introduction

c-*myc* is a protooncogene that encodes a 64 kDa nuclear protein containing carboxy-terminal leucine zipper and helix-loop-helix domains [1]. These two structural features predict a role for the Myc oncoprotein as a transcription factor requiring a protein partner. Blackwell and colleagues [2] demonstrated that Myc binds DNA in a sequence specific fashion by recognizing the sequence CAC(G/A)TG. This same group also isolated Max, a leucine zipper and helix-loop-helix protein partner for Myc [3]. Although Myc and Max homodimers can bind CAC(G/A)TG motifs with weak affinity [2, 3], the Myc:Max heterodimers demonstrate a much higher binding affinity, indicating that relative cellular levels of both these phosphoproteins is important. Max, but not Myc, is present in quiescent cells, and functions as a transcription repressor [4, 5]. Therefore, the induction of Myc expression as cells enter the cell cycle not only countermands the repression of gene expression elicited by the Max homodimers, but also results in the gradual increase in Myc:Max heterodimers that initiate growth-related gene expression. Two growth related genes known to be regulated by Myc are ornithine decarboxylase [6] and cdc25A phosphatase [7]. The appearance of Myc:Max heterodimers not only occur as cells progess into the G_1 stage of the cell cycle, but are required for cells to progress through the G_1 cell cycle stage [8]. Thus, unlike other oncoproteins that appear early during cell cycle progression, such as Fos, both c-*myc* mRNA and Myc protein are expressed at multiple cell cycle stages [9-11]. This indicates that the protein products of Myc regulated genes are available during the entire mammalian cell cycle.

Myc Expression during Normal Lymphocyte Activation

As mentioned above, Myc is not expressed by truely quiescent cells. Therefore, signals that elicit cell cycle progression must induce and regulate expression of the c-*myc* gene. Both mitogenic [12-15] or antigenic [9] stimulation of resting B cells elicits the initial appearance of c-*myc* mRNA 1-2 hours poststimulation. Although stimulation with either phorbol esters [15-17] or a calcium ionophore [15] invoke modest increases in c-*myc* mRNA in resting lymphocytes, maximum expression requires the addition of both stimulants. This finding suggests that at least one of the calcium-dependent PKC isoforms functions as a critical component in this signal transduction pathway. Even though the use of selective PKC inhibitors provided additional experimental support for the role of PKC in receptor-mediated induction of c-*myc* [15, 16, 18, 19], it is not clear which calcium-dependent PKC isoforms participate in this process. The results are consistent with the possibility that occupancy of either the T (TCR) or B (BCR) cell receptors for antigens induces c-*myc* transcription early during the activation cascade [9, 15, 20].

Since a calcium-dependent PKC appears to mediate the increase in c-*myc* gene transcription seen within hours of stimulating resting B or T cells by antigen, the question remains as to how the active, membrane-associated PKC is able to regulate a distal process, such as transcription in the nucleus. The occupancy of either the TCR or BCR results in active phosphatidylinositol metabolism, and the resultant increases in calcium fluxes enables the activation of calcium-dependent enzymes, such as calpains [21]. The activation of calpain, a neutral protease, results in the cleavage of membrane-associated PKC, releasing the proteolytic fragment PKM into the cytosol [15, 22]. Since calpain cleaves calcium-dependent PKC isoforms at the junction between the regulatory and catalytic domains, PKM exhibits constitutive kinase activity. This may be the only time that a PKC-like kinase activity exists free within the cytosol, resulting in the phosphorylation of non-membrane associated proteins, such as transcription factors. Thus, the inhibition of calpain activity blocks BCR-induced c-*myc* mRNA accumulation in resting B cell preparations [15].

NF-κB binding sites are present upstream of the c-*myc* promoter [23], and signaling through the BCR induces both active NF-κB and c-*myc* expression [24-26]. NF-κB exists as an inactive heterodimer with IκB in the cytosol. The phosphorylation of IκB on serine or threonine residues targets it for destruction in a ubiquitin-proteasome-dependent process [27, 28]. IκB serves as a substrate for PKC [29-31], and therefore, will also be a substrate to released PKM. Recent studies have indicated that this scenario may not be the only way that signaling cascades can induce transcription of c-*myc*. For example, signaling through the PDGF receptor elicits a *src* kinase-dependent induction of c-*myc* expression in NIH-3T3 cells. This signaling pathway activates NF-κB via protein tyrosine kinases, such as Src [32] and Fyn [33]. PDGF signaling appears to involve a mechanism distinct from the one described above, because the tyrosine phosphorylated IκB subunits are not degraded in a ubiquitin-proteasome-dependent fashion [34]. Moreover, the dissociation of NF-κB-IκB complexes can be mediated by Raf-1 phosphorylation of IκB [35, 36]. The implications of these additional means for activating NF-κB transcriptional activity remain to be resolved. It is possible that these alternative means for increasing NF-κB-mediated transcription might be involved in regulating c-*myc* transcription as cells move into later stages of the cell cycle.

Since quiescent cells transcribe c-*myc* at a low rate [37], cells receiving activation stimuli must either upregulate constitutive or initiate new mechanisms that allow for the accumulation of c-*myc* mRNA. Signaling through the BCR elicits increased initiation of transcription [38], and this is followed by both the removal of a constitutive block to transcriptional elongation through the c-myc gene and changes in c-*myc* mRNA stability [37, 39]. Besides the possible role of NF-κB in the initiation of c-*myc* transcription, little is known concerning how signaling mechanisms impact on cellular accumulation of c-*myc* mRNA and protein.

Even though cellular accumulation of Myc is not sufficient for passage of G_1 cells into the S phase [9], the genes regulated by Myc, such as ornithine decarboxylase [6, 40], are absolutely required for successful cell cycle progression. Not surprisingly, antisense experiments show that Myc expression is essential for cell proliferation [41]. However, cellular accumulation of Myc at inappropriate times can result in the induction of apoptosis. The consequences of this are discussed in the following sections.

Myc Expression and Induction of Apoptosis

Programmed cell death is a regulatory mechanism used by all vertebrate cellular systems, including the immune system. Naive or cycling B and T cells receiving either partial or inappropriate growth-related signals commit suicide, thereby protecting the host. This regulatory mechanism is operative during both peripheral clonal deletion of T cells binding antigen in the absence of costimulation and death of cycling follicular B cells not competitive for antigen.

Since lymphocyte apoptosis is elicited after inappropriate or partial signaling, it is not surprising that expression of some growth-related proteins is found to occur during induction of apoptosis. As might be expected, the pattern of growth-related proteins correlating with induction of apoptosis differs depending on the cell type, the activation or differentiation stage of the cells, or the apoptotic signal itself [42-45]. As described below, this is certainly found to be true when considering Myc expression as a component of apoptosis.

Myc-dependent apoptosis was initially reported by Askew and colleagues [46] studying hematopoietic cell lines cultured in either the absence or low levels of necessary growth factors. Their results confirmed previous experiments showing a correlation between elevated c-*myc* expression and apoptosis in a rodent tumors [47]. The inclusion of c-*myc* antisense oligonucleotides blocks anti-TCR-induced apoptosis in T cell hybridomas [48], clearly showing that Myc is a critical component of receptor-induced T cell death. Myc is also found expressed in follicular B cell subpopulations most susceptible to cell death in the absence of appropriate survival signals [49]. Finally, Evan and colleagues [50] demonstrated that blocking the cell cycle progression of immortalized rat fibroblasts expressing heightened Myc levels initiates the apoptotic process. Interestingly, this induction of apoptosis occurs regardless of where in the cell cycle the cells are arrested and in the absence of protein synthesis [51]. Cytokines that protect the Myc-expressing, growth factor-deprived cells from apoptosis could do so without having to re-initiate cell growth. This rules out the possibility that only cells receiving full growth stimuli become resistent to Myc-dependent apoptosis [51]. Finally, transcriptionally active Myc [50] and the presence of Max [52] are both required for the initiation of Myc-dependent apoptosis.

Recently, a 'dual signal' hypothesis has been put forward to explain Myc-dependent apoptosis [50, 51, 53]. This hypothesis predicts that accumulation of Myc during cell cycle progression elicits two cellular programmes, one involved with proliferation and the other with apoptosis. The timely appearance of either viability factors or signals promoting cell cycle progression always override the Myc-induced apoptotic pathway. In the absence of such factors or signals, the apoptotic pathway predominates and the cells die. This represents, therefore, an automatic protective mechanism in place every time the cell increases Myc levels. This includes partially activated normal B cells, as well as preneoplastic B cells exhibiting translocated c-*myc*.

Cdc25A is an integral component of the Myc-dependent apoptotic pathway [7]. Cdc25 is a dual specific phosphatase originally discovered in fission yeast as a phosphatase that activates cyclin:Cdc2 complexes by dephosphorylating tyr15 of Cdc2 [54]. This dephosphorylation is absolutely essential for optimal Cdc2 kinase activity. The same tyr residue is found to regulate the activity of both G_1 kinases, cdk4 and cdk2 [55, 56]. There are three Cdc25 homologs expressed by mammalian cells, and they are referred to as Cdc25A, Cdc25B, and Cdc25C [57-59]. In contrast to Cdc25B and Cdc25C, which function similarly to the sole yeast phosphatase by regulating cell mitosis, Cdc25A is expressed early during G_1 progression [60]. This suggests that Cdc25A functions to activate cdk4 and/or cdk2 after they bind their cyclin partners. The first hint at a possible connection between Myc expression and apoptosis came from the observation that Myc expression results in the activation of both cyclin D:cdk4 and cyclin E:cdk2 kinase complexes [61]. Galaktionov and colleagues subsequently showed that Myc expression elicits induction of Cdc25A expression [7]. It is thought that cycling cells maintain a reservoir of cyclin D:cdk4 and cyclin E:cdk2 as inactive complexes that can be quickly activated by either releasing them from inhibitory proteins [61], or by cdc25A-mediated dephosphorylation of the tyr15 residue of the kinases. The study by Galaktionov and colleagues [7] suggests that the inappropriate activation of these kinase complexes, or the activation of the complexes in the absence of addition signals, initiates a cell death pathway.

Myc and the Lymphomagenesis Process

The process of lymphomagenesis requires multiple genetic lesions [62], each providing the transforming cell with a selective survival advantage over normal lymphocytes co-localized to the same secondary lymphoid tissue. A common genetic lesion seen in many lymphoid neoplasias is the translocation of the c-*myc* protooncogene into the immunoglobulin heavy gene locus [63, 64]. This results in the constitutive expression of Myc, and the affected clones exhibit altered growth characteristics. However, transgenic mice expressing a deregulated c-*myc* gene exclusively in B lymphocytes exhibit polyclonal pre-B cell expansion without a dramatic increase in total B cells [65]. Even though this polyclonal B cell activation is detected in young transgenic mice, the appearance of pre B and B cell lymphomas does not occur until the animals are 3-4 months of age. Although B cell clones with deregulated c-*myc* display altered growth characteristics during the initial 3 or 4 months, most of these B cells seem to be short-lived. This is probably due to Myc-dependent apoptosis of those B cells not receiving required viability or growth factors. A second translocated protooncogene found in many B cell neoplasias is *bcl-2* [66]. In contrast to mice constitutively expressing Myc, mice with deregulated expression of Bcl-2 have increased numbers of small, resting B cells in their secondary lymphoid organs. This increase results from Bcl-2-dependent blockage of normal B cell turnover typically mediated by programmed cell death mechanisms [64, 67]. The *bcl-2* transgenic mice do not exhibit B cell neoplasias until 15 months of age, suggesting that constitutive expression of Bcl-2 is not, by itself, transforming [68]. Interestingly, over 50% of the B cell neoplasias isolated from 15-month old *bcl-2* transgenic mice have a translocated *c-myc* gene. The simultaneous appearance of both c-*myc* and *bcl-2* translocations is also seen in isolated human B cell neoplasias [69, 70], validating the findings with transgenic mice. The extended times required for appearance of B cell neoplasias in mice constitutively expressing either Myc or Bcl-2 exclusively in their B cells clearly supports the idea that a single genetic lesion is insufficient to establish a transformation phenotype.

Translocation of oncogenes, such as *bcl-2*, into the immunoglobulin heavy chain locus can be detected in apparently normal B cells isolated from secondary lymphoid tissues [71-73]. It is thought that during the process of VDJ rearrangement some pre B cells inadvertently undergo translocations resulting in constitutive expression of oncogenes, such as *bcl-2* or c-*myc*. Although such isolated genetic accidents are not sufficient to transform the affected B cell clones, these clones are considered to be in a preneoplastic state. If the translocation involves *bcl-2*, the affected clone has a definite survival advantage over sister clones, but such clones are not proliferative in the absence of stimulants that normally regulate B cell expansion. The antigen-mediated activation of such clones will initiate clonal expansion, and this also provides the opportunity for secondary translocations to occur. If, for example, c-*myc* undergoes secondary translocation, the affected clone adds a growth advantage to the already existing survival advantage, resulting in a transformed cell. Conversely, if the first translocation involves c-*myc*, the affected clone receives a selective growth advantage over its sister clones. This advantage is countermanded by the c-*myc*-dependent death cascade described above [50, 51]. As long as such clones continue to receive either growth or survival signals from their environment, they will survive. Because of biological limitations there is an increased probability that such clones will be deleted. However, a secondary translocation of *bcl-2* blocks the c-*myc*-induced death pathway [74, 75] providing the clone, again, with both a growth and survival advantage.

The above considerations suggest that normal antigenic stimulation of B cells may contribute to the transformation of B cell clones that have undergone a single translocation of a protooncogene during their developmental period. Thus, sequence analyses of immunoglobulin heavy chain genes isolated from B cell neoplasias reveal nucleotide substitutions consistent with clonal selection being involved during the lymphomagenesis process [76-79]. This means that signaling through the BCR may contribute to the continued expansion of these transformed B cells. The problem with this interpretation is that cross-linking BCR expressed by B lymphoma cells typically induces apoptosis [80-82]. Since T cell-mediated signals can rescue anti-BCR stimulated B lymphoma cells [83-86], it appears that in many cases the antigen-stimulated preneoplastic and neoplastic B cells must recruit appropriate T helper (Th) cell activity to survive.

A histopathologic examination of human lymphomas revealed that $CD4^+$ T cells are routinely seen to infiltrate sites of B lymphoma cell accumulation within secondary lymphoid tissues [87]. In addition, both murine [82, 83] and human [88, 89] B cell lymphomas require T cells and/or their soluble mediators to proliferate *in vitro*. Based on these experiments, it is reasonable to suggest that normal Th cells can participate in both the lymphomagenesis process and serve as a continuing sources of growth and viability signals for the neoplastic B cells.

If neoplastic B cells require Th cell-induced survival or growth signals, a mechanism must exist for the transformed cells to continuously recruit Th cell activity. Possible ways include recruiting either T cells specific for the same autoantigen as the neoplastic B cell [90] or T cells that recognize idiotypic determinants of the neoplastic B cell's BCR [76]. It is important to remember that the Th cells recruited by the neoplastic B cells are normal, and, therefore, subject to the regulatory mechanisms in place that limit T cell immune responses. This makes it unlikely that either of these mechanisms can provide the requisite long-term Th cell activity. A third possibility is that the transformed B cells express a dormant, retrovirally encoded superantigen (vSAG) [91].

A Model for the Transformation of B Cells

This model is based on the assumption that the first step in the transformation of normal B cells into lymphoma cells is the translocation of either *bcl-2* or c-*myc* into the heavy chain locus during VDJ rearrangement. The available information seems to indicate that *bcl-2* translocations are more frequently seen in B cells that survive long enough to migrate into secondary lymphoid tissues [71-73]. This probably is less a reflection of the actual frequency of c-*myc* translocations, and more the result of constitutive Myc expression initiating apoptosis in B cells not receiving additional signals. Lymphomagenesis continues when a B cell clone expressing a *bcl-2* translocation becomes activated in an antigen-dependent fashion, with the initial process similar to that seen when any B cell clone encounters its specific antigen. The difference is that the expanded, antigen reactive clones constitutively express Bcl-2 are not subject to the usual antigen-mediated clonal selection mechanism. This occurs because Bcl-2 blocks the ability of these B cells to die in the absence of antigen- or Th cell-derived signals. Although long-lived, these clones are basically harmless in the absence of either additional genetic translocations or the appearance of some form of continuous stimulation. Even if the preneoplastic clone is specific for an autoantigen, it is unlikely that appropriate Th cell activity can be recruited over an extended time as the result of Th cell directed regulatory mechanisms.

We have previously suggested [91] that one way to continuously provide recruitable Th cell activity is for the preneoplastic B cell to express a dormant vSAG. This prediction is based on studies by Thorbecke and colleagues [92, 93] that looked at spontaneously arising B cell lymphomas in SJL mice. Their results demonstrated that lymphoma infiltrating T cells expressed restricted V_β usage, and that the B lymphoma cells could stimulate both expansion and lymphokine secretion of T cell hybridomas prepared from these tumor infiltrating T cells. Finally, they went on to clone mouse mammary tumor virus encoded vSAG from some of these B cell lymphomas, and showed that these vSAG are responsible for the ability of the B lymphoma cells to stimulate the T hybridoma cells.

The accidental expression of a dormant vSAG during antigen-mediated expansion of a B cell clone bearing a translocated protooncogene has profound implications. First, such B cells can recruit Th cell activity from up to 20% of all available T cells. Second, the Th cell recruitment has the potential to be long-term because the vSAG expressing B cells can continue to recruit new Th cells bearing the appropriate V_β chain(s) indefinitely. The process is independent of normal regulatory mechanisms aimed at controlling Th cell activity, since the loss of any particular Th cell reactivity occurs in an antigen specific manner. This will not effect the other Th cells present that happen to express the same V_β chain(s) but have distinct antigenic reactivity. Third, the continuous focusing of Th cell activity onto these B cells will initiate a lymphoproliferative disorder. The uncontrolled expansion of these B cells exposes them to the danger of developing additional genetic lesions, such as the translocation of c-*myc* into the immunoglobulin heavy chain locus. Finally, a role for specific antigen is not required, except for initiating the process. However, if the transformed cell is specific for an autoantigen, a role for signaling through the BCR over an extended time is possible. The consequences of this are not clear.

This same mechanism can be used to transform B cell clones that initially translocate c-*myc* into the heavy chain locus, except that the Myc expressing clones will require the immediate recruitment of continuous Th cell activity to survival. Alternatively, if the initial genetic lesion is the activation of a dormant vSAG, then c-*myc* or *bcl-2* translocation could occur during the ensuring lymphoproliferative disorder.

It is important to recall that it is improbable that B cells with a single genetic lesion survive. A reflection of this is that the frequency of inappropriate chromosomal rearrangements seen in peripheral B cells is much higher than the observable frequency of B cell neoplasias [71, 72]. Although not absolutely required for B cell transformation, the expression of a dormant vSAG greatly enhances the probability that the B cell will proliferate with sufficient intensity to increase the chances for the appearance of single or multiple genetic lesions. An additional benefit is that vSAG expressing, transformed B cells can continuously focus growth and survival signals onto themselves, therefore, maintaining a long-term competitive growth and survival advantage over co-localized sister clones.

Aknowledgments. I thank Dr. Thomas Roszman and Mr. Brian Pittner for their helpful comments on the manuscript.

References

1. Luscher B, Eisenman RN (1990) New light on Myc and Myb. Part I. Myc. Genes Dev 4*:*2025-2035.
2. Blackwell TK, Kretzner L, Blackwood EM, Eisenman RN, Weintraub H (1990) Sequence-specific DNA binding by the c-*myc* protein. Science 250*:*1149-1151.
3. Blackwood EM, Eisenman RN (1991) Max: a helix-loop-helix zipper protein that forms a sequence-specific DNA-binding complex with Myc. Science 251*:*1211-1217.
4. Kretzner L, Blackwood EM, Eisenman RN (1992) Myc and Max proteins possess distinct transcriptional activities. Nature 359*:*426-429.
5. Gu W, Cechova K, Tassi V, Dalla-Favera R (1993) Opposite regulation of gene transcription and cell proliferation by c-*myc* and Max. Proc Natl Acad Sci USA 90*:*2935-2939.
6. Bello-Fernandez C, Packham G, Cleveland JL (1993) The ornithine decarboxylase gene is a transcriptional target of c-*myc*. Proc Natl Acad Sci USA 90*:*7804-7808.
7. Galaktionov K, Chen X, Beach D (1996) Cdc25 cell-cycle phosphatase as a target of c-*myc*. Nature 382*:*511-517.
8. Roussel MF, Cleveland JL, Shurtleff SA, Sherr CJ (1991) Myc rescue of a mutant CSF-1 receptor impaired in mitogenic signalling. Nature 353*:*361-363.
9. Shipp MA, Reinherz EL (1987) Differential expression of nuclear proto-oncogenes in T cells triggered with mitogenic and nonmitogenic T3 and T11 ctivation signals. J Immunol 139*:*2143-2148.
10. Hann SR, Thompson CB, Eisenman RN (1985) c-*myc* oncogene protein synthesis is independent of the cell cycle in human and avian cells. Nature 314*:*366-369.
11. Thompson CB, Challoner PB, Neiman PE, Groudine M (1993) Levels of c-*myc* oncogene mRNA are invariant throughout the cell cycle. Nature 314*:*363-366.

12. Smeland E, Godal T, Ruud E, Beiske K, Funderud S, Clark EA, Pfeifer-Ohlsson S, Ohlsson R (1985) The specific induction of *myc* protooncogene expression in normal human B cells is not a sufficient event for acquisition of competence to proliferate. Proc Natl Acad Sci USA 82*:*6255-6259.
13. Snow EC, Fetherston JD, Zimmer S (1986) Induction of the c-*myc* protooncogene after antigen binding to hapten-specific B cells. J Exp Med 164*:*944-949.
14. Kelly K, Cochran BH, Stiles CD, Leder P (1983) Cell-specific regulation of the c-*myc* gene by lymphocyte mitogens and platelet-derived growth factor. Cell 35*:*603-610.
15. Pollok KE, Snow EC (1991) The proteolysis of membrane-associated protein kinase C as a possible component of the signalling pathway leading to c-*myc* induction. Cell Signalling 3*:*435-452.
16. Coughlin SR, Lee WMF, Williams PW, Giels GM, Williams LT (1985) c-*myc* gene expression is stimulated by agents that activate protein kinase C and does not account for the mitogenic effect of PDGF. Cell 43*:*243-251.
17. Morris DR, Allen ML, Rabinovitch PS, Kuepfer CA, White MW (1988) Mitogenic signaling pathways regulating expression of c-*myc* and ornithine decarboxylase genes in bovine T-lymphocytes. Biochemistry 27*:*8689-8693.
18. Wright TC, Pukac LA, Castellot JJ, Karnovsky MJ, Levine RA, Kim-Park H-Y, Campisi J (1989) Heparin suppresses the induction of c-*fos* and c-*myc* mRNA in murine fibroblasts by selective inhibition of a protein kinase C-dependent pathway. Proc Natl Acad Sci USA 86*:*3199-3203.
19. Spangler R, Bailey SC, Sytkowski AJ (1991) Erythropoietin increases c-*myc* mRNA by a protein kinase C-dependent pathway. J Biol Chem 266*:*681-684.
20. Reed JC, Nowell PC, Hoover RG (1985) Regulation of c-*myc* mRNA levels in normal human lymphocytes by modulators of cell proliferation. Proc Natl Acad Sci USA 82*:*4221-4224.
21. Mellgren RL (1987) Calcium-dependent proteases: an enzyme system active at cellular membranes. FASEB J 1*:*110-115.
22. Cressman CM, Mohan PS, Nixon RA, Shea TB (1995) Proteolysis of protein kinase C: mM and μM calcium-requiring calpains have different abilities to generate, and degrade the free catalytic subunit, protein kinase M. FEBS 367*:*223-227.
23. Duyao MP, Buckler AJ, Sonenshein GE (1990) Interaction of an NF-κB-like factor with a site upstream of the c-*myc* promoter. Proc Natl Acad Sci USA 87*:*4727-4731.
24. Liu J, Chiles TC, Sen R, Rothstein TL (1991) Inducible nuclear expression of NF-κB in primary B cells stimulated through the surface Ig receptor. J Immunol 146*:*1685-1691.
25. Lee H, Arsura M, Wu M, Duyao M, Buckler AJ, Sonenshein GE (1995) Role of Rel-related factors in control of c-*myc* gene transcription in receptor-mediated apoptosis of the murine B cell WEHI 231 line. J Exp Med 181*:*1169-1177.
26. Schauer SL, Wang Z, Sonenshein GE, Rothstein TL (1996) Maintenance of nuclear factor-κB/Rel and c-*myc* expression during CD40 ligand rescue of WEHI 231 early B cells from receptor-mediated apoptosis through modulation of IκB proteins. J Immunol 157*:*81-86.
27. Palombella VJ, Rando OJ, Goldberg AL, Maniatis T (1994) The ubiquitin-proteasome pathway is required for processing the NF-κB1 precursor protein and the activation of NF-κB. Cell 78*:*773-785.
28. Alkalay I, Yaron A, Hatzubai A, Orian A, Ciechanover A, Ben-Neriah Y (1995) Stimulation-dependent IκBα phosphorylation marks the NF-κB inhibitor for degradation via the ubiquitin-proteasome pathway. Proc Natl Acad Sci USA 92*:*10599-10603.
29. Shirakawa F, Mizel SB (1989) *In vitro* activation and nuclear translocation of NF-κB catalyzed by cyclic AMP-dependent protein kinase and protein kinase C. Mol Cell Biol 9*:*2424-2430.
30. Ghosh S, Baltimore D (1990) Activation *in vitro* of NF-κB by phosphorylation of its inhibitor IκB. Nature 344*:*678-682.
31. Bomsztyk K, Rooney JW, Iwasaki T, Rachie NA, Dower SK, Sibley CH (1991) Evidence that interleukin-1 and phorbol esters activate NF-κB by different pathways: role of protein kinase C. Cell Regul 2*:*329-335.
32. Eicher DM, Tan T-H, Rice NR, O'Shea JJ, Kennedy ICS (1994) Expression of v-*src* in T cells correlates with nuclear expression of NF-κB. J immunol 152*:*2710-2717.
33. Hohashi N, Hayashi T, Fusaki N, Takeuchi M, Higurashi M, Okamoto T, Semba K, Yamamoto T (1995) The protein tyrosine kinase Fyn activates transcription from the HIV promoter via activation of NF-κB-like DNA-binding proteins. Inter Immunol 7*:*1851-1859.
34. Imbert V, Rupec RA, Livolsi A, Pahl HL, Traenckner EB-M, Mueller-Dieckmann C, Farahifar D, Rossi B, Auberger P, Baeuerle PA, Peyron J-F (1996) Tyrosine phosphorylation of IκB-α activates NF-κB without proteolytic degradation of IκB-α. Cell 86*:*787-798.
35. Finco TS, Baldwin AS (1993) κB site-dependent induction of gene expression by diverse induces of nuclear factor κB requires Raf-1. J Biol Chem 268*:*17676-17679.
36. Li S, Sedivy JM (1993) Raf-1 protein kinase activates the NF-κB transcription factor by dissociating the cytoplasmic NF-κB-IκB complex. Proc Natl Acad Sci USA 90*:*9247-9251.
37. Lindsten T, June CH, Thompson CB (1988) Multiple mechanisms regulate c-*myc* gene expression during normal T cell activation. EMBO J 7*:*2787-2794.

38. Buckler AJ, Rothstein TL, Sonenshein GE (1990) Transcriptional control of c-*myc* gene expression during stimulation of murine B lymphocytes. J Immunol 145*:*732-736.
39. Reed JC, Alpers JD, Nowell PC (1987) Expression of c-*myc* proto-oncogene in normal human lymphocytes. Regulation by transcription and posttranscriptional mechanisms. J Clin Invest 80*:*101-106.
40. Pollok KE, O'Brien V, Marshall L, Olson JW, Noelle RJ, Snow EC (1991) The development of competence in resting B cells. The induction of cyclic AMP and ornithine decarboxylase activity after direct contact between B and T helper cells. J Immunol 146*:*1633-1641.
41. Heikkila R, Schwab G, Wickstrom E, Loke SL, Pluznik DH, Watt R, Neckers LM (1987) A c-*myc* antisense oligodeoxynucleotide inhibits entry into S phase but not progress from G0 to G1. Nature 328*:*445-449.
42. Fotedar R, Flatt J, Gupta S, Margolis RL, Fitzgerald P, Messier H, Fotedar A (1995) Activation-induced T-cell death is cell cycle dependent and regulated by cyclin B. Mol Cell Biol 15*:*932-942.
43. Wang Q, Worland PJ, Clark JL, Carlson BA, Sausville EA (1995) Apoptosis in 7-hydroxystaurospurine-treated T lymphoblasts correlates with activation of cyclin-dependent kinases 1 and 2. Cell Growth Different 6*:*927-936.
44. Takata M, Homma Y, Kurosaki T (1995) Requirement of phospholipase C-γ2 activation in surface immunoglobulin M-induced B cell apoptosis. J Exp Med 182*:*907-914.
45. Anderson KL, Anderson G, Michell RH, Jenkinson EJ, Owen JJT (1996) Intracellular signaling pathways involved in the induction of apoptosis in immature thymic T lymphocytes. J Immunol 156*:*4083-4091.
46. Askew D, Ashmun R, Simmons B, Cleveland J (1991) Constitutive c-*myc* expression in IL-3-dependent myeloid cell line suppresses cycle arrest and accelerates apoptosis. Oncogene 6*:*1915-1922.
47. Wyllie AH, Rose KA, Morris RG, Steel CM, Foster E, Spandidos DA (1987) Rodent fibroblast tumours expressing human *myc* and *ras* genes: growth, metastasis and endogenous oncogene expression. Br J Cancer 56*:*251-259.
48. Shi Y, M. GJ, Guibert LJ, Cotter TG, Bissonnette RP, Green DR (1992) Role for c-*myc* in activation-induced apoptotic cell death in T cell hybridomas. Science 257*:*212-214.
49. Martinez-Valdez H, Guret C, de Bouteiller O, Fugier I, Banchereau J, Liu Y-J (1996) Human germinal center B cells express the apoptosis-inducing genes Fas, c-*myc*, P53, and Bax but not the survival gene Bcl-2. J Exp Med 183*:*971-977.
50. Evan GI, Wyllie AH, Gilbert CS, Littlewood TD, Land H, Brooks M, Waters CM, Penn LZ, Hancock DC (1992) Induction of apoptosis in fibroblasts by c-*myc* protein. Cell 69*:*119-128.
51. Harrington EA, Bennett MR, Fanidi A, Evan GI (1994) c-Myc-induced apoptosis in fibroblasts is inhibited by specific cytokines. EMBO J 13*:*3286-3295.
52. Amati B, Littlewood TD, Evan GI, Land H (1993) The c-Myc protein induces cell cycle progression and apoptosis through dimerization with Max. EMBO J 12*:*5083-5087.
53. Evan GL, Littlewood TD (1993) The role of c-*myc* in cell growth. Curr Opin Genet Dev 3*:*44-49.
54. Labib K, Nurse P (1993) Bring on the phosphatases. Curr Biol 3*:*164-166.
55. Gu Y, Rosenblatt J, Morgan DO (1992) Cell cycle regulation of CDK2 activity by phosphorylation of Thr160 and Tyr15. EMBO J 11*:*3995-4005.
56. Matsushime H, Ewen ME, Strom DK, Kato JY, Hanks SK, Roussel MF, Scherr CJ (1992) Identification and properties of an atypical catalytic subunit ($p34^{psk-J3}$/cdk4) for mammalian D type G1 cyclins. Cell 71*:*323-334.
57. Sadhu K, Reed SI, Richardson H, Russel P (1990) Human homolog of fission yeast cdc25 mitotic inducer is predominately expressed in G2. Proc Natl Acad Sci USA 87*:*5139-5143.
58. Galaktionov K, Beach D (1991) Specific activation of cdc25 tyrosine phosphatases by B-type cyclins: evidence for multiple roles of mitotic cyclins. Cell 67*:*1181-1194.
59. Nagata A, Igarashi M, Jinno S, Suot K, Okayama H (1991) An additional homolog of the fission yeast cdc25+ gene occurs in humans and is highly expressed in some cancer cells. New Biol 3*:*959-968.
60. Jinno S, Suto K, Nagata A, Igarashi M, Kanaoka Y, Nojima H, Okayama H (1994) Cdc25A is a novel phosphatase functioning early in the cell cycle. EMBO J 13*:*1549-1556.
61. Steiner P, Philipp A, Lukas J, Godden-Kent D, Pagano M, Mittnacht S, Bartek J, Eilers M (1995) Identification of a Myc-dependent step during the formation of active G1 cyclin-cdk complexes. EMBO J 14*:*4814-4826.
62. Magrath I (1992) Molecular basis of lymphomagenesis. Cancer Res (Suppl) 52*:*5529s-5540s.
63. Klein G, Klein E (1985) Myc/Ig juxtaposition by chromosomal translocations: some new insights, puzzles and paradoxes. Immunol Today 6*:*208-215.
64. Cory S (1986) Activation of cellular oncogenes in hemopoietic cells by chromosomal translocations. Adv Cancer Res 47*:*189-234.
65. Langdon WY, Harris AW, Cory S, Adams JM (1986) The c-*myc* oncogene perturbs B lymphocyte development in Eu-myc transgenic mice. Cell 47*:*11-18.

66. Tsujimoto Y, Cossman J, Jaffe E, Croce CM (1985) Involvement of the *bcl-2* gene in human follicular lymphoma. Science 228*:*1440-1443.

67. McDonnel TJ, Deane N, Platt FM, Nunez G, Jaeger U, McKearn JP, Korsmeyer SJ (1989) *bcl-2*-immunoglobulin transgenic mice demonstrate extended B cell survival and follicular lymphoproliferation. Cell 57*:*79-88.

68. McDonnell TJ, Korsmeyer SJ (1991) Progression from lymphoid hyperplasia to high-grade malignant lymphoma in mice transgenic for the t(14; 18). Nature 349*:*254-256.

69. Gauwerky CE, Haluska FG, Tsujimoto Y, Nowell PC, Croce CM (1988) Evolution of B-cell malignancy: Pre-B-cell leukemia resulting from MYC activation in a B-cell neoplasm with a rearranged BCL2 gene. Proc Natl Acad Sci USA 85*:*8548-8552.

70. de Jong D, Voetdijk BMH, Beverstock GC, van Ommen GJB, Willemze R, Kluin PM (1988) Activation of the c-*myc* oncogene in a precursor-B-cell blast crisis of follicular lymphoma, presenting as composite lymphoma. N Engl J Med 318*:*1373-1378.

71. Limpens J, de Jong D, van Krieken JHJM, Price CGA, Young BD, Van Ommen GJB, Kluin PM (1991) *Bcl-2*/Jh rearrangements in benign lymphoid tissues with follicular hyperplasia. Oncogene 6*:*2271-2276.

72. Price CGA, Tuszynski A, Watt SM, Murdoch SJ, Lister TA, Young BD (1991) Detection of additional JH/BCL2 translocations in follicular lymphoma. Leukemia 5*:*548-554.

73. Aster JC, Kobayashi Y, Shiota M, Mori S, Sklar J (1992) Detection of the t(14; 18) at similar frequencies in hyperplastic lymphoid tissues from Americans and Japanese patients. Am J Pathol 141*:*291-299.

74. Bissonnette RP, Echeverri F, Mahboubi A, Green DR (1992) Apoptotic cell death induced by c-*myc* is inhibited by *bcl-2*. Nature 359*:*552-554.

75. Fanidi A, Harrington EA, Evan GI (1992) Cooperative interaction between c-*myc* and *bcl-2* proto-oncogenes. Nature 359*:*554-556.

76. Friedman DF, Cho EA, Goldman J, Carmack CE, Besa EC, Hardy RR, Silberstein LE (1991) The role of clonal selection in the pathogenesis of autoreactive human B cell lymphoma. J Exp Med 174*:*525-537.

77. Zelenetz AD, Chen TT, Levy R (1991) Histologic transformation of follicular lymphoma to diffuse lymphoma represents tumor progression by a single malignant B cell. J Exp Med 173*:*197-207.

78. Bahler DW, Levy R (1992) Clonal evolution of a follicular lymphoma: evidence for antigen selection. Proc Natl Acad Sci USA 89*:*6770-6774.

79. Zelenetz AD, Chen TT, Levy R (1992) Clonal expansion in follicular lymphoma occurs subsequent to antigenic selection. J Exp Med 176*:*1137-1148.

80. Boyd AW, Schrader JS (1981) The regulation of growth and differentiation of a murine B cell lymphoma. II. The inhibition of WEHI-231 by anti-immunoglobulin. J Immunol 126*:*2466-2469.

81. Jakway JP, Usinger WR, Gold MR, Mishell RI, DeFranco AL (1986) Growth regulation of the B lymphoma cell line WEHI-231 by anti-immunoglobulin, lipopolysaccharide, and other bacterial products. J Immunology 137*:*2225-2231.

82. Udhayakumar V, Brodeur PH, Rajagopalan MS, Zimmer S, Pollok KE, Subbarao B (1989) Isolation and immunological characterization of a group of new B lymphomas from CBA mice. Clin Immunol Immunopath 51*:*240-251.

83. Ales-Martinez JE, Silver L, LoCascio N, Scott DW (1991) Lymphoma models for B-cell activation and tolerance. IX. Efficient reversal of anti-Ig-mediated growth inhibition by an activated Th2 clone. Cell Immunol 135*:*402-409.

84. Valentine MA, Licciardi KA (1992) Rescue from anti-IgM-induced programmed cell death by the B cell surface proteins CD20 and CD40. Eur J Immunol 22*:*3141-3148.

85. Sumimoto SI, Heike T, Kanazashi SI, Shintaku N, Jung EY, Hata D, Katamura K, Mayumi M (1994) Involvement of LFA-1/intracellular adhesion molecule-1-dependent cell adhesion in CD40-mediated inhibition of human B lymphoma cell death induced by surface IgM crosslinking. J Immunol 153*:*2488-2496.

86. Muthukkumar S, Bondada S (1995) Involvement of CD5 in Th1 and Th2 contact-mediated rescue of anti-μ and ionomycin induced growth inhibition in a B cell lymphoma. Int Immunol 7*:*305-315.

87. Dvoretsky P, Wood GS, Levy R, Warnke RA (1982) T lymphocyte subsets in follicular lymphomas compared with those in non-neoplastic lymph nodes and tonsils. Hum Path 13*:*618-625.

88. Tweeddale ME, Lim B, Jamal N, Robinson JM, Zalcberg J, Lockwood G, Minden MD, Messner HA (1987) The presence of clonogenic cells in high-grade malignant lymphoma: a prognostic factor. Blood 69*:*307-314.

89. Umetsu DT, Esserman L, Donlon TA, DeKruyff RH, Levy R (1990) Induction of proliferation of human follicular (B type) lymphoma cells by cognate interaction with $CD4^+$ T cell clones. J Immunol 144*:*2550-2557.

90. Bahler DW, Zelenetz AD, Chen TT, Levy R (1992) Antigen selection in human lymphomagenesis. Cancer Res (Suppl) 52*:*5547s-5551s.

91. Snow EC, Pittner B, Reid S (1994) T helper cell regulation of normal and neoplastic B cell growth. Sem Immunol 6:311-326.
92. Tsiagbe VK, Asakawa J, Miranda A, Sutherland RM, Paterson Y, Thorbecke GJ (1993) Syngeneic response to SJL follicular center B cell lymphoma (reticular cell sarcoma) cells is primarily in $V_{\beta}16^{+}$ $CD4^{+}$ T cells. J Immunol 150:5519-5528.
93. Tsiagbe VK, Yoshimoto T, Asakawa J, Cho SY, Meruelo D, Thorbecke GJ (1993) Linkage of superantigen-like stimulation of syngeneic T cells in a mouse model of follicular center B cell lymphoma to transcription of endogenous mammary tumor virus. EMBO J 12:2313-2320.

Lymphomas and Plasmacytomas in Transgenic Mice Involving *Bcl2*, *Myc* and v-*Abl*

A. W. HARRIS, A. STRASSER, M. L. BATH, A. G. ELEFANTY and S. CORY
The Walter and Eliza Hall Institute of Medical Research, PO Royal Melbourne Hospital, Melbourne 3050, Australia

Introduction

During the past twelve years, our laboratory has been analyzing the tumorigenic potential of oncogenes in the lymphoid system of transgenic mice (for reviews see Adams and Cory 1991, 1992). Tissue specific expression of the oncogenes in these animals was achieved by including in the transgene constructs an enhancer sequence (Eμ) from the mouse immunoglobulin heavy chain locus. In most individual strains resulting from the introduction of such constructs, expression was confined to the B lymphoid lineage while a small minority of strains showed expression in both T and B lineages or only in T cells. The pattern for each strain has proved to be stable over many generations of breeding.

A single activated oncogene added to the mouse germline may alter the behavior of the cells that express it (e.g. see Langdon et al. 1986, Strasser et al. 1991), but it does not directly render those cells tumorigenic. To become malignant, a cell must acquire multiple genetic alterations in cooperatively acting oncogenes and tumor-suppressor genes. Thus, the single introduced oncogene will appear more or less strongly predisposing to tumorigenesis in the transgenic mouse, according to the likelihood that one of its oncogene-expressing cells will acquire a cooperative set of additional mutations during a practically feasible observation period, typically 12-18 months. In some cases, the activity of an oncogene that appears weak by this criterion can be revealed more clearly by combining the gene with a second, cooperating oncogene or inactivated tumor-suppressor gene through a genetic cross with appropriate transgenic or gene knockout mice. Another means of altering the apparent tumorigenic activity is to vary the genetic background of a transgenic strain by introducing the transgene into mice of different inbred strains. Examples of both of these will be described here.

Spontaneous Lymphoid Tumors in *bcl2* mice

The *bcl2* gene was first identified as the locus juxtaposed to the *Igh* locus by the t(14;18) chromosome translocation in human follicular lymphoma (Tsujimoto et al. 1984). While it has a viability-sustaining action on cells that express it as a transgene in mice or in cultured cell lines of various types (for reviews see Cory 1995, Korsmeyer 1996), its lymphoma-predisposing action seems to be weak. B cells bearing the chromosome translocation are detectable by polymerase chain reaction-based assay in the blood of most normal individuals (Limpens et al. 1995), only a tiny proportion of whom would eventually develop lymphoma. In *bcl2* transgenic mice, the tumor incidence is low and the tumor latent period is long. Our initial work on *bcl2* mice with a (C57BL/6 × SJL)F2 genetic background, monitored up to one year of age, found a tumor incidence of less than 10% (Strasser et al. 1993). Pooled data from several independent Eμ-*bcl2*-transgenic strains that expressed the transgene in B cells yielded a crude incidence of 3% for plasmacytomas and 5% for early B-lineage tumors. The plasmacytomas carried rearrangements of the *myc* gene, implying that spontaneous *myc*-activating chromosome translocations played a role in their transformation to malignancy. The low figures for incidence were significant because neither plasmacytomas nor early B cell tumors were seen at all in non-transgenic littermates. For T cell-expressing strains, on the other hand, the incidence of T cell lymphoma of only 2% at 12 months of age was not significantly different from that found in non-transgenic (C57BL/6 × SJL)F2 mice.

Longer-term monitoring of tumor formation in several independently derived *bcl2*-Ig and *lck^{pr}-bcl2* mouse strains with a (C57BL/6 × C3H)F2 background has been carried out in the Korsmeyer laboratory. The *bcl2*-Ig strains produced some diffuse large cell lymphomas, mostly in the second year of life (McDonnell et al. 1991). These lymphomas were morphologically similar to the tumors we designated plasmacytomas from the associated clonal immunoglobulins in the serum of affected mice. Again like the plasmacytomas, the diffuse large cell lymphomas often carried a rearranged *myc* gene. Among the *lck^{pr}-bcl2* strains, peripheral T cell lymphomas were found in the second year of life. The incidence was 13% at 18 months, progressing to 26% at 2 yr (Linette et al. 1995).

To produce genetically uniform transgenic strains and to test for genetic polymorphism of tumor susceptibility, we transferred our Eμ-*bcl2* transgenes by serial backcrossing into inbred strains. On a C57BL/6 (B6, N9-10) background, the tumor incidence at 12 months was insignificant (one case of lymphoma among 97 mice), and even at 18 months only five mice in a cohort of 56 developed lymphoid tumors (four lymphoblastic lymphomas and one plasmacytoma). Thus, the B6 constitution is less prone to support *bcl2*-initiated tumorigenesis than that of B6-SJL (or B6-C3H) mice. This result is similar to those we have obtained by transferring more strongly tumor-predisposing transgenes such as Eμ-*myc*, Eμ-*Nras* and Eμ-v-*abl* from their initial B6-SJL context into inbred B6 mice (Sidman et al. 1988; our unpublished observations, and see below). In each case, the rate at which tumors appeared was reduced, implying a degree of general resistance to lymphoid tumorigenesis in the B6 strain.

Relative to B6 mice, BALB/c mice seem generally to be more prone to support the development of lymphoid malignancy. A long-established example can be found in the generation of plasmacytomas by intraperitoneally administered irritants such as mineral oil or pristane (Potter et al. 1975). Further examples come from our own work on spontaneous pre-B and B cell lymphomas provoked by an Eμ-*myc* transgene, and pre-B and T cell lymphomas by an Eμ-v-*abl* transgene (Harris 1991, and see below). To test whether such a susceptible genetic background would hasten the emergence of plasmacytomas and lymphomas in *bcl2* mice, we serially backcrossed the Eμ-*bcl2*-22 transgene into the BALB/c strain. In the 10th and 18th generations of such backcrossing, only a single lymphoblastic lymphoma developed in a group of 72 mice observed to 12 months of age. Extending the monitoring period on 30 mice to 18 months yielded only one lymphoma and one plasmacytoma. This very low incidence was unexpected, particularly since the accumulation of B lymphocytes induced by transgene expression in the BALB/c mice was about twice as great as that induced in the B6-SJL mice (Harris, 1993). Thus, even with the putatively tumor-permissive BALB/c strain, we have been unable so far to generate an inbred model for *bcl2*-initiated lymphoid tumorigenesis that produces a useful incidence of tumors in a reasonable observation period.

Cooperative Tumorigenesis by *bcl2* and *myc* Transgenes

The plasmacytomas arising spontaneously in *bcl2*-transgenic mice frequently bear rearrangements of *myc* (see above), and aggressive tumors that develop from indolent, t(14;18)-bearing follicular lymphomas in humans are sometimes found to have acquired an additional 8;14 (*Igh–myc*) chromosome translocation (e.g. see de Jong et al. 1988). These findings, together with experiments showing transformation of mouse pre-B cells in culture by enforced coexpression of *myc* and *bcl2* (Vaux et al. 1988), indicated that the two genes could cooperate in promoting malignancy at each of the three major stages of B lymphoid differentiation. Cooperation was also demonstrated in doubly transgenic *bcl2–myc* mice, but the malignancy that developed in these animals was composed of a previously unrecognized cell type, initially postulated to be a lymphoid progenitor or stem cell (Strasser et al. 1990). The tumor picture was remarkably uniform for the two strains of Eμ-*bcl2* mice (strains 22 and 36) tested in crosses with Eμ-*myc* mice; by 5 weeks of age all of the mice that inherited both a *bcl2* and a *myc* transgene developed terminal, widely disseminated tumors with the microscopic morphology of lymphoblastic lymphoma. None was a pre-B lymphoma or a plasmacytoma. All of the tumors analyzed from more than a dozen bi-transgenic mice had the same surface-marker phenotype (Table 1), which did not correspond to that of any known T or B lymphoid cell.

The novelty of the tumor cell type prompted us to grow the cells in culture so that their character could be assessed in more detail. This proved to be much more difficult than establishing cell lines from pre-B, B or T lymphomas. Given the overexpression of Bcl2 protein and the rapid growth of the tumors on transplantation in mice, it was surprising that the *bcl2–myc* tumor cells died rapidly in culture. They could not be rescued by supplementing the medium with cytokines and growth factors, singly or in multiple combinations. After many tests on transplanted tumor cells, however, conditions were identified that could sustain viability, and some interesting cell lines were developed (Strasser et al. 1996).

In cultures initiated with $>10^6$ tumor cells in the absence of added cytokines, almost all of the tumor cells died, but a few growing cells emerged and subsequently proliferated as continuous lines. These cells no longer displayed the distinctive markers of the initial tumor cells, Thy 1 (low), Sca-1, Gr-1 and CD4, but expressed CD19 and HSA (as well as B220) and bore *Igh* rearrangements, identifying them as pre-B cells. Differentiation further down the B lymphoid lineage was seen in tumor cells that survived culture on monolayers of the bone marrow-derived stromal cell line AC-6. The continuous cell lines developed from these cultures had undergone both *Igh* and *Igk* rearrangement and the cells expressed IgM on their surface, defining them as B cells.

Table 1. Surface phenotype of tumor cells from bi-transgenic *bcl2–myc* mice

Cell surface marker	Expression*
B220	+
CD4	+
Thy-1	+ (low)
Sca-1	+
class II MHC	+
NK-1.1	–
IgM, CD19, CD43, BP-1	–
CD25, CD8, CD3	–
Mac-1	–

* assayed by flow cytometric analysis of immunofluorescence (Strasser et al. 1996)

Another type of cell could be grown from the *bcl2–myc* tumors by culture in medium supplemented with a mixture of either lipopolysaccharide and leukemia inhibitory factor, or interleukins 1, 3 and 6. As in the previous cultures, most of the cells died in the first few days, but then the cultures spawned larger, semi-adherent, proliferating cells that lacked B lymphoid markers but had acquired myeloid cell character. Their *Igh* and *Tcrb* genes were unrearranged and they expressed Mac-1, F4/80 and *fms*. Under treatment with IL-3, GM-CSF and M-CSF some of them differentiated into macrophages. Hence, the *bcl2–myc* tumor cells represent hematopoietic progenitors that have the potential to develop into both B lymphoid cells and macrophages.

Although hematopoietic differentiation is conventionally envisaged as proceeding through progenitor cells that are separately and exclusively committed to lymphoid (B and T) or to myeloid (granulocyte and macrophage) cell production, there have been indications of the existence of progenitors with alternative commitments. In addition to somewhat indirect evidence from chemical treatment or virus infection experiments on continuous cell lines (e.g. Boyd and Schrader 1982; Klinken et al. 1988), a bi-potential progenitor of B cells and macrophages has been detected in normal mouse fetal liver (Cumano et al. 1992). Is there a normal counterpart of the *bcl2–myc* tumor cell in normal mouse bone marrow? A cell expressing B220 and CD4 was recently identified as constituting about 1% of nucleated bone marrow cells (Rolink et al. 1996) so we compared this cell with undifferentiated *bcl2–myc* tumor cells for additional markers (Strasser et al. 1996). In surface phenotype, the normal $B220^{+}CD4^{+}$ cells had all of the same characteristics as those shown in Table 1 for the tumor cells. The developmental potential of the normal cells is presently unknown. In their expression of B220, they differ from the bi-potential progenitor cells of Cumano et al. (1992) that have recently been analyzed for growth factor dependence of lineage commitment (Kee and Paige 1996).

Genetics of Susceptibility to v-*abl* Tumorigenesis

Abelson murine leukemia virus carries the v-*abl* oncogene, comprising a fusion between the 5' region of the Moloney virus *gag* gene and a mutant derivative of the tyrosine kinase-encoding gene c-*abl*, which enables the virus to rapidly induce pre-B or T cell lymphomas depending on the route of infection (for review see Rosenberg and Witte 1988). The virus also accelerates the development of plasmacytomas bearing *Ig–myc* translocations in pristane-treated BALB/c mice (Ohno et al. 1984).

Several years ago, to generate a v-*abl*-initiated system of tumorigenesis that would be independent of mouse strain variations in susceptibility to retrovirus infection, we established four strains of Eμ-v-*abl*-transgenic mice with a (B6 × SJL)F2 background (Rosenbaum et al. 1990; Harris et al. 1990). Three strains developed plasmacytomas (mostly bearing rearrangements of *myc*) to an incidence of 30-60% at 12 months of age; one of these, v-*abl* 40, was perpetuated for long-term studies. The other strain, v-*abl* 1, developed pre-B lymphomas and thymic T cell lymphomas, but no plasmacytomas. After several generations of propagation and characterization as (B6 × SJL)F2 stocks, strains 1 and 40 were serially crossed with B6 and BALB/c inbred strains to test for genetic variation in tumor susceptibility. A substantial number of generations of such crosses has now been achieved, and a large divergence in susceptibility is apparent. Our recent results of tumor monitoring will be described here.

Lymphomagenesis in v-*abl* 1 Mice

Mice of the v-*abl* 1 strain with a B6-SJL background developed two types of lymphoma to a total incidence of 70% by 12 months of age. Pre-B cell lymphomas occurred between 3 weeks and 11 weeks, and accounted for 18% of the tumors. The remaining 82% of tumors were T cell lymphomas, which started to appear at 7 weeks and developed sporadically thereafter with a median latency of 16 weeks in the cohort of 73 transgenic animals that we monitored (Harris et al. 1990). Unlike the plasmacytomas that developed in the v-*abl* 40 strain, neither the T nor the pre-B lymphomas carried a rearranged *myc* gene (our unpublished results).

When the v-*abl* 1 transgene was crossed into the BALB/c strain for several generations, tumors developed more rapidly, the median latent period being only 5-6 weeks and the incidence reaching 100% by 16 weeks (Fig. 1). In addition, the balance of tumor types swung markedly in favor of pre-B cell lymphomas. These now constituted 60% of all the tumors. The BALB/c-backcrossed line of v-*abl* 1 was terminated after seven generations because lymphoma onset was too rapid to allow continued breeding. By contrast, serial crossing with B6 mice has resulted in a greatly reduced tumor incidence, longer latent periods and a reduction in (or perhaps elimination of) pre-B lymphomas (Fig. 1). Further characterization of the B6-backcrossed stock is proceeding with a view to using it to initiate crosses with BALB/c mice to determine the pattern of susceptibility inheritance.

Plasmacytomagenesis in v-*abl* 40 Mice

Our observations on successive generations of this strain over a number of years have involved the diagnosis of over 300 independently arising tumors by histology and by monitoring tumor-bearing mouse serum by electrophoresis for clonal immunoglobulin. In every case, the tumor was a plasmacytoma; not a single pre-B or T cell lymphoma was found. In the B6-SJL-v-*abl* 40 line, 60% of the animals developed terminal tumors before 12 months of age. The majority of these

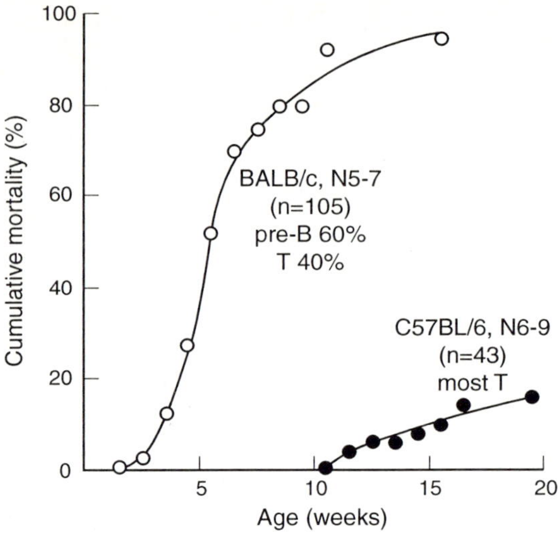

Fig. 1. Differential susceptibility to lymphomagenesis by the Eμ-v-*abl* 1 transgene in BALB/c (open circles) and C57BL/6 (filled circles) mice. The animal were monitored weekly and killed when they became ill. Tumors were verified by autopsy, histology and immunophenotyping.

plasmacytomas carried a rearranged *myc* gene, implying that a spontaneous translocation deregulating *myc* expression contributed to the malignant transformation, just as in Abelson virus-induced plasmacytomas in pristane-treated mice (Ohno et al. 1984). Some of the transgenic B6-SJL mice showed two additional kinds of pathology that occur in some human cases of multiple myeloma. About 20% of the mouse tumors were associated with 'myeloma kidney' in which renal function is impaired by extensive deposition of intratubular casts of immunoglobulin-related protein. A largely independent 20% of tumor cases showed amyloidosis, predominantly in the spleen. Examples are shown in our previous papers (Rosenbaum et al. 1990, Harris et al. 1990).

Introducing the v-*abl* 40 transgene into the inbred BALB/c and B6 mouse strains had a similar effect on tumor incidence to that seen with the v-*abl* 1 transgene. In BALB/c it was increased and in B6 it was decreased (Fig. 2). The tumor type remained the same; on both inbred backgrounds, all of the tumors assessed to date in the v-*abl* 40 mice have been plasmacytomas. In BALB/c-backcrossed mice, the tumors arose relatively synchronously, most appearing at 10-20 weeks. However, the incidence did not continue to rise to 100%. Consistently over successive generations of backcrossing (now more than 20), 10-20% of the transgenic animals survived without tumors for at least a year. Their transgenic genotype was confirmed by re-testing, and in some cases by their production of transgenic progeny that developed plasmacytomas early in life. Thus, their survival did not represent the persistence of some heritable resistance factor from the original B6-SJL background. Rather, it suggests that there is a time window of high susceptibility early in the adult life of the BALB/c mouse. Perhaps it is a time during which there is the most rapid production of plasma cells, with an attendant high probability of such a cell undergoing a *myc–Ig* translocation and other genetic alterations that will cooperate with v-*abl* expression to produce malignant transformation.

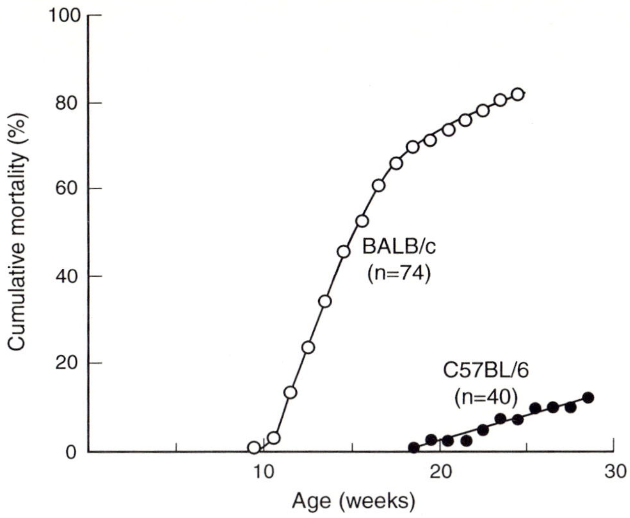

Fig. 2. Differential susceptibility to plasmacytomagenesis by the Eμ-v-*abl* 40 transgene in BALB/c (N10, 11 & 21) (open circles) and C57BL/6 (N5-9) (filled circles) mice. The animals were monitored weekly and killed when they became ill. Tumors were verified by autopsy, histology and the presence of a clonal immunoglobulin in the serum.

These experiments showed clearly that susceptibility to v-*abl* tumorigenesis is strongly determined by genetic constitution. They also showed incidentally that the other types of pathology sometimes associated with plasmacytoma, amyloidosis and myeloma kidney, were also determined by genetic background. From histologic examination of more than 50 cases of plasmacytoma-bearing v-*abl* 40 mice of the BALB/c-backcrossed subline, we have seen none with amyloidosis and only two or three with some renal tubular casts; none with compromised renal function. Hence, these conditions must have been dependent on the SJL or the B6 component (or both) of the original mixed B6-SJL genetic constitution.

As the first step in further characterizing the genetics of plasmacytoma susceptibility, we recently determined the incidence of tumors in F1 hybrids made by crossing BALB/c-v-*abl* 40 and normal B6 mice. The results showed that the incidence depended on whether the transgenic parent was the father or the mother (Fig. 3). In transgenic F1 hybrid progeny of transgenic BALB/c fathers, the tumor incidence at 12 months was 82%, similar to that seen in BALB/c backcross mice, although the median latent period was somewhat longer at 23 weeks versus 15 weeks. These data suggested that a major genetic determinant of high susceptibility to tumorigenesis in the BALB/c genome was dominant over its resistant allele in the B6 genome. However, F1 hybrids that inherited the transgene from their BALB/c mothers developed tumors to an incidence of only 21%. This result implies that susceptibility is subject to genomic imprinting, a feature of a small subset of genetic loci which causes male and female alleles to be expressed unequally (for review see Barlow 1995). In principle, the relevant imprinted locus could be either the transgene itself or a normal constitutional determinant of tumor susceptibility. The former seems unlikely because the F1 hybrids bearing a maternally transmitted transgene did produce a few plasmacytomas with a short latent period.

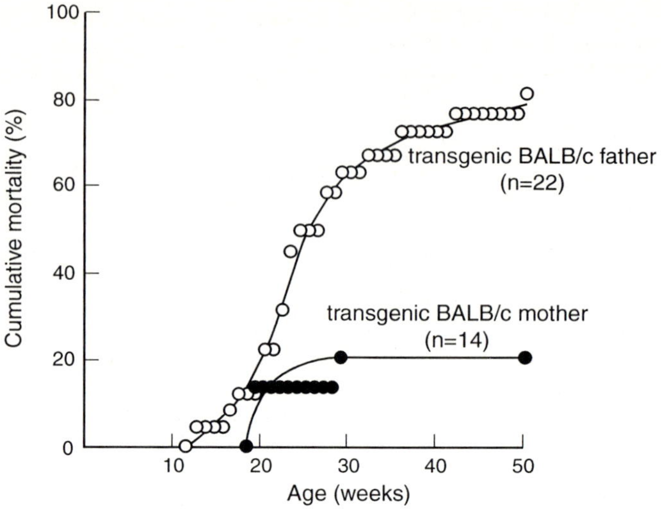

Fig. 3. Plasmacytomagenesis in v-*abl* 40 transgenic F1 hybrids produced by crossing transgenic BALB/c (N16) males with normal C57BL/6 females (open circles), or transgenic BALB/c (N16) females with normal C57BL/6 males (filled circles). The animals were monitored weekly and killed when they became ill. Tumors were verified by autopsy, histology and the presence of a clonal immunoglobulin in the serum.

Furthermore, tumor incidence within the BALB/c and B6 backcross strains has not shown a substantial dependence on whether the transgene was maternally or paternally derived (AWH and MLB unpublished data). Hence, the susceptibility factor subject to imprinting seems to be a normal mouse gene with an allelic difference between the BALB/c and B6 inbred strains. We are presently monitoring tumor formation in (B6 × BALB/c) and (BALB/c × B6) F1 hybrids in which the transgene is derived from the B6 parents rather than the BALB/c parents. This should test whether the imprinting of susceptibility occurs in both strains or is strain-specific.

Concluding Remarks

Expression of a transgenic oncogene in mouse lymphocytes can be more or less predisposing to lymphoid tumorigenesis depending on the nature of the oncogene and the mouse strain carrying the transgene. We have shown here that two inbred strains, B6 and BALB/c, differ markedly in their propensity to develop pre-B and T lymphomas or plasmacytomas when carrying either of two different integrations of an Eμ-v-*abl* transgenic construct. The susceptibility difference between the strains seems to be sufficiently large that rapid tumor formation could be used as a criterion for mapping the gene or genes responsible. Similar strain differences in tumor incidence have been used by others to identify two chromosomal regions that affect the inducibility of plasmacytomas by pristane treatment (Mock et al. 1993).

Preliminary results from monitoring the rate of plasmacytoma appearance in v-*abl* 40-transgenic B6–BALB/c F1 hybrids suggest that a major component of susceptibility is subject to genomic imprinting. This was not seen in the pristane induction system (Potter et al. 1975). In subsequent crosses to make F2 or backcross v-*abl* 40 animals, we plan to attempt genetic mapping of plasmacytoma susceptibility genes by their co-segregation with known polymorphic DNA markers. A parallel analysis of similar genetic segregants carrying the v-*abl* 1 transgene should indicate whether the same susceptibility genes are involved in the development of pre-B and T cell lymphomas.

Acknowledgments

We thank M Stanley and M Santamaria for technical assistance, and K Patane and J De Winter for supervising animal husbandry. AS was the recipient of a fellowship from the Leukemia Society of America; SC is an International Scholar of the Howard Hughes Medical Institute. This work was supported by the NHMRC (Canberra), the US National Cancer Institute (CA43540) and the Howard Hughes Medical Institute (75193-531101).

References

Adams JM, Cory S (1991) Transgenic models of tumor development. Science 254:1161-1167

Adams JM, Cory S (1992) Oncogene cooperation in leukemogenesis. Cancer Surv 15:119-141

Barlow DP (1995) Gametic imprinting in mammals. Science 270:1610-1613

Cory S (1995) Regulation of lymphocyte survival by the bcl-2 gene family. Annu Rev Immunol 13:513-543

Cumano A, Paige CJ, Iscove NN, Brady G (1992) Bipotential precursors of B cells and macrophages in murine fetal liver. Nature 356:612-615

de Jong D, Voetdijk MH, Beverstock GC, van Ommen GJB, Willemze R, Kluin PM (1988) Activation of the c-*myc* oncogene in a precursor-B-cell blast crisis of follicular lymphoma, presenting as composite lymphoma. New Engl J Med 318:1373-1378

Harris AW, Bath ML, Rosenbaum H, McNeall J, Adams JM, Cory S (1990) Lymphoid tumorigenesis by v-*abl* and *BCR*-v-*abl* in transgenic mice. Curr Top Microbiol Immunol 166:165-173

Harris AW (1991) Untitled. In: Mechanisms of B Cell Neoplasia 1991, Roche, Basel, pp 367-372

Harris AW (1993) Untitled. In: Mechanisms of B Cell Neoplasia 1993, Roche, Basel, pp 371-374

Kee BL, Paige CJ (1996) *In vitro* tracking of IL-7 responsiveness and gene expression during commitment of bipotent B-cell/macrophage progenitors. Curr Biol 6:1159-1169

Korsmeyer SJ (1995) Regulators of cell death. Trends Genet 11:101-105

Langdon WY, Harris AW, Cory S, Adams JM (1986) The c-*myc* oncogene perturbs B lymphocyte development in Eμ-*myc* transgenic mice. Cell 47:11-18

Limpens J, Stad R, Vos C, de Vlaam C, de Jong D, van Ommen G-JB, Schuuring E, Kluin PM (1995) Lymphoma-associated translocation t(14;18) in blood B cells of normal individuals. Blood 85:2528-2536

Linette GP, Hess JL, Sentman CL, Korsmeyer SJ (1995) Peripheral T-cell lymphoma in *lck*^{pr}-*bcl-2* transgenic mice. Blood 86:1255-1260

McDonnell TJ, Korsmeyer SJ (1991) Progression from lymphoid hyperplasia to high-grade malignant lymphoma in mice transgenic for the t(14;18). Nature 349:254-256

Mock BA, Krall MM, Dosik JK (1993) Genetic mapping of tumor susceptibility genes involved in mouse plasmacytomagenesis. Proc Natl Acad Sci USA 90:9499-9503

Ohno S, Migita S, Weiner F, Babonits M, Klein G, Mushinski JF, Potter M (1984) Chromosomal translocations activating *myc* sequences and transduction of v-*abl* are critical events in the rapid induction of plasmacytomas by pristane and Abelson virus. J Exp Med 159:1762-1777

Potter M, Pumphrey JG, Bailey DW (1975) Genetics of susceptibility to plasmacytoma induction. I. BALB/cAnN (C), C57BL/6N (B6), C57BL/Ka (BK), (C × B6)F1, (C × BK)F1, and C × B recombinant-inbred strains. J Natl Cancer Inst 54:1413-1417

Rolink A, ten Boekel E, Melchers F, Fearon DT, Krop I, Andersson J (1996) A subpopulation of $B220^+$ cells in murine bone marrow does not express CD19 and contains natural killer cell progenitors. J Exp Med 183:187-194

Rosenberg N, Witte ON (1988) The viral and cellular forms of the Abelson (abl) oncogene. Adv Virus Res 35:39-81

Rosenbaum H, Harris AW, Bath ML, McNeall J, Webb E, Adams JM, Cory S (1990) An Eμ-v-*abl* transgene elicits plasmacytomas in concert with an activated *myc* gene. EMBO J 9:897-905

Sidman C, Marshall JD, Harris AW (1988) Genetic studies on Eμ-*myc* transgenic mice. Curr Top Microbiol Immunol 141:94-99

Strasser A, Harris AW, Bath ML, Cory S (1990) Novel primitive lymphoid tumours induced in transgenic mice by cooperation between *myc* and *bcl*-2. Nature 348: 331-333

Strasser A, Whittingham S, Vaux DL, Bath ML, Adams JM, Cory S, Harris AW (1991) Enforced *BCL2* expression in B-lymphoid cells prolongs antibody responses and elicits autoimmune disease. Proc Natl Acad Sci USA 88:8661-8665

Strasser A, Harris AW, Cory S (1993) Eμ-*bcl*-2 transgene facilitates spontaneous transformation of early pre-B and immunoglobulin-secreting cells but not B cells. Oncogene 8:1-9

Strasser A, Elefanty AG, Harris AW, Cory S (1996) Progenitor tumours from Eμ-*bcl-2–myc* transgenic mice have lymphomyeloid differentiation potential and reveal developmental differences in cell survival. EMBO J 15: 3823-3834

Tsujimoto Y, Finger LR, Yunis J, Nowell PC, Croce CM (1984) Cloning of the chromosome breakpoint of neoplastic B cells with the t(14;18) chromosome translocation. Science 226:1097-1099

Vaux DL, Cory S, Adams JM (1988) *bcl*-2 gene promotes haemopoietic cell survival and co-operates with c-*myc* to immortalize pre-B cells. Nature 335:440-442

Molecular Pathogenesis of *myc*-initiated B-cell Lymphomas in the Bursa of Fabricius

P. E. Neiman[1,2,3], B. E. Clurman[1,2] and V. V. Lobanenkov[1]
Fred Hutchinson Cancer Researech Center[1] and the Departments of Medicine[2] and Pathology[3], University of Washington, Seattle, Washington, USA

The Transformed Bursal Follicle

Constitutive over-expression of *myc* oncogenes in the stem cell compartment of the bursa-of Fabricius of chickens provides an *in-vivo* model system for analysis of the mechanisms of *myc*-induced, multi-staged neoplastic change. The biology, molecular biology and genetics of this system has recently been reviewed (Neiman 1994a). Briefly, the lymphoid population of embryonic follicles of the bursa is composed of large cycling lymphoblasts expressing surface IgM (Thompson et al. 1987a) This population includes a compartment of stem cells that can clonally reconstitute ablated bursal follicles in transplantation experiments (Pink et al. 1985). Deregulated expression of a *myc* oncogene within this stem cell compartment, either due to integration of an avian leukosis virus (ALV) near c-*myc* (Hayward et al. 1981) or due to *ex-vivo* infection of embryonic bursal lymphoblasts with a v-*myc* transducing myelocytomatosis virus (HB1)(Neiman et al. 1985; Thompson et al. 1987a), initiates neoplastic change in bursal follicles. This change is signaled by the replacement of the lymphoid cells of the follicle with a monomorphic population of pyroninophilic lymphoblasts producing a histologically distinctive lesion called a transformed follicle (TF)(Cooper et al. 1960; Neiman et al. 1980a, b; Baba and Humphries 1985). TF cells demonstrate the cardinal properties of bursal stem cells in that they reconstitute bursal follicles efficiently in transplantation experiments and diversify their light chain immunoglobulin genes by gene conversion at a rate similar to that of the immunoglobulin genes of normal bursal follicles (Neiman et al. 1985; Thompson et al. 1987a, b). Unlike normal bursal stem cells they persist after hatching and are preneoplastic giving rise to invasive bursal lymphomas. Therefore deregulated expression of *myc* genes appears to produce an arrest of B-cell maturation in the bursa at the stem cell stage and either permits or induces overgrowth of bursal stem cells within the follicular architecture. In this paper we summarize what we have learned about the mechanisms which lie down stream of *myc*-deregulation in the further development of neoplastic change as well as about a novel gene, CTCF, which may be a tumor suppressor acting directly upstream of *myc*.

Role of Apoptotic Cell Death

One process we believe is critical in neoplastic progression of *myc*-induced TF is the exceptionally active apoptotic cell death pathway present bursal follicles. Only a small percentage of cells produced there ever leave the bursa. We have observed that DNA damaging agents , such as gamma radiation, as well as disruption of cell-cell contact by dispersion of bursal follicles in short term tissue culture, induces apoptotic cell death in virtually all of the bursal lymphoid population within a few hours (Neiman et al., 1991). In addition analysis by the

TdT DNA break labeling technique (TUNEL)(Gavrieli et al., 1992) revealed that normal follicles from 18 day embryos contained relatively few apoptotic cells while TF demonstrated high rates of spontaneous apoptosis by this technique (Neiman et al. 1994b). This finding was entirely consistent with our earlier observation that TF were hypersensitive (in comparison with normal embryonic bursal populations) to induction of apoptosis induced by either dispersion or gamma-radiation Neiman et al. 1991) as well as to the observation of *myc* enhancement of apoptotic cell death in cultured cell lines (Askew et al. 1991; Evan et al. 1992). Of importance to this discussion is the observation that this hypersensitivity to induction of apoptosis is significantly reduced when TF cells progress to form invasive bursal lymphomas (Neiman et al. 1991). We interpret these observations to indicate that normal bursal lymphoblasts and preneoplastic TF cells live with a hair trigger cell death response held in check by survival signals dependent upon close cell-cell contact within the follicular architecture. Progression of TF cells to invasive tumor cells which can survive away from such contacts requires suppression of this apoptotic pathway, at least to the point where rates of cell division exceed those of cell death.

For that reason we have been seeking evidence of the activation of a suppressor of cell death as part of the complex of changes required for tumor progression in this system. A screen of the expression of the bcl-2 family of genes demonstrated that bcl-2 itself was not expressed in either normal bursa or bursal tumors and therefore did not seem to play a role. Bcl-x was expressed at low levels in normal bursa, but did not show changes in levels of expression either during tumorigenesis or in apoptotic bursal cells. Therefore it does not seem an attractive candidate for a central role in regulation of apoptosis in normal or neoplastic bursal cells. In contrast, preliminary studies of a newly characterized member of the bcl-2 family called NR-13 seem to implicate this gene. NR-13 is induced in avian neuroretinal by the *src* gene of Rous sarcoma virus, is normally expressed during avian neural development (Gillet et al. 1995), and will protect a human marrow derived cell line Baf-3 from IL-3 withdrawal-induced apoptosis (Mangeney et al. 1996). In preliminary studies, conducted in collaboration with Germain Gillet, we find that NR-13 RNA is expressed at ample levels in embryonic bursal follicles and decreases progressively after hatching (as levels of spontaneous apoptosis increase). Furthermore, mature NR-13 mRNA disappears within 15 minute after induction of apoptosis in embryonic bursal lymphoblasts by dispersion in culture medium. Finally, NR-13 mRNA is expressed in metastatic bursal lymphomas at levels comparable to that of normal embryonic bursal cells. Thus current studies focus on NR-13. We plan to determine whether constitutive over expression of NR-13 in bursal stem cells will block apoptosis, and accelerate *myc*-induced tumorigenesis, in the bursa.

Mechanisms and Targets of Progression

Bursal transplantation assay. The basic technique used for these studies was reconstitution of cyclophosphamide-ablated bursal follicle populations with donor cells transduced with a retrovirus expressing a v-*myc* oncogene. The methodology for this approach has been previously described(Neiman et al. 1985; Thompson et al., 1987a) and is outlined in Figure 1.

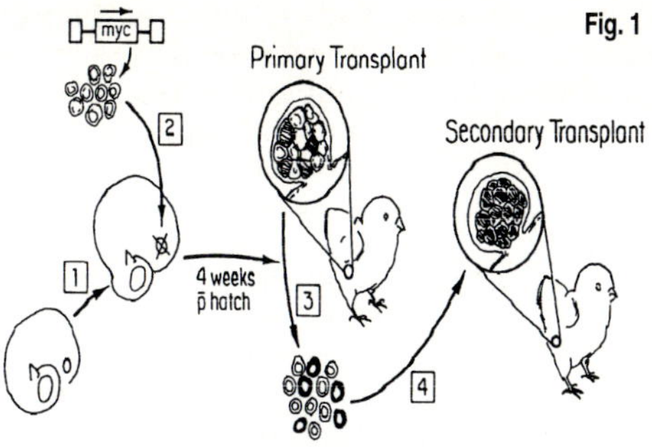

Fig. 1

Fig. 1. Schematic of the bursal transplant technique (1). Recipient chick embryos between 18 days of embryogenesis and day-of-hatch are treated with cyclophosphamide to induce apoptosis in the bursal lymphoid population (Eskola and Toivanen, 1974). (2). Bursal follicles from syngeneic 18 day chick embryo donors are dispersed and co-cultivated for 8-16 hours on adherent monolayers producing the v-*myc* transducing retrovirus and injected intravenously into the cyclophosphamide prepared recipients. (3) Stem cells in the donor population reconstitute the ablated follicles. Those successfully transduced and expressing v-*myc* show TF morphology (dark cross hatch). (3). By four weeks after hatching normal stem cells have disappeared and the only transplantable stem cells in the bursal are in TF. These can be dispersed in culture and transplanted again (4) into secondary cyclophosphamide ablated recipients. Reconstituted follicles in these secondary transplants are composed only of TF. Tumors invading between follicles in the bursa, and metastatic to the liver, can be observed following both primary and secondary transplants.

Induction of transformed follicles and bursal lymphomas with helper-free retroviral vectors. The retroviral system we have used previously to introduce v-*myc* into bursal follicles by the transplantation technique (figure 1) has been a "recovered" avian myelocytomatosis virus called HB1 (Enrietto et al. 1983). HB1 is defective and requires a subgroup C helper-virus (tdB-77). Co cultivation of embryonic bursal lymphoblasts on monolayers producing high titers (about 10^6 focus forming units per ml) of HB1(tdB-77) yielded 20-60% TF in primary transplants and, essentially, 100% TF in secondary transplants. Invasive lymphomas were observed in the bursa in 6% of primary transplants examined 4 weeks after hatching and about 20% of secondary transplants in which the serially transplanted populations represented bursal cells about 8 weeks after the original infection with HB1. Since HB1(tdB-77) is a spreading viral complex which causes a variety of lethal tumors in other organs (Enrietto et al. 1983) we could not analyze the effects of metastatic disease arising from the bursal lymphomas separately from primary HB1-induced neoplasia. Furthermore, since the replication competent helper virus could act as an insertional mutagen, we could not determine whether tumor progression in the bursa was the result of genetic instability generated by deregulated *myc* expression or reflected mutagenic activity of the spreading helper virus.

In order to address the relative roles of v-*myc* and helper virus on tumor progression in the bursa we constructed a helper-free vector, LXSN-HB1, in the vector system LXSN (Miller and Rosman 1989) to use for transducing the HB1 v-*myc* gene into bursal stem cells. The transplantation assay (Fig. 1) was then carried out following cocultivation of embryonic bursal lymphoblasts on monolayers producing LXSN-HB1. The results showed the development of TF primary bursal tumors and metastatic lymphomas with the same timing and frequency as we observed in the presence of helper virus (Neiman et al. 1994b). Therefore, neoplastic progression of v-*myc*-induced bursal stem cells occurred rapidly in the absence of spreading retroviral infection, presumably as an inevitable consequence of deregulated v-*myc* expression.

Are the same genes targeted during progression in the presence and absence of retroviral insertional mutagenesis? Multiple proviral insertions provide a mechanism for activation of cooperating oncogenes in multistage neoplasia induced by "non-acute" retroviruses. In the case of bursal lymphomas arising after infection by avian leukosis virus (ALV), integration of ALV causing transcriptional activation of a locus called *bic* was observed in a significant proportion of these tumors by Clurman and Hayward (1989). These authors found the *bic* locus to be transcriptionally silent in normal bursa and bursal tumors lacking retroviral insertions near *bic*. We were curious to learn what happened to gene expression at *bic* in our experimental system where, once the v-*myc* gene transfer vector was integrated in bursal stem cells, no further retroviral insertions could occur. A cloned *bic* cDNA probe was obtained through the generosity of Walter Tam, Bill Hayward and Peter Bessmer (Memorial Sloan Cancer Center, New York). As shown by northern blot-hybridization analysis (Fig. 2), this probe detected only very low levels of *bic* RNA in normal bursal lymphocytes at various times in bursal development. In contrast high levels of *bic* RNA were detected in metastatic bursal lymphomas. Three examples are shown, but we detected ample levels of *bic* RNA in all eight tumors we have analyzed.

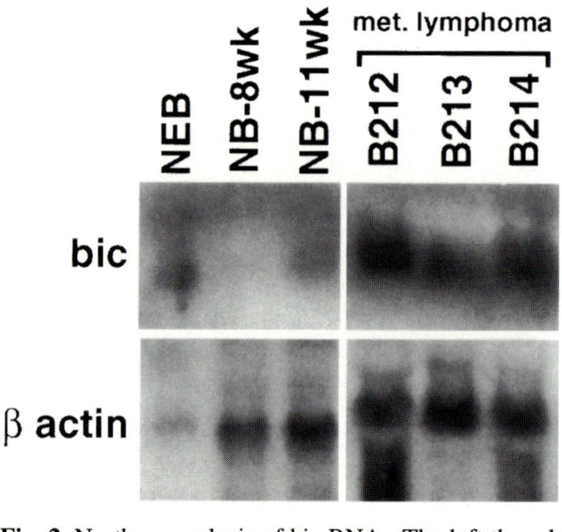

Fig. 2. Northern analysis of bic RNA. The left three lanes show RNA from day hatch (NEB) and 8 and 11 week normal bursas (NB). The right three lanes show RNA from hepatic metastases of bursal lymphomas. The blot was first probed with the *bic* probe, washed and reprobed with a chicken beta actin probe as a loading control.

These results suggest a consistent selection of cooperating oncogenes regardless of the underlying genetic mechanism of activation. Current studies are directed at determining how bic is transcriptionally activated in these tumors as a clue to underlying mechanisms of genetic instability induced by *myc* in bursal stem cells. Co-expression of *myc* and *bic* from a viral vector in bursal stem cells should allow us to determine if this leads to accelerated tumorigenesis, a finding which would suggest that *bic* expression is rate limiting for *myc*-induced multi-staged tumorigenesis in this model system.

CTCF is a Candidate Tumor Suppressor Which Can Act Directly on c-*myc*.

Fig. 3 summarizes the oncogenic effects of deregulated *myc* oncogene expression in bursal stem cells. As indicated in the figure *myc* deregulation in this compartment does not affect all functions. Preimmune immunoglobulin gene diversification and transplantation functions are apparently not perturbed. However, maturation arrest, abnormal proliferation and enhancement of an active cell death pathway are profound effects of constitutive *myc* over expression in these cells. These changes are not sufficient for the full malignant phenotype. Somehow these cells are highly susceptible to additional (presumably genetic) change, involving regulators of cell death and additional cooperating oncogenes (NR-13 and *bic*, respectively, being candidate direct or indirect targets).

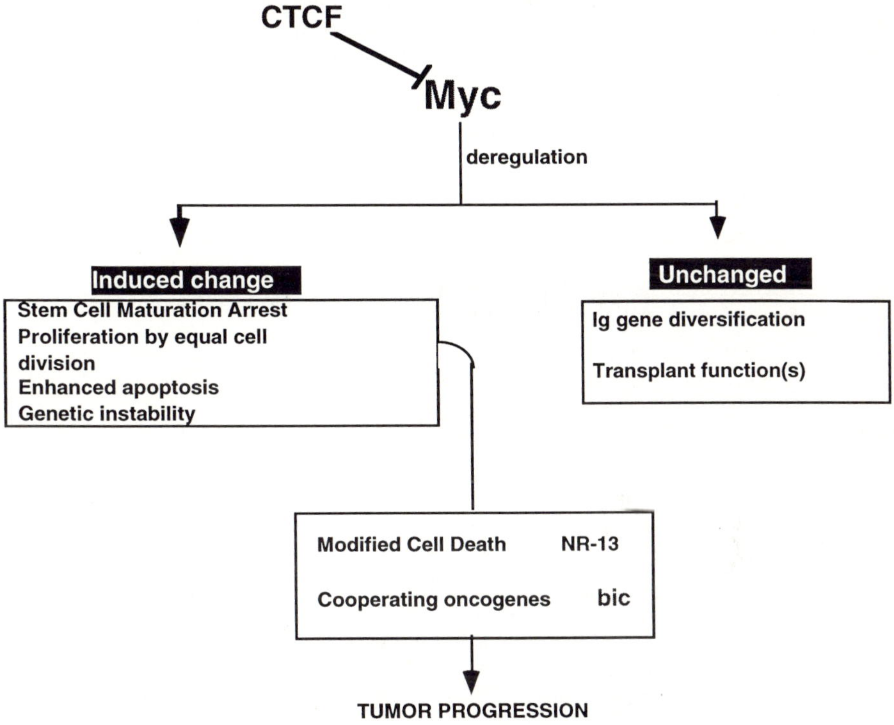

Fig 3. Deregulation of *myc*: effects in bursal stem cells.

This experimental system, and most of those discussed at this conference, are based on *myc* deregulation caused by either engineered, or virus-induced or naturally occurring structural change at the *myc*-locus. An alternative scenario, which may be important in many human neoplasms, could involve the loss of function of upstream normal repressors of *myc* expression. Although not yet demonstrated in the bursal lymphoma model, Fig. 3 indicates the presence of one candidate, called CTCF, which may play such a role. CTCF was originally isolated as a protein which bound specifically to a large (about 45 bp) GC rich sequence within a DNase I footprint region at a promoter-proximal site in the chicken c-*myc* promoter (Lobanenkov et al. 1986, 1990). The chicken (Klenova et al, 1993) and human (Filippova et al. 1996) homologues of CTCF have now been cloned and characterized. They encode 728 and 727 amino acid polypeptides respectively which demonstrate 93% identity at the amino acid level. Fig. 4 summarizes some of the features of CTCF. About the middle third of the protein is comprised of an 11 Zn-finger DNA binding domain which is totally conserved in amino acid sequence between mammals and birds. CTCF is ubiquitously expressed as a nuclear phosphoprotein in all of the animal cell types in culture we have tested. In addition to binding in footprint V(Lobanenkov et al. 1986, 1990) of chicken c-*myc*, CTCF binds, via its Zn-finger domain, to very divergent P1 and P2 promoter proximal sites in human c-*myc* . It binds to these three different site by use of different combinations of Zn-fingers contacting different nucleotides (Filippova et al 1996). Recent screening of multiple segments of the human c-*myc* locus detected CTCF specific binding at two additional previously characterized DNase hypersensitivity sites: one at -2020 from P2 and the other in the first intron. All four of the mammalian CTCF binding sites at the c-*myc* locus, while different from each other, are conserved between mouse and man. All are bound by different subsets of CTCF Zn-fingers. We conclude that this highly conserved DNA binding protein is a "multivalent" factor with extensive binding capability at all vertebrate c-*myc* loci.

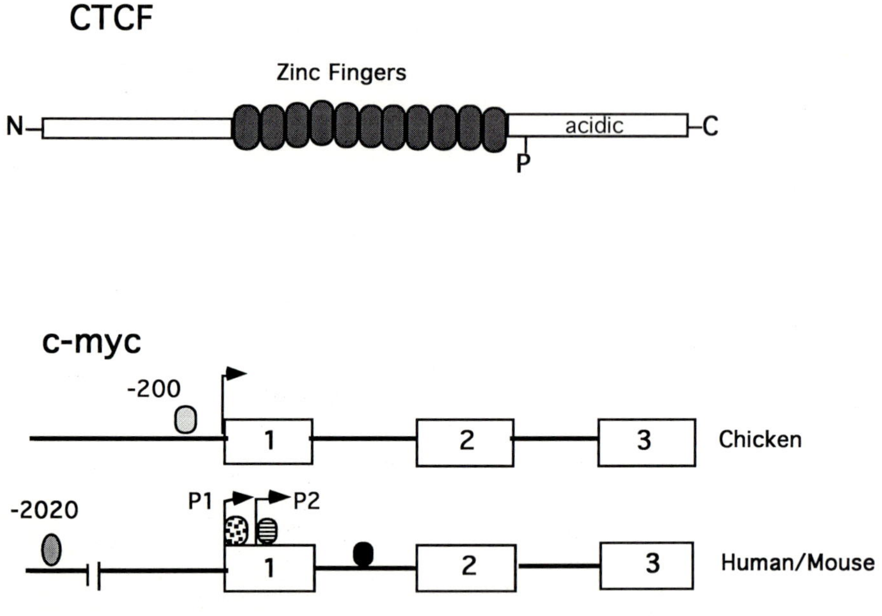

Fig. 4. Schematic representation of the CTCF polypeptide (top) and the CTCF binding sites (filled ovals) on chicken human and murine c-*myc* genes

The evidence we have accumulated so far implicates CTCF as a repressor of c-*myc* transcription. There are three pieces of evidence which suggest this conclusion (Filippova et al. 1996). First, both the amino terminal and carboxy terminal CTCF domains are transferable repressor domains. They will, in transient transfection assays, strongly repress transcription from a test promoter (thymidine kinase gene promoter) when grafted onto a heterologous DNA binding domain (GAL-4) specific for an engineered binding site (UAS) upstream of the test promoter-reporter construct. Second, a mutation, which selectively abrogates CTCF binding at human P2, results in significantly increased transcription from a P2-dependent c-*myc* promoter-reporter construct in stable transfection assays. Finally, transient cotransfection assays with a CTCF expression vector and a c-*myc* promoter-dependent target construct demonstrate significant repression of P2-dependent transcription.

As has been emphasized several times at this conference, ectopically expressed c-*myc* constructs may not behave like c-*myc* loci *in-situ.* Therefore, we are seeking to determine the effects of CTCF on endogenous *myc* gene expression. We have found that constitutive over-expression of wild-type CTCF from both viral vectors and transfected plasmid constructs is incompatible with growth of selected colonies in several types of cell culture. Thus, current studies are exploring conditional expression systems to more conveniently observe these effects. Furthermore chromosomal mapping and mutational analyses of CTCF are being carried out with DNA from human neoplasms in which deregulated c-*myc* gene expression has been implicated. These studies are intended to obtain more definitive evidence of a role for CTCF as a tumor suppressor and determine whether or not such a role can be attributed to its effects on c-*myc*. In this connection we are characterizing putative dominant negative mutants of CTCF which can be introduced on viral vectors and expressed in bursal stem cells. In this fashion we hope to determine if interruption of CTCF function will produce the oncogenic phenotypes which result specifically from deregulated *myc* expression in this experimental system.

References

Askew DS, Ashmun RA, Simmons BC, Cleveland L (1991) Constitutive *c-myc* expression in an IL-3 dependant myeloid cell line supresses cell cycle arrest and accelerates apoptosis. Oncogene 6:1915-1922

Baba TW Humphries EH (1985) Formation of a transformed follicle is necessary but not sufficient for development of an avian leukosis virus-induced lymphoma. Proc. Natl. Acad. Sci. USA 82:213-216

Clurman BE, Hayward WS (1989) Multiple proto-oncogene activations in avian leukosis virus-induced lymphomas: Evidence for stage specific events. Mol. Cell. Biol. 9:2657-2664

Cooper MD, Payne LN, Dent PB, Burmester BR, Good RA (1960) Pathogenesis of avian lymphoid leukosis. 1. Histogenesis. J. Natl. Cancer Inst. 41:373-389

Evan GI, Wyllie AH, Gilbert CS, Littlewood TD, Land H, Brooks M,Waters CM, Penn LZ, Hancock DC (1992) Apoptosis in fibroblasts by *c-myc* protein. Cell 69:119-128

Eskola J, Toivanen P (1974) Cell transplantation in immunodeficient chickens. Cell. Immunol. 13:459-471

Enrietto PJ, Payne LN, Hayman MJ (1983) A recovered avian myelocytomatosisvirus that induces lymphomas in chickens: pathologic properties and their molecular basis. Cell 35:369-379

Filippova G, Fagerlie S, Klenova EM, Myers C, Dehner Y, Goodwin G, Neiman PE, Colllins SJ, Lobanenkov VV (1995) An exceptionally conserved transcriptional repressor, CTCF, employs different combinations of zinc fingers to bind diverged promoter sequences of avian and mammalian c-*myc* oncogenes. Mol. Cell Biol. 16:2802-2813

Gavrieli Y, Sherman,Y, Ben-Sasson, SA (1992): Identification of programmed cell death *in-situ* via specific labeling of nuclear DNA fragmentation. J. Cell Biol. 119, 493-501

Gillet G, Guerin M, Trembleau A, Brun G (1995) A BCL-2 related gene is activated in avian cells transformed by Rous sarcoma virus. EMBO J. 14:1372-1381

Hayward WS, Neel BG, Astrin SM (1981) Activation of a cellular *onc* gene by promoter insertion in ALV-induced lymphoid leukosis. Nature 290:475-480

Klenova E, Nicolas RH, Paterson HF, Carne AF, Heath CM, Goodwin GH, Neiman PE, Lobanenkov VV (1993) CTCF, a conserved nuclear factor required for optimal transcriptional activity of the chicken c-*myc* gene, is an 11-zinc-finger protein differentially expressed in multiple forms. Mol. Cell. Biol. 13:7612-7624

Lobanenkov VV, Nicolas RH, Adler VV, Paterson H, Klenova EM, Polotskaja AV, Goodwin GH (1990) A novel sequence specific DNA binding protein which interacts with three regularly spaced direct repeats of the CCCTC-motif in the 5'-flanking sequence of the chicken c-*myc* gene. Oncogene 5:1743-1753

Lobanenkov VV, Nicolas RH, Plumb MA, Wright CA, Goodwin GH (1986) Sequence specific DNA binding proteins which interact with G+C-rich sequences flanking the chicken c-*myc* gene. Eur. J. Biochem. 159:159-188

Mangeney M, Schmiitt J-R, Leverrier Y, Thomas J, Marvel J, Brun G, Gillet G (1996) The product of the v-*src* inducible gene *nr*-13 is a potent anti-apoptotic factor. Oncogene 13:1-6

Miller AD, Rossman GJ (1989) Improved retroviral vectord for gene transfer and expresssion. Biotechniques 7:980-990

Neiman PE (1994) Retrovirus-induced B-cell neoplasia in the bursa of Fabricius. Adv. Immunol. 56:467-484

Neiman PE; Jordan L, Weiss RA, Payne LN (1980) Malignant Lymphoma of the Bursa of Fabricius: Analysis of Early Transformation. In: Essex M; Todaro G; Zur Hausen H (eds) Viruses in Naturally Occurring Cancer. Cold Spring Harbor Laboratory, Cold Spring Harbor, NY, pp 519-528 (Cold Spring Harbor Conferences on Cell Proliferation, vol. 7)

Neiman P, Payne LN, Weiss RA (1980) Viral DNA in bursal lymphomas induced by avian leukosis viruses. J. Virol. 34:178-186

Neiman PE, Summers J, Thomas SJ, Xuereb S, Loring G (1994): Genetic instability and apoptotic cell death during neoplastic progression of *v-myc* initiated B-cell lymphomas in the bursa of Fabricius. In: Stillman B (ed) Molecular Genetics of Cancer. Cold Spring Harbor Laboratory, Cold Spring Harbor, NY, pp 509-515 (Cold Spring Harbor Symposium on Quantitative Biology, vol 56)

Neiman PE, Thomas SJ, Loring G (1991) Induction of apoptosis during normal and neoplastic development in the bursa of Fabricius. Proc. Natl. Acad. Sci. USA 88:5857-5861

Neiman P, Wolf C, Enrietto PJ, Cooper GM (1985) A retroviral *myc* gene induces preneoplastic transformation of lymphocytes in a bursal transplantation assay. Proc. Natl. Acad. Sci. USA 82:222-236

Thompson CB, Humphries EH, Carlson LM, Chen C-LH, Neiman PE (1987) The effect of alterations in *myc* gene expression on B-cell development in the bursa of Fabricius. Cell 51, 371-381

Thompson CB, Neiman PE (1987) Somatic diversification of the chicken immunoglobulin light chain gene is limited to the rearranged gene segment. Cell 48:369-378

Pink JR, Vaino O, Rijinbeek A-M (1985) Clones of B lymphocytes in individual bursal follicles of the bursa of Fabricius. Eur. J. Immunol. 15:83-90

C-Myc in Multiple Myeloma Plasmacytomagenesis

Genetic Recombinations Between c-*myc* and Ighμ as Precursors for Recombinations Between c-myc and Ighα in BALB/c Plasmacytomas

S. Janz, A. L. Kovalchuk, J. R. Müller and M. Potter
Laboratory of Genetics, Division of Basic Sciences, NCI, NIH, Bethesda, MD, USA

Abstract

In this paper we present evidence that primary plasmacytomas harboring a balanced chromosomal translocation t(12;15) may consist of a mosaic of neoplastic clones of tumor cells, in which some of the clones are derived from common progenitors by large additional deletions which alter or "remodel" the fine structure of the t(12;15) on the c-*myc*-deregulating chromosome. This finding is based on the molecular analysis of the t(12;15) in three plasmacytomas, TEPC 1194, PCT 4127 and PCT 4132, in which primary clones of tumor cells with recombinations between the Ig heavy-chain (Igh) μ locus (Ighμ) and c-*myc* were found to be related to secondary clones of tumor cells with recombinations between the Igh α locus (Ighα) and c-*myc*. Clonal relatedness was based on unique junction fragments between Sμ and c-*myc* that were found to be identical in Ighμ/c-*myc* and Ighα/c-*myc* breakpoint regions. Sμ/c-*myc* breakpoints with adjoining sequences can thus be used as clonotypic markers, providing molecular fingerprints for the evolution of precursor cells with Ighμ/c-*myc* recombinations into progenitor cells with Ighα/c-*myc* recombinations. We propose that aberrant isotype switch recombination or illegitimate rearrangement in switch regions converts Ighμ/c-*myc* rearrangements, which are found very rarely in established plasmacytomas, into Ighα/c-*myc* rearrangements, which are present in about 80% of plasmacytomas with t(12;15). Remodeling of the t(12;15) results in closer juxtaposition of c-*myc* to the 3'-Cα locus control region and probably in enhanced transcription of c-*myc*. We suggest that remodeling of c-*myc*-deregulating rearrangements constitutes a novel progression mechanism in malignant B-cell development.

Introduction

In pristane-induced BALB/c plasmacytomas, c-*myc*-deregulating genetic recombinations usually take the form of reciprocal chromosomal translocations t(12;15) that recombine c-*myc*, residing on chromosome (chr.) 15, with genes of the Ig heavy-chain gene cluster on chr. 12. At the molecular level, the t(12;15) is characterized by juxtaposition of the 5' region of c-*myc*, stretching from about 1 kbp upstream of exon 1 to the 3' end of intron 1, to an Igh switch region (S) or the intervening sequence between a S region and the first exon of the pertaining Igh gene (C_H1). Of importance, the seven S regions (Sμ, Sγ3, Sγ2a, Sγ2b, Sγ1, Sε, Sα) and the pseudo switch region of the Ighδ locus do not participate equally in recombinations with c-*myc*. Instead, there is a strong bias toward Sα which is utilized in about 80% of the t(12;15)-positive plasmacytomas so far studied [20]. The reason for the preferred usage of Sα is currently unclear, but we propose that it may be caused, in part, by the novel remodeling mechanism that has been unveiled in this study on three primary plasmacytomas, TEPC 1194, PCT 4127 and PCT 4132. In these tumors, clones with initial recombinations between Ighμ and c-*myc* were found to co-exist with related clones harboring secondary exchanges between Ighα and c-*myc*. Thus, remodeling appears to transform Ighμ/c-*myc* precursor lesions into Ighα/c-*myc* product lesions. The mechanism of the remodeling process is not known, but its result, a composite switch region with a clonotypic junction between c-*myc* and Sμ, can most readily been explained by abnormal heavy-chain class switching or illegitimate recombination in switch regions. Remodeling may have biological significance in malignant B-cell transformation, because it repositions c-*myc* over a distance of about 170 kbp from the most upstream gene of the Igh gene cluster, Ighμ, to the most downstream one, Ighα, placing the recombined c-*myc* gene in close proximity to the strong 3'-Cα enhancer elements.

Results

Long range and high fidelity PCR techniques were developed as part of our continuing effort to better understand the balanced chromosomal translocation t(12;15) [8, 16]. We were particularly interested to distinguish the t(12;15) at the molecular level with respect to illegitimate recombinations of c-*myc* with either Ighμ or Ighα and decided therefore to analyse a panel of pristane-induced primary plasmacytomas for the occurrence of both types of recombinational fragments. That approach was successful in three tumors, TEPC 1194, PCT 4127 and PCT 4132, in which the fine structure of the t(12;15) had been elucidated in part in previous studies [11, 17]. In these plasmacytomas, different genomic fragments harboring both Ighμ/c-*myc* and Ighα/c-*myc* recombinations were detected. Subsequent DNA sequence determination of the junction fragments revealed in all three tumors precursor product-relationship between both types of Igh/c-*myc* exchanges and established Ighμ/c-*myc* junctions as molecular precursors for Ighα/c-*myc* recombinations. The findings suggesting such a precursor and product relationship are summerized in Fig. 1.

Fig. 1 shows structural schemas of chr. 12+-typical recombinational fragments between c-*myc* and Ighμ or Ighα that were detected by PCR in three primary pristane-induced plasmacytomas: TEPC 1194 at the top, PCT 4127 in the center, and PCT 4132 at the bottom. All recombination structures are aligned at the postulated cross-over point of the t(12;15) that is indicated by a dashed vertical line. The map of the 5' portion of the recombined c-*myc* gene is shown to the left, and the map of the upstrem part of the involved Igh locus is illustrated to the right of the translocation breakpoint. Note that the t(12;15) joins c-*myc* with Igh in a head-to-head recombination with respect to the transcriptional orientation of the genes. Exons 1 and 2 of c-*myc* are designated by open numbered boxes, while Ig switch regions and the first exons of the Ighμ and Ighα genes are illustrated by striped and filled boxes that are labeled. Since the Igh gene cluster maps to the telomeric end of chr. 12, the acromere of chr. 12+, denoted by a filled circle at the right end of the map, is separated from the translocation breakpoint region by a very large distance that is indicated by an oblique double line to the left of the acromere. PCR indicator fragments that were used for DNA sequencing and to differentiate between Ighμ/c-*myc* and Ighα/c-*myc* recombinations are depicted by horizontal bars below the gene maps. Tumor-specific, clonotypic Sμ/c-*myc* junctions and 60 bp of adjoining sequences are given for each tumor below the bottom most PCR fragment, where 30 bp of both c-*myc* and Igh sequence are shown in capital and lower letters, respectively. For all three plasmacytomas, the initial genetic exchange between c-*myc* and Ighμ is illustrated on top of the secondary, remodeled exchange between c-*myc* and Ighα. Importantly, initial and remodeled recombinations share clonotypic Sμ/c-*myc* breakpoint regions indicating their clonal relatedness.

In TEPC 1194 and PCT 4127, the breaksite in c-*myc* occurred upstream of exon 1, whereas the breakpoint in PCT 4132 was located in intron 1. The break in Igh occurred in the Sμ region in PCTs 4127 and 4132, but in the near 5' flank of Sμ in TEPC 1194. Secondary Ighα/c-*myc* recombinations are characterized by additional rearrangement of Sμ with a downstream switch acceptor region. This results in creation of a compound switch region, a Sμ/Sα region in TEPC 1194 and PCT 4127 and a Sμ/Sγ2b/Sα region in PCT 4132. Bipartite and tripartite switch regions may reflect remodeling events that take place as single-step and sequential rearrangements, respectively. In the Sμ/c-*myc* junction observed in PCT 4127, a 2-bp homology was found at the breaksite and has been arbitrarily assigned to c-*myc* (underlined). In PCT 4132, a characteristic base substitution mutation in c-*myc* was detected next to the translocation breakpoint in both Ighμ/c-*myc* and Ighα/c-*myc* fragments. That mutation is illustrated by a star and lends additional support for clonal relatedness. In TEPC 1194, two subclones of tumor cells with chr. 12+-typical Ighα/c-*myc* recombinations were detected. However, DNA sequence analysis does not allow to distinguish whether the clone with the secondary rearrangment between 5'-Sμ and Sα (designated #2, shown at the bottom) has been derived from the initial clone by an independent remodeling event or from the secondary Ighα/c-*myc*-positive clone with the rearrangement between Sμ and Sα (denoted #1, shown in the center) by an internal deletion in the breakpoint region.

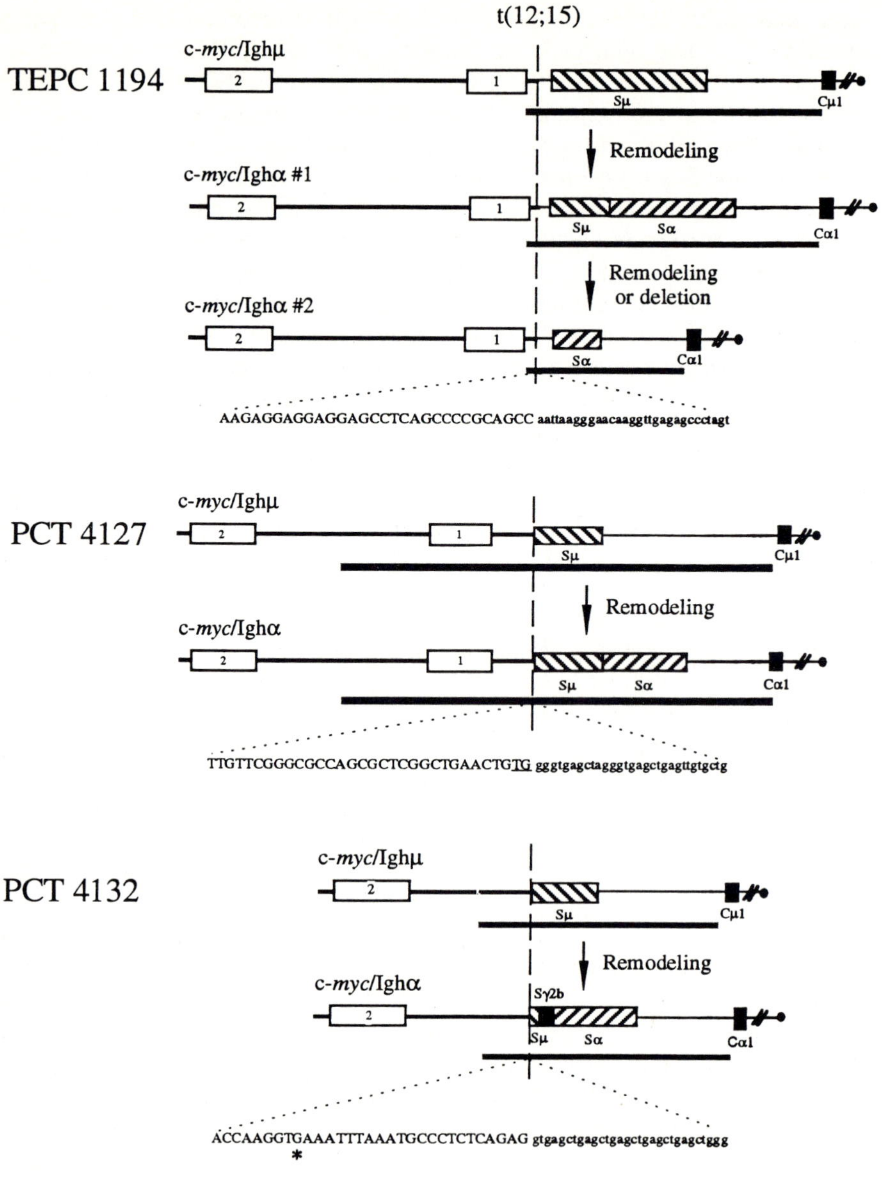

Fig. 1. Structure of initial recombinations between c-*myc* and Ighμ and remodeled recombinations between Ighα and c-*myc*

Discussion

The basic finding described in this paper is the identification of three plasmacytomas, TEPC 1194, PCT 4127 and PCT 4132, in which primary clones of tumor cells with Ighμ/c-*myc* recombinations were found to be precursors of secondary clones of tumor cells with Ighα/c-*myc* recombinations. Clonal relatedness was based on identical clonotypic junction fragments between Sμ and c-*myc* that occurred in both Ighμ/c-*myc* and Ighα/c-*myc* breakpoint regions. During clonal evolution, the tumor-characteristic Sμ/c-*myc* junctions, which were established during the initial genetic exchange between Ighμ and c-*myc*, were preserved in the composite switch regions of Ighα/c-*myc* fragments, where they served as molecular fingerprints to trace back clonal relationship. We interpret this finding to indicate that plasmacytoma cells harboring Ighα/c-*myc* recombinations can be derived from precursor cells with Ighμ/c-*myc* recombinations. Additional support for the presence of such a precursor product-relationship was obtained in PCT 4132 in which the clonotypic Sμ/c-*myc* junction was further defined by a specific base substitution mutation in c-*myc* that was co-detected in recombinational fragments with Ighμ and Ighα.

We propose that remodeling of primary Ighμ/c-*myc* recombinations into secondary Ighα/c-*myc* recombinations was accomplished by aberrant isotype switching according to the looping-out-and-deletion model. However, a number of alternative mechanisms warrants consideration, too. For example, DNA sequence analysis of composite switch regions does not allow to distinguish between abnormal switch recombination and illegitimate recombination in switch regions [4], which could take place as rejoining of DNA double strand breaks in switch regions or by unequal sister chromatid exchange. Furthermore, additional and more complex mechanisms may be invoked, such as i) intrachromosomal recombinations subsequent to amplifications of genomic regions on chr. 12+ involving the combined Igh/c-*myc* locus, ii) duplications of chr. 12+ followed by trans-chromosomal rearrangements, and iii) unequal crossing over between homologous chromosomes 12 and 12+. We favor, but can not prove at present, the idea that initial Ighμ/c-*myc* rearrangements are remodeled by aberrant class switching, since i) recombination breakpoints in participating switch regions (Sμ, Sγ2b and Sα) occurred in the repetitive region which is typical for normal switch recombination, ii) the composition of the compound switch regions, Sμ/Sα in PCT 4127 and Sμ/Sγ2b/Sα in PCT 4132, is indistinguishable from structures resulting from normal switching, and iii) switching to Cα in PCT 4132 involved an intermediate switch acceptor region, Sγ2b, in a sequential class switch recombination event, which is known to take place in normal B cells [2, 7].

Precedence for illegitimate genetic recombinations in B cells that appear to be mediated by aberrant isotype switching has been reported by other investigators. To appreciate these events, it is useful to review the diversity of normal and aberrant rearrangements that have been observed in B lymphocytes and ascribed to activities of the still elusive switch recombinase. This examination suggests that switching can either occur in cis or trans and can either take place legitimately as part of a normal antibody response or illegitimately as part of an abnormal genetic exchange. Normal heavy-chain isotype switching is known to occur in cis in most species, but has recently been shown to take place in trans in rabbits, in which Igh genes encoding a substantial fraction of the normal α heavy-chain response are apparently recombined by isotype trans-switching [9]. Another well-documented example of interchromosomal switch recombination can be found in the reciprocal chromosomal translocation t(5;12) that results when a human Cμ transgene, residing on mouse chr. 5, is recombined with one of the mouse C_H genes on chr. 12 [6]. Further cases of aberrant and probably trans-chromosomal rearrangements that are suggestive of involvement of switch recombinase are provided by the integration of a long interspersed nuclear element (LINE) next to the Sε region in a rat plasmacytoma [19] and the interruption of the Sγ2a region in a mouse plasmacytoma by an early transposon-like element, E.Tn [5]. Examples in which switch recombinase was apparently instrumental in generating inappropriate intrachromosomal rearrangements include the findings of this study and the recombination of a LINE-1 element with the expressed Igh cluster in a subline of mouse plasmacytoma MPC 11 [1]. Illegitimate recombinations in cis that are generated by aberrant isotype switching may also occur in humans, specifically on the translocated chr. 14q32 in B-cell lymphomas, in which some circumstantial evidence suggests that abnormal class switching modifies the fine structure of two types of reciprocal chromosomal translocations involving chr. 14q32, the t(14;18) [22] and the t(14;19) [3].

The biological significance of remodeling of c-*myc*-deregulating translocations is not known, but we speculate that it may be related to an upregulation of c-*myc* message that is postulated to be accomplished by conversion of c-*myc*/Ighμ into c-*myc*/Ighα rearrangements. According to this hypothesis, we propose that the initial Ighμ/c-*myc* exchange results in modest, at the most, transcriptional activation of c-*myc* on chr. 12^+. Failure to transcriptionally activate the rearranged c-*myc* gene is also conceivable, and in this situation c-*myc* would likely be transcribed from the germ-line allele on chr. 15. It is further surmised that in the presence of survival signals, such as IL-6, the Ighμ/c-*myc*-positive B cell may survive, undergo further differentiation, and accumulate secondary oncogenic changes that have been postulated to occur during plasmacytoma development. The nature of the proposed secondary mutations in plasmacytomagenesis has not been defined yet, but it seems possible that they include mutations rendering plasmacytoma precursor cells tolerant against the effects of high levels of c-*myc* message, which can be anticipated when remodeling of Ighμ/c-*myc* into Ighα/c-*myc* rearrangements has been completed. From a selection-of-the-fittest-clone point of view, it would make sense for a B cell to aquire mutations that protect against high levels of c-*myc* message, since strong and abrupt upregulation of c-*myc* has been shown to be deleterious in lymphocytes, in which it can, for example, induce apoptosis [18].

The validity of the hypothesis outlined above has not been tested yet, and it is presently not known whether c-*myc* is transcribed after juxtaposition to Ighμ. However, we note that recombination of c-*myc* with Sμ removes all known upstream Igh enhancer and promoter elements from chr. 12+, including the intronic Igh enhancer, regulatory regions 3' of the intronic Igh enhancer [21], the DQ52 enhancer/promoter [10] and additional promoters that are associated with D elements and V_H genes. Thus, no strong regulator of c-*myc* expression appears to be available in the 5' portion of the heavy-chain gene complex after genetic exchange with Ighμ. In this situation, transcription of c-*myc* could only be accomplished by enhancer elements that might be present in the 3' flank of c-*myc*. However, 3'-c-*myc* enhancers have not been identified thus far, and the two candidate enhancer elements that were recently found in a molecular analysis of the 30-kbp downstream region of the human c-*myc* gene [13] have been shown in subsequent studies to be insufficient to upregulate c-*myc* expression in vivo [14]. In contrast to the situation of poor c-*myc* expression after juxtaposition of c-*myc* to Ighμ, the transfer of c-*myc* from Ighμ to Ighα is likely to result in a more stable and vigorous deregulation of c-*myc*. This is due to the close approximation of c-*myc* to the powerful locus control region (LCR) 3' of Cα. The 3'-Cα LCR contains several strong enhancers that are known to be active in late B cells, such as plasma cells. What is more, the enhancers have been shown to activate c-*myc* expression efficiently in transfected reporter constructs and thus appear to provide perfect control elements for the deregulation of c-*myc* after exchange with Ighα [12, 15].

It is tempting to combine the postulated changes in the expression of c-*myc* that are caused by remodeling of t(12;15) with a general model on clonal evolution during plasmacytomagenesis. Such a model is illustrated in Fig. 2, in which a mature B cell is shown at the top that has undergone productive VDJ rearrangement on chr. 12, resulting in production of μ and δ heavy-chains and surface expression of IgM and IgD. The other chr. 12 is available for translocation with chr. 15 that is likely to take place in a B cell at a later developmental stage, possibly a germinal center B cell, in which the Ighμ locus is rendered accessible in preparation for class switching. In that cell, the trans-chromosomal exchange between c-*myc* on chr. 15 and Ighμ on chr. 12 is carried out, resulting in formation of the two derivative chromosomes, chr. 12+ and chr. 15-, and generation of an abnormal, tumor-initiated B cell. The initiated cell is assumed to i) undergo isotype switching to Cα on the productive allele, followed by production of IgA, ii) differentiate into a plasma cell, iii) accumulate secondary genetic changes as indicated above, and iv) finally develop into a plasmacytoma precursor cell. Then, at some later point in the course of oncogenesis, remodeling of the Ighμ/c-*myc* exchange on chr. 12+ takes place, approximating c-*myc* to the 3'-Cα enhancer. It is speculated that this event provides an important step to complete malignant transformation and to arrive at the stage of a primary plasmacytoma cell. In some primary plasmacytomas, e. g. in TEPC 1194, PCT 4127 and PCT 4132, the mosaic of evolving clones can be detected, if the tumor is sampled at an appropriate time, at which early clones harboring initial Ighμ/c-*myc* exchanges co-exist with more progressed clones

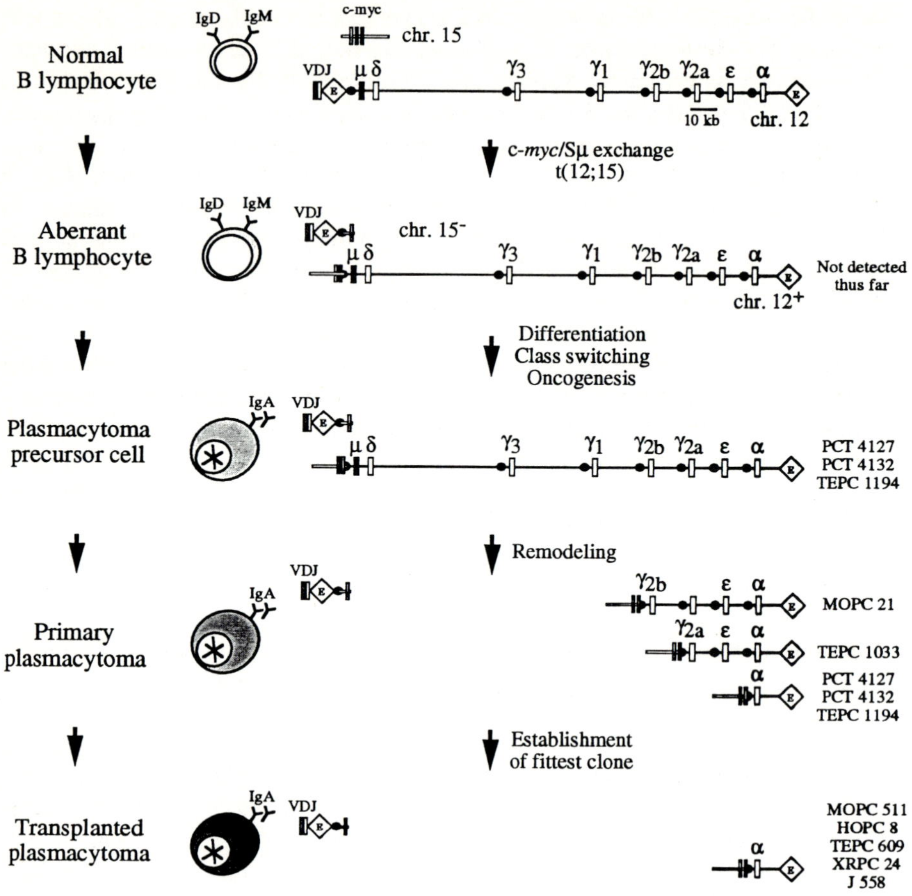

Fig. 2. Proposed schema on clonal evolution of Ighμ/c-*myc* recombinations during plasmacytoma development in BALB/c mice

carrying remodeled, secondary Ighα/c-*myc* exchanges. Several intermediate clones can be expected to be generated during remodeling, and the chr.12+-typical recombination structures between c-*myc* and Ighγ2b and c-*myc* and Ighγ2a that were detected in MOPC 21 and TEPC 1033, respectively, may represent such "frozen" intermediates. Finally, when primary plasmacytomas have been propagated by serial transplantation or after cell lines have been established, the tumor cell with the Ighα/c-*myc* rearrangement on the c-*myc*-deregulating allele will frequently have emerged as the fittest clone. This situation can apparently be encountered in a large number of BALB/c plasmacytomas and is exemplified in Fig. 2 by MOPC 511, HOPC 8, TEPC 609, XRPC 24, J558. In summary, we suggest that remodeling of Ighμ/c-*myc* recombinations provides a novel, yet not the exclusive (unpublished data), pathway for the molecular evolution of c-*myc*-deregulating chromosomal translocations, contributing to the plasmacytoma-typical predominance of genetic exchanges between Ighα and c-*myc* on chr. 12+.

References

1. Bard JA, Birshtein BK (1995) Rearrangement of a VH-associated LINE-1 element with the expressed IgH cluster in a murine myeloma cell line. J Immunol 154:201-208
2. Coffman RL, Lebman DA, Rothman P (1993) Mechanism and regulation of immunoglobulin isotype switching. Adv Immunol 54:229-270
3. Crossen PE, Kennedy MA, Heaton DC, Morrison MJ (1993) Cloning and sequencing of a t(14;19) breakpoint that involves the Cμ switch region. Genes Chromosomes Cancer 8:60-62
4. Dunnick W, Hertz GZ, Scappino L, Gritzmacher C (1993) DNA sequences at immunoglobulin switch region recombination sites. Nucleic Acids Res 21:365-372
5. Elenich LA, Dunnick WA (1991) Sequence at insertion site of E.Tn retrotransposon into an immunoglobulin switch region suggests a role for switch recombinase. Nucleic Acids Res 19:396
6. Gerstein RM, Frankel WN, Hsieh CL, Durdik JM, Rath S, Coffin JM, Nisonoff A, Selsing E (1990) Isotype switching of an immunoglobulin heavy chain transgene occurs by DNA recombination between different chromosomes. Cell 63:537-548
7. Harriman W, Volk H, Defranoux N, Wabl M (1993) Immunoglobulin class switch recombination. Annu Rev Immunol 11:361-384
8. Janz S, Müller J, Shaughnessy J, Potter M (1993) Detection of recombinations between c-*myc* and immunoglobulin switch α in murine plasma cell tumors and preneoplastic lesions by polymerase chain reaction. Proc Natl Acad Sci USA 90:7361-7365
9. Knight KL, Kingzette M, Crane MA, Zhai SK (1995) Transchromosomally

derived Ig heavy chains. J Immunol 155:684-691
10. Kottmann AH, Zevnik B, Welte M, Nielsen PJ, Köhler G (1994) A second promoter and enhancer element within the immunoglobulin heavy chain locus. Eur J Immunol 24:817-821
11. Kovalchuk AL, Potter M, Janz S (1996) DNA sequence analysis of the genetic recombination between *Igh*6 and *Myc* in an uncommon BALB/c plasmacytoma, TEPC 1194. Immunogenetics 44:151-156
12. Madisen L, Groudine M (1994) Identification of a locus control region in the immunoglobulin heavy-chain locus that deregulates c-*myc* expression in plasmacytoma and Burkitt's lymphoma cells. Genes Dev 8:2212-2226
13. Mautner J, Joos S, Werner T, Eick D, Bornkamm GW, Polack A (1995) Identification of two enhancer elements downstream of the human c-*myc* gene.Nucleic Acids Res 23:72-80
14. Mautner J, Behrends U, Hortnagel K, Brielmeier M, Hammerschmidt W, Strobl L, Bornkamm GW (1996) c-*myc* expression is activated by the immunoglobulin kappa-enhancers from a distance of at least 30 kb but not by elements located within 50 kb of the unaltered c-*myc* locus in vivo. Oncogene 12:1299-1307
15. Michaelson JS, Giannini SL, Birshtein BK (1995) Identification of 3'α-hs4, a novel Ig heavy chain enhancer element regulated at multiple stages of B cell differentiation. Nucleic Acids Res 23:975-981
16. Müller JR, Potter M, Janz S (1994) Differences in the molecular structure of c-*myc*-activating recombinations in murine plasmacytomas and precursor cells. Proc Natl Acad Sci USA 91:12066-12070
17. Müller JR, Janz S, Potter M (1995) Differences between Burkitt's lymphomas and mouse plasmacytomas in the immunoglobulin heavy chain/c-*myc* recombinations that occur in their chromosomal translocations. Cancer Res 55:5012-5018
18. Packham G, Cleveland JL (1995) c-Myc and apoptosis. Biochim Biophys Acta 1242:11-28
19. Pear WS, Nelson SF, Axelson H, Wahlstrom G, Bazin H, Klein G, Sumegi J. (1988) Aberrant class switching juxtaposes c-*myc* with a middle repetitive element (LINE) and an IgH intron in two spontaneously arising rat immunocytomas. Oncogene 2:499-507
20. Potter M, Wiener F (1992) Plasmacytomagenesis in mice: model of neoplastic development dependent upon chromosomal translocations. Carcinogenesis 13:1681-1697
21. Sigurdardottir D, Sohn J, Kass J, Selsing E (1995) Regulatory regions 3' of the immunoglobulin heavy chain intronic enhancer differentially affect expression of a heavy chain transgene in resting and activated B cells. J Immunol 154:2217-2225
22. Zelenetz AD, Cleary ML, Levy R (1993) A submicroscopic interstitial deletion of chromosome 14 frequently occurs adjacent to the t(14;18) translocation breakpoint in human follicular lymphoma. Genes Chromosom Cancer 6:140-150

Generation of Immunoglobulin/c-*myc* Recombinations in Murine Peyer's Patch Follicles

J. R. Müller, E. B. Mushinski, G. M. Jones, J. A. Williams, S. Janz, P. F. Hausner and M. Potter
Laboratory of Genetics, National Cancer Institute, National Institutes of Health, Bethesda, MD, USA

Introduction

Plasmacytoma can be induced by the intraperitoneal injection of pristane in susceptible BALB/c mice. Most inbred strains of mice, however, are resistant to this type of plasmacytoma induction (Potter & Wiener, 1992).

Virtually all BALB/c plasmacytoma carry characteristic chromosomal translocations that deregulate c-*myc* by juxtaposing immunoglobulin enhancer sequences and the c-*myc* gene. Most frequently, c-*myc* is joined to the immunoglobulin heavy chain (IgH) locus within the IgHα switch region (Janz et al., 1993; Müller et al., 1995). Plasmacytomas with IgHμ/c-*myc* are only occasionally observed.

Using polymerase chain reaction (PCR) as a detection method, we recently found cells with IgH/c-*myc* recombinations in preneoplastic tissues of pristane-treated mice (Müller et al., 1994, 1996). However, the origin of these genetically aberrant cells remains obscure. Here we describe the detection of IgH/c-*myc* recombination-harboring cell clones in secondary lymph tissues of normal mice, and we show the migration of these cells in response to pristane in plasmacytoma-resistant and -susceptible mice.

Results and Discussion

IgH/c-*myc* recombinations occur in secondary lymph tissues of normal mice.
To investigate the origin of cells with IgH/c-*myc* rearrangements in untreated BALB/c mice, we studied a number of DNAs from different tissues by PCR (Fig. 1A). Bone marrows and fetal livers did not harbor

detectable IgH/c-*myc* fusion products. In contrast, we found c-*myc* recombinations in secondary lymphoid tissues, chiefly in the gut-associated lymphoid tissues. Plasmacytoma-resistant strains of mice did harbor recombination-positive cells, although at lower frequency (not shown). Using in situ PCR, we detected IgH/c-*myc* recombination-positive cells in Peyer's patch follicles (Fig. 2) as well as within the intestinal lamina propria (not shown). Based on the identification of clonotypic IgH/c-*myc* fusion sequences, we observed a migration of these cells within the intestinal tissues (Fig. 3).

Tissue Distribution of IgH/c-*myc* Recombination-Carrying Cells in Response to Pristane.

Treatment with pristane induces plasmacytoma development within an oil granuloma that forms on mesenteric surfaces in BALB/c mice (Potter & Wiener, 1992). Whereas the mesenteries of untreated BALB/c mice were negative for cells with IgH/c-*myc* recombinations, half of the developing mesenteric oil granulomas harbored these cells 7 days after pristane injection (Fig. 1B), indicating that recombination-positive cells had migrated into the granuloma. Analysis of IgH/c-*myc* fusion sequences revealed a trafficking of these cells between intestinal tissues and spleen as well as between spleen and oil granuloma (not shown).

To investigate a possible correlation between genetically determined resistance to plasmacytoma development and the occurrence of cells with IgH/c-*myc* fusions, three resistant inbred strains of mice were analyzed (DBA/2N, C3H/HeJ, C57BL/6). Mice that are resistant to pristane-induced plasmacytoma development harbored fewer IgH/c-*myc*-positive clones in general (Fig. 1B). In addition, these cells were not detected in either spleen or oil granuloma, suggesting that the tendency to migrate is a

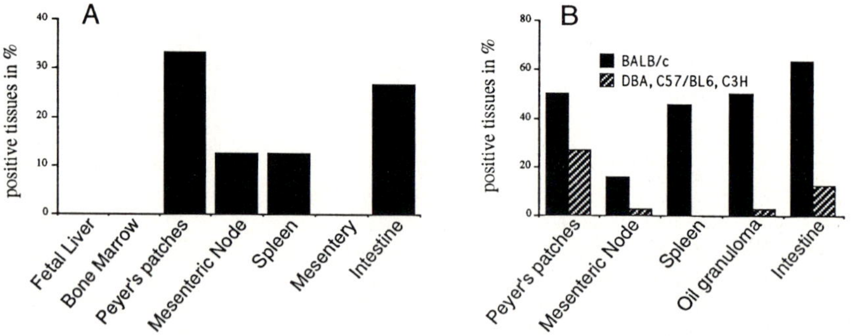

Fig. 1. Tissue distribution of IgH/c-*myc* recombinations in untreated BALB/c mice (A) and in plasmacytoma-susceptible and -resistant mice 7 days after pristane treatment (B) as detected by PCR. Bars represent the percentage of tissues where at least one recombination was amplified.

pronounced feature of IgH/c-*myc*-positive cells in BALB/c mice. The absence of cells with IgH/c-*myc* recombinations in the oil granuloma of resistant mice may be one factor that determines the resistance phenotype.

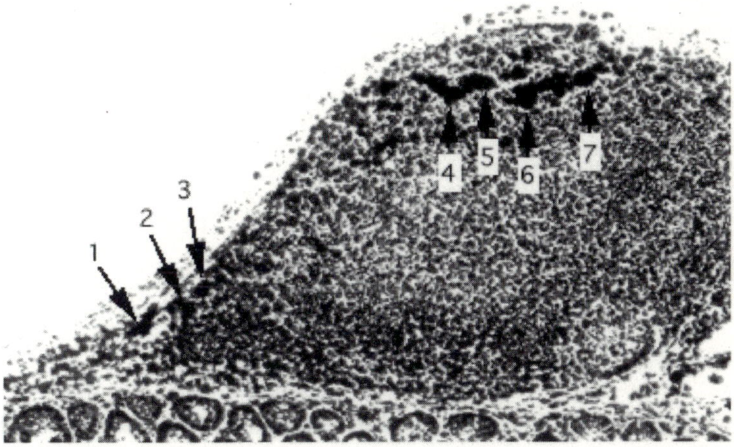

Fig. 2. Detection of IgH/c-*myc* recombinations by in situ PCR. A Peyer's patch follicle is shown. Tissue sections were treated by two rounds of PCR followed by a hybridization with riboprobes that contain a pseudonucleotide. After treatment with an enzyme-tagged antibody that recognizes the pseudonucleotide, sections were stained with alkaline phosphatase. To confirm the presence of c-*myc* recombinations, darkly stained cells (#1-#7) were microdissected, and IgH/c-*myc* fusion products were reamplified using conventional PCR and were sequenced.

Fig. 3. Migration of cells with IgH/c-*myc* recombinations within gut-associated lymphoid tissues. Following removal of Peyer's patches, the intestine was dissected into ten segments (# 1/2, duodenum; #19/20, colon). Duplicate PCR analysis resulted in the amplification of a number of different IgH/c-*myc* fusion products (arrows). Reactions #1/#8/#11 and #13/#14/#18 revealed identical recombination sequences, indicating that a IgH/c-*myc*-positive cell had undergone proliferation and migration between these parts of the intestine.

Specificity of IgH Loci in Recombinations with c-*myc*.
The PCR technology used in these studies permits the detection of fusion products that involve c-*myc* and either the IgHα or IgHμ locus. Sequence analysis of recombination products revealed a high frequency of c-*myc* recombinations with the IgHα locus in BALB/c mice (72%, Fig. 4). In contrast, two of the plasmacytoma-resistant strains of mice, DBA/2N and C57BL/6, had predominantly IgHμ involved (67%). The fusion of the IgHα locus to c-*myc* juxtaposes the immunoglobulin 3' enhancer to c-*myc*, possibly leading to a stronger transcriptional upreglation of c-*myc* compared to recombinations with the IgHμ locus. Therefore, the fusion of c-*myc* to different IgH loci may have different oncogenic potentials, and the failure of inbred strains of mice to generate IgHα/c-*myc* rearrangements may count in part for their resistance to develop plasmacytoma.

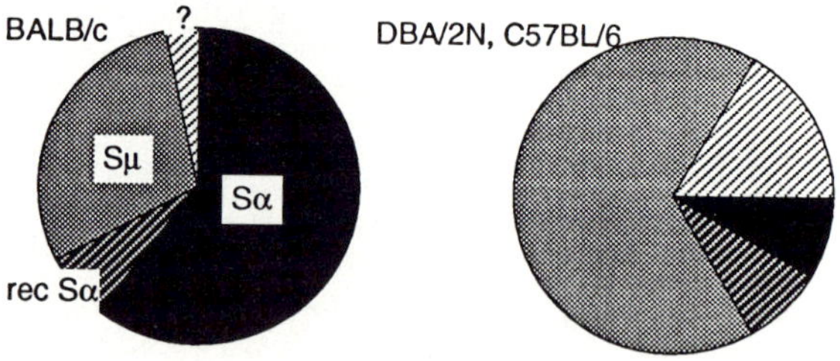

Fig. 4. Inbred strain-specific involvement of IgH regions in c-*myc* recombinations. Whereas the IgHα locus (Sα-switchα region; rec Sα-recombined switchα region) is predominantly juxtaposed to c-*myc* in BALB/c mice, Sμ is more often found in DBA/2N and in C57BL/6 mice. Several fusion sequences could not be aligned to germ-line (?).

Conclusions

Ig/c-*myc* recombinations are generated in secondary lymphoid tissues of untreated plasmacytoma-susceptible and -resistant mice, chiefly in the gut-associated lymphoid tissues.

In BALB/c mice, cells with c-*myc* recombinations can be detected migrating within the gut-associated lymphoid tissues, into other lymphoid organs and into the oil granuloma in response to pristane treatment.

Plasmacytoma-resistant strains of mice (DBA/2N, C3H/HeJ, C57BL/6) differ in that: i) they harbor fewer IgH/c-*myc*-positive clones; ii) these cells are largely excluded from the developing oil granuloma; iii) Igμ rather than Igα is more frequently involved in recombinations with c-*myc* (DBA/2N and C57BL/6).

References

Janz S, Müller J, Shaughnessy J, Potter M (1993) Detection of recombinations between c-*myc* and immunoglobulin switch α in murine plasma cell tumors and preneoplastic lesions by polymerase chain reaction. Proc Natl Acad Sci USA 90: 7361-7365

Müller JR, Potter M, Janz, S (1994) Differences in the molecular structure of c-*myc*-activating recombinations in murine plasmacytomas and precursor cells. Proc Natl Acad Sci USA 91: 12066-12070

Müller JR, Janz S, Potter M (1995) Differences between Burkitt's lymphomas and mouse plasmacytomas in the immunoglobulin heavy chain/c-*myc* recombinations that occur in their chromosomal translocations. Cancer Res 55: 5012-5018

Müller JR, Jones GM, Potter M, Janz S (1996) Detection of immunoglobulin/c-*myc* recombinations in mice that are resistant to plasmacytoma induction. Cancer Res 56: 419-423

Potter M, Wiener F (1992) Plasmacytomagenesis in mice: model of neoplastic development dependent upon chromosomal translocations. Carcinogenesis 13: 1681-1697

Myc/Max Family of Transcription Factors and bcl-2 are Involved in Drug-induced Apoptosis of Myeloma Cells

D. S. Siegel, J. A. Terry, J. Koury, B. Barlogie, J. Epstein and R. Feinman
Division of Hematology and Oncology, University of Arkansas for Medical Sciences, Little Rock, AR, USA

Introduction

Cell homeostasis is controlled by a balance between proliferation, growth arrest and apoptosis. It is becoming increasingly evident that dysregulation of genes that control apoptosis contributes to the pathogenesis of disease such as cancer and autoimmune disease (1). In multiple myeloma, myeloma cells are terminally differentiated and fail to apoptose. Glucocorticoids such as dexamethasone (Dex) are often used in the treatment of myeloma, either alone or in combination with cytotoxic agents (2,3). Similarly, IL-6 in the bone marrow environment protects immature myeloma cells form Dex-induced apoptosis (4). However, with prolonged treatment, patients develop resistance to these agents. It is well established that both glucocorticoids and chemotherapeutic drugs are potent inducers of cell death, by apoptosis (1). In fact, recent studies have demonstrated that Dex-induced apoptosis in several human myeloma cell lines and that interleukin-6 (IL-6), a B cell differentiation/survival factor, protected them from Dex-induced apoptosis (5,6,Epstein J personal communication) The molecular mechanisms that govern these processes are not fully understood. Restoration of the apoptopic response in myeloma cells could lead to the development of effective therapy for multiple myeloma.

Bcl-2 and Bcl-X_L Confer Resistance to Drug-Induced Apoptosis

In numerous lymphoid model systems, glucocorticoids have been shown to induce lymphoid cells to either undergo growth arrest or apoptosis. Yet, very little is known about glucocorticoids' mode of action. Recent reports in the literature have proposed that steroids such as glucocorticoids and estrogen induce apoptosis by repressing transcription of *survival* genes (7,8). Dysregulation of both c-myc and bcl-2 gene expression, two major *survival* genes, have been implicated in the pathogenesis of myeloma. (9-11). Our preliminary studies have demonstrated that glucocorticoid susceptibility and bcl-2 expression are related inversely in several myeloma cell lines. Stable parental, bcl-2 and bcl-X_L transfectants of the human multiple myeloma cell line ARP-1 were generated and characterized for their susceptibility to Dex-induced apoptosis. The expression vectors used in these studies were pSFFV-neo and pSFFV-bcl-2-neo (kindly provided by S. Korsmeyer, Washington University, St. Louis, MO), and pCDNA3 and pCDNA-bcl-X_L. Western blot analysis confirmed that both bcl-2 and bcl-

X_L transfected cells expressed higher levels of bcl-2 and bcl-X_L proteins relative to their parental counterparts. In agreement with earlier reports by Hardin and coworkers (5) and Xhang and coworkers (12), Dex and hexamethylene bisacetamide (HMBA), a potent inducer of differentiation were able to induce apoptosis in the parental ARP-1 transfectants within 48 hour of treatment, as determined by in situ end labeling. Overexpression of bcl-2 protected ARP-1 cells from undergoing both Dex- and HMBA-mediated apoptosis. Overexpression of bcl-X_L also conferred resistance to Dex-mediated apoptosis.

Bcl-2 Prevents the Downmodulation of Mad1 and Max proteins by either Dex or HMBA

Genes involved in cell cycle progression have been shown to serve as intracellular targets for glucocorticoids action. In T cell lymphoma and leukemia cell lines, Dex induces G0/G1 growth arrest in cells grown in the presence of fetal bovine serum, whereas in serum-free medium, Dex induces apoptosis (13). More recently, Dex has been demonstrated to inhibit c-myc E2F, cyclin-dependent kinase 4, and cyclin D3 gene expression in these cell lines. Overexpression of both cyclin D3 and c-myc in a murine T cell lymphoma conferred resistance to Dex-induced apoptosis (14). Decreased transcription of c-myc was also associated with etoposide-induced apoptosis in a wide variety of cancers (15) and with anti-sIgM- or phorbol ester-triggered apoptosis in the murine B cell lymphoma, WEHI231 (16).

Myc/max family of basic helix-loop-helix leucine zipper (bHLHzip) transcription factors appear to serve as intracellular targets for glucocorticoids' suppressive effects. Both Dex and HMBA decreased c-myc expression in parental ARP-1 cells within 12 and 4 hrs of treatment, respectively. Bcl-2 overexpressing ARP-1 cells had higher constitutive levels of c-myc protein compared to their parental counterpart. Whereas overexpression of bcl-2 delayed the onset of Dex-mediated downregulation of c-myc proteins, no effects were seen on the HMBA-mediated decline of c-myc expression. Treatment of the parental ARP-1 transfectants with either Dex or HMBA downregulated mad1 and max levels within 24 hours. Overexpression of bcl-2 prevented the Dex- and HMBA-mediated downregulation of mad1 and max. These results suggest that the difference in the sensitivity to Dex and HMBA cytotoxic effects between the parental and bcl-2 ARP-1 transfectants was due to the differential expression of the myc/max family members.

Bcl-2 Blocks the Downmodulation of E Box DNA binding activities by Dex and HMBA

As discussed earlier, very little is known about the molecular mechanisms by which Dex induces apoptosis in myeloma cells, and the mechanism by which bcl-2 suppresses drug-induced apoptosis. Myc/max, mad/max, and mxi/mad heterodimers as well as max/max, USF, and TFE3 homodimers have been reported to activate or repress the transcription from E box containing promoters (17). To examine the DNA binding factors that interact with the E box, electrophoretic mobility shift assay (EMSA) was performed using the CM-1 probe probe (identical to the E box nucleotide sequence reported in 18). Both Dex and HMBA inhibited E box DNA complex formation in extracts of parental ARP-1 transfectants. Reduced E box binding was observed within 4 hr and 12 hr of Dex and HMBA treatment respectively. The absence of E box complex formation was evident within 12 hr and 24 hr of Dex and HMBA treatment, respectively. Perhaps more interestingly, overexpression of bcl-2 blocked the downmodulation of E box DNA binding by Dex and HMBA. In a related experiment, ectopic expression of Bcl-X_L also blocked downregulation of E box binding.

In electrophoretic mobility supershift assays, anti-mad antibody abrogated E box complex formation while anti-max antibody markedly reduced E box complex formation by extracts of both parental and bcl-2 transfected ARP-1 cells (antibodies kindly provided by R.N. Eisenman, Fred Hutchinson Cancer Research Center, Seattle, WA). The upstream stimulatory factor (USF), a member of this family of bHLH-zip transcription factors, binds to this DNA sequence and is part of the slower migrating complex (18). We found that USF is part of this complex that remained constant in the absence and presence of Dex.

To determine the clinical significance of these findings, freshly-obtained patient myeloma cells were studied. The ability of Dex to downregulate E-box DNA binding activity by extracts of purified myeloma plasma cells (19) *in vitro*, correlated with the clinical response of the patients to Dex treatment.

Conclusion

On the basis of these observations, it is tempting to speculate that activation of E box DNA binding activity protects myeloma cells from undergoing drug-induced apoptosis. Both Dex and HMBA appear to downregulate mad1 and max expression which in turn prevents E box complex formation. Conversely, increased Bcl-2 or Bcl-X_L expression enables mad1 and max to heterodimerize and bind to E box in the presence of Dex or HMBA. Whether E box activation in myeloma is important in the differentiation process and/or in the repression of major target molecules involved in the apoptotic pathway, remains to be resolved.

References

1. Thompson CB (1995) Apoptosis in the pathogenesis and treatment of disease. Science 267:1456-1462
2. Barlogie B, Epstein J (1990) Multiple myeloma:biology and therapy. J. Cancer Res. & Clin. Oncol. 116:109-111
3. Alexanian R, Dimopoulos MA, Delasalle K, Barlogie B (1992) Primary dexamethasonetreatment of multiple myeloma. Blood 80:887-890
4. Grigorieva I, Thomas X, Woodliff J, Epstein J (1995) The bone marrow environment contributes to dexamethasone resistance in multiple myeloma. Blood 86(Suppl 1): 728
5. Hardin J, Macleod S, Grigorieva I, Chang R, Barlogie B, Xiao H, Epstein J (1994) Interleukin-6 prevents dexamethasone-induced myeloma cell death. Blood 84:3063- 3070
6. Lichtenstein A, Tu Y, Fady C, Vescio R, Berenson J (1995) Interleukin-6 inhibits apoptosis of malignant plasma cells. Cell. Immunol. 162:248-255
7. Helmberg A, Auphan N, Caelles C, Karin M (1995) Glucocorticoid-induced apoptosis of human leukemic cells is caused by the repressive function of the glucocorticoid receptor. EMBO J. 14:452-460
8. Blobel GA, Orkin SH (1996) Estrogen-induced apoptosis by inhibition of the erythroid transcription factor GATA-1. Mol. Cell Biol. 16:1687-1694
9. Petersson M, Jernberg-Wiklund, Larssin LG, Sundstrom C, Givol I, Tsujimoto Y, Nilsson K (1992) Expression of the bcl-2 gene in human multiple myeloma cell lines and normal plasma cells. Blood 79:495-502

10. Skopelitou A, Hadiyannakis M, Tsenga A, Theocharis S, Alexopoulou V, Kittas C, Agnantis N (1993) Expression of c-myc p62 oncoprotein in multiple myeloma: An immunohistochemical study of 180 cases. Anticancer Res. 13:1091-1095
11. Selvanyagam P, Blick M, Narni F, van Tuinen P, Ledbetter DH, Alexanian R, Saunders F, Barlogie B (1988) Alteration and abnormal expression of the c-myc oncogene in human multiple myeloma. Blood 71:30-35
12. Zhang X, Siegel D, Pearse R, Michaeli J (1995) Distinct apoptotic pathways in human myeloma cells in response to dexamethasone and the differentiation inducer hexamethylene bisacetamide. Blood 86, Suppl 1:237
13. Thulasi R, Harbour DV, Thompson EB (1993) Suppression of c-myc is a critical step in glucocorticoid-induced human leukemic cell lysis. J.Biol.Chem. 268:18306-18312
14. Rhee K, Bresnaham W, Hirai A, Hirai M, Thompson EA (1995) c-Myc and cyclin D3 (CcnD3) genes are independent targets for glucocorticoid inhibition of lymphoid cell proliferation. Cancer Res. 55:4188-4195
15. Eliot HE, Borner MM, Sinha BK (1995) Differential oncogene expression and susceptibility to apoptosis in the human leukemia HL60 cell lines:implications for etoposide resistance. Anticancer Res. 15:729-734
16. Lee H, Arsura M, Wu M, Duyao M, Buckler AJ, Sonenshein GE (1995) Role of Rel-related factors in control of c-myc gene transcription in receptor-mediated apoptosis of the murine B cell WEHI 231 line. J. Exp. Med. 181:1169-1177
17. Ryan KM, Birnie GD (1996) Myc oncogenes: the enigmatic family. Biochem. J. 14:713-721
18. Blackwood EM, Eisenman RN (1991) Max: A helix-loop-helix zipper protein that forms a sequence-specific DNA binding complex with myc. Science 251:1211-1217
19. Hata H, Xiao H, Petrucci MT,Woodliff J, Chang R, Epstein J (1993) Interleukin-6 gene expression in multiple myeloma: a characteristic of immature tumor cells. Blood 81:3357-3364

Effects of Interferon Alpha on Myeloma Cells: Mechanisms of Differential Responsiveness

D. F. Jelinek and T. Arora
Department of Immunology, Mayo Clinic Foundation, Rochester, Minnesota 55905, USA

Introduction

Multiple myeloma is a progressive and fatal disease characterized by the accumulation of malignant plasma cells in the bone marrow. We have been interested in understanding the mechanisms of growth control in myeloma cells. By way of introduction, Figure 1 is a schematic depiction of the proposed progression from monoclonal gammopathy of undetermined significance (MGUS) into myeloma. The incidence of MGUS over the age of 60 has been shown to be approximately 1% and incidence increases to 3% in individuals over the age of 70 (reviewed in 1). Importantly, it has been shown that a significant proportion of MGUS patients will progress into myeloma over time (2). The key distinguishing features between MGUS and myeloma include the absence of lytic bone lesions (MGUS; 3) and differences in the proliferative index of the monoclonal plasma cell population. Thus, a well-documented change that occurs during the progression from MGUS to myeloma is an increase in the plasma cell labeling (proliferative index) of the plasma cell (LI; 4,5). Because of the key differences between the growth properties displayed by benign (MGUS) and malignant (myeloma) plasma cells, we have had a keen interest in understanding the mechanisms of growth control. Figure 1 suggests that key changes that may occur during this progression include alterations in cytokine responsiveness, acquisition of autocrine growth factor expression, or alterations in cytokine receptor expression.

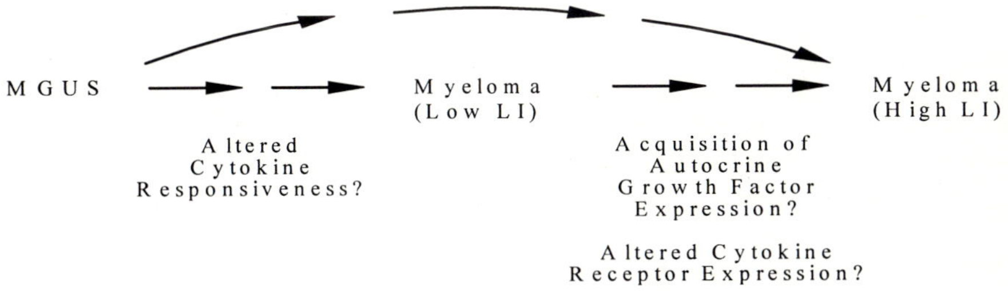

Fig 1. Speculative model of tumor progression in the monoclonal gammopathies.

One means to study growth control of myeloma cells is to use agents that have been shown to function as negative regulators of cellular growth. In this respect, interferon alpha (IFN-α) has been identified as a negative regulator of myeloma cell growth and because of this it has been a commonly employed chemotherapeutic agent for the treatment of multiple myeloma (6-9). The effectiveness of IFN-α, however, is variable as is its effects on *in vitro* cultured myeloma cells (10-13). The reason(s) for this variability is not yet understood, nor is the mechanism by which IFN-α inhibits myeloma cell growth. In this study, we have utilized a panel of human myeloma cell lines that are uniformly growth-responsive to interleukin 6 (IL-6) yet vary remarkably in responsiveness to IFN-α. Because IFN-α disrupts IL-6 stimulated proliferation of myeloma cells, we reasoned that an analysis of the mechanism(s) by which IFN-α mediated this disruption of signal transduction would similarly be informative about growth control of myeloma cells. We have therefore examined key signaling events that are known to be associated with growth control and that are induced following stimulation with either IL-6 or IFN-α.

Materials and Methods

Cell lines and proliferation assays

The myeloma cell lines ANBL-6 (14), KAS-6/1, and DP-6 (15) were derived in our laboratory and maintained in the presence of IL-6 as previously described. Before assaying the effects of cytokines on cellular DNA synthesis, cells were washed three times and resuspended in media lacking cytokines prior to culturing cells in round-bottomed 96-well microtiter plates. Cultures were conducted in triplicate in the presence of the indicated additions for 3 days at 37° C in the presence of 5% CO_2. One microcurie of [^{3}H]thymidine was added to the cultures 18 hours before harvesting and [^{3}H]thymidine incorporation was quantitated by liquid scintillation spectroscopy. Values represent the mean of triplicate samples.

Cytokine induction

Before assaying cytokine-mediated signaling events, viable myeloma cells were first isolated with sodium diatrizoate/Ficoll gradients (Isolymph; Gallard-Schlesinger), washed with saline, and recultured without IL-6 for 24-48 hrs in RPMI 1640 containing 1% FCS. Immediately prior to cytokine stimulation, cells were washed and recultured in cytokine-free media at a density of 5 x 10^6 cells/ml. IL-6 (kindly provided by the Immunex Corporation, Seattle, WA) or IFN-α2b (Schering Corporation) were added at a final concentration of 30 ng/ml. Stimulation with cytokine was terminated by the addition of ice-cold PBS and immediate centrifugation. Nuclear extracts were prepared as previously described (16). Electrophoretic mobility shift assays (EMSA) using the serum-inducible element (SIE) of the c-fos promoter as a probe were also performed as previously described (16).

Analysis of c-myc mRNA and protein expression

To determine the effects of IFN-α on induction of c-myc mRNA expression, reverse transcription PCR was utilized. The ANBL-6 and KAS-6/1 cell lines were stimulated with cytokines for various lengths of time, total RNA was isolated as previously described (15), and primers specific for c-myc (Clontech, Palo Alto, CA) were used to amplify c-myc mRNA. For analysis of c-myc protein expression, the ANBL-6 and KAS-6/1 cell lines were stimulated with cytokines and total cellular lysates were prepared using a 50 mM Tris, pH 8.0 based lysis buffer that was supplemented with 10% v/v glycerol, 0.5% NP-40, 0.1 mM EDTA, 1 mM Na_3VO_4, 1 mM DTT, 200 μM PMSF, and protease inhibitors. Protein levels for c-myc were detected by Western analysis using c-myc-specific antibodies obtained from UBI, Lake Placid, NY. The ECL detection system (Amersham) was used to visualize protein levels.

Results

Myeloma cell line responsiveness to IFN-α is heterogeneous

Previous results from our group have demonstrated that myeloma cell line responsiveness to IFN-α is heterogeneous (14-16). Table 1 demonstrates that each cell line is stimulated by IL-6 to synthesize DNA. By contrast, however, IFNα did not stimulate DNA synthesis by the ANBL-6 or KP-6 cell lines and furthermore, significantly inhibited IL-6 stimulated DNA synthesis. Of interest, IFN-α was directly stimulatory for the KAS-6/1 cell line. These results suggest that myeloma cell line responsiveness to IFN-α is heterogeneous.

Table 1. Effects of IL-6 and IFN-α on Myeloma Cell Line DNA Synthesis

	Stimulus			
Cell Line	Nil	IL-6	IFN-α	IL-6 + IFN-α
	[^{3}H] Thymidine Incorporation (cpm x 10^{-3})			
ANBL-6	9.6	128.1	0.6	4.4
KP-6	12.0	129.1	0.4	1.2
KAS-6/1	29.8	143.1	104.8	140.5

Myeloma cells were cultured at a density of 2.5 x 10^4 cells per microtiter well. Cells were stimulated with 1 ng/ml IL-6 or 1000 u/ml IFN-α. DNA synthesis was assayed on day 3.

STAT factor activation

Both IL-6 and IFN-α have both been shown to utilize a direct signal transduction pathway to the nucleus that involves phosphorylation and activation of cytoplasmic STAT proteins via JAK family kinases (reviewed in 17, 18). Detection of the presence of activated STAT factors is possible by incubation of nuclear extracts with an oligonucleotide probe that contains a mutant high-affinity version of the SIE from the c-fos promoter (19). This element has been shown to serve as a high-affinity target sequence for STAT factors activated in response to both IL-6 and IFN-α. The next experiments were designed to analyze the ability of IL-6 and IFN-α to induce STAT factor activation in the three myeloma cell lines.

Figure 2 depicts the results obtained when the three cell lines were stimulated with IL-6, IFN-α, or the combination of the two cytokines and the nuclear extracts were assayed for the presence of activated STAT factors. It may be seen, however, that there were no discernible differences between patterns of STAT activation between the cell lines. In experiments not shown, we have identified the slowest migrating complex as consisting of STAT3 homodimers, the fastest migrating complex as consisting of STAT1 homodimers, and the intermediate complex as consisting of STAT1/STAT3 heterodimers. These results suggest that the differential responsiveness to IFN-α does not result from differential STAT factor activation.

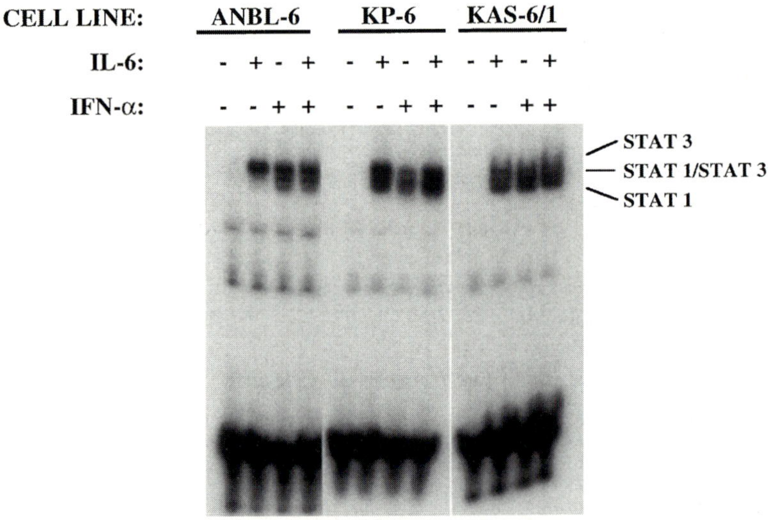

Fig. 2. STAT factor activation. Nuclear extracts were prepared from unstimulated or cytokine stimulated (15 minutes) myeloma cells and 5 μg of extract was incubated with a ^{32}P-labeled SIE probe. Following co-incubation of probe with nuclear extract, samples were electrophoresed on non-denaturing 4.5% acrylamide gels, gels were dried down, and subsequently exposed to film.

Effects of IFN-α on c-myc mRNA or protein expression

Other investigators have demonstrated that IFN-α-mediated growth inhibition can be correlated with decreases in levels of c-myc expression (20). Our next experiments, therefore, were designed to determine if the differential responsiveness of myeloma cells to IFN-α could be explained by differences in c-myc expression. In our first experiments, we utilized RT-PCR to assess the ability of IFN-α to either increase or decrease c-myc mRNA expression. It may be seen in Figure 3, however, that both cell lines express constitutively high levels of c-myc mRNA and that neither IL-6 nor IFN-α significantly altered mRNA expression levels.

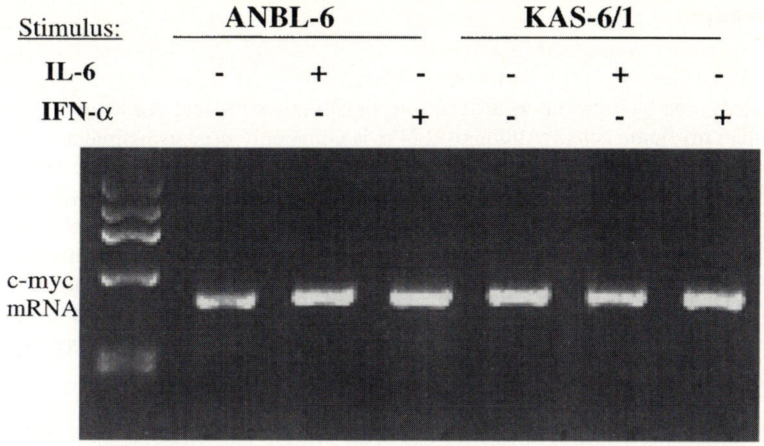

Fig. 3. Analysis of c-myc mRNA expression. ANBL-6 and KAS-6/1 cells were deprived of IL-6 overnight before stimulating the cells with cytokines. After a 24 hr cytokine stimulation, total RNA was isolated and RT-PCR was performed utilizing primers specific for c-myc. PCR products were visualized by agarose gel electrophoresis and ethidium bromide staining.

Similar experiments were performed to assess the effects of IFN-α on c-myc protein levels in the ANBL-6 and KAS-6/1 cell lines. Consistent with the results shown in Figure 3 suggesting that c-myc expression may be elevated and deregulated in these myeloma cell lines, the results shown in Figure 4 similarly demonstrated that both cell lines express constitutively high levels of c-myc protein. Thus, even after depriving both cell lines of cytokines for a period of 48 hrs, c-myc levels remained elevated. IFN-α was essentially without effect in modulating c-myc expression in either cell line. These results suggest that the differential responsiveness of myeloma cells to IFN-α does not appear to result from differences in c-myc expression.

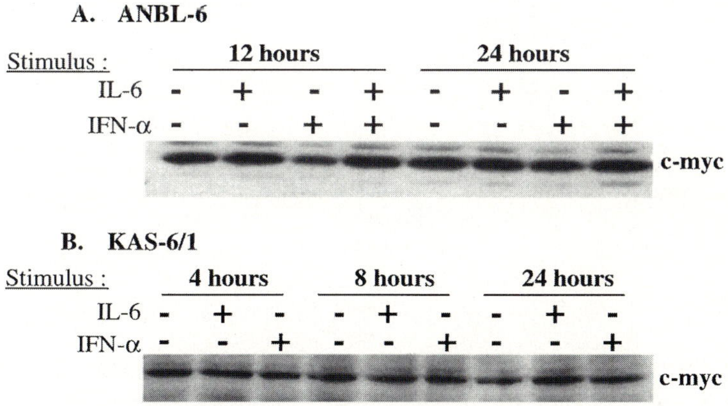

Fig. 4. Analysis of c-myc protein expression. ANBL-6 and KAS-6/1 cells were deprived of IL-6 overnight before stimulating the cells for the indicated periods of time with IL-6 or IFN-α. Total cellular lysates were prepared and 50 μg of protein were electrophoresed on 7.5% polyacrylamide gels, transferred to Immobilon P, and probed with an antibody specific for c-myc.

Discussion

In this study, we have begun to analyze the signaling events that are triggered by IFN-α in human myeloma cells. Although IFN-α is commonly used as maintenance therapy for myeloma patients, there are a number of reports in the literature that IFN-α may actually aggravate disease via its ability to stimulate myeloma cell growth (21, 22). However, this result is controversial in that reports also exist in which IFN-α has been clearly demonstrated to inhibit myeloma cell growth (12, 13). Because we have established a panel of human myeloma cell lines that capture the heterogeneity that has been published in the literature, we were in a unique position to begin to identify the molecular differences that may underly differential myeloma cell responsiveness to IFN-α.

Although the work described in this report has not identified the mechanism that accounts for these differences, we have presented data which suggest that the differences do not derive from differential STAT factor activation or c-myc expression. It is important to note, however, that we have not yet examined the expression levels of other members of the c-myc family. Thus, it remains possible that differences in mad or max expression may be playing a role in determining whether the outcome of IFN-α signaling is cellular growth or growth cessation. It is also important to acknowledge that although STAT activation appeared to be comparable between the two cell lines, it remains possible that there may be differences between the two cell lines with respect to expression of genes that are transcriptionally activated by STAT factors (Figure 5). Finally, the Ras/MAP kinase pathway has also been shown to be activated by these two cytokines (Figure 5). It likewise remains possible that differential myeloma cell

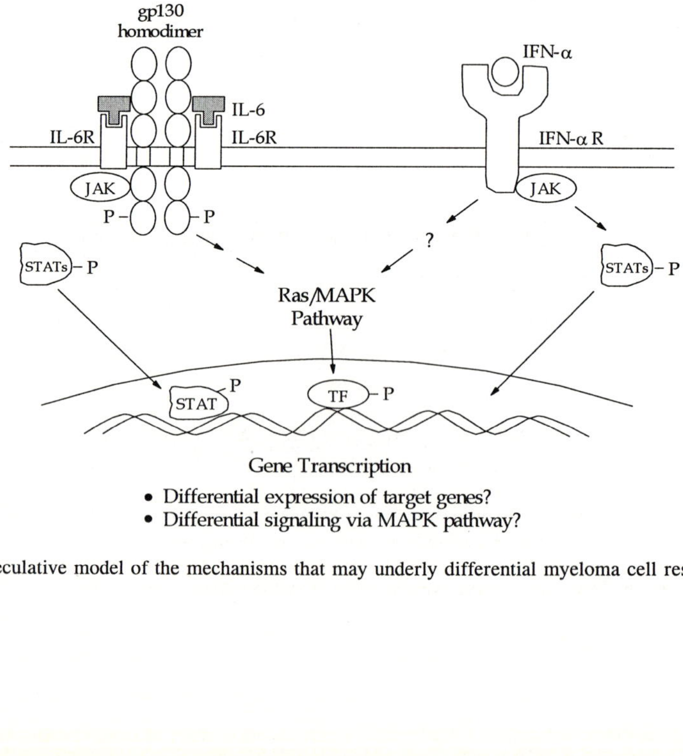

Fig. 5. Speculative model of the mechanisms that may underly differential myeloma cell responsiveness to IFN-α.

responsiveness to IFN-α may result from alterations in this pathway. This possibility is currently being explored.

In summary, we have described a model system that provides a mechanism to address a number of interesting issues. First, because IFN-α is typically anti-proliferative in action, the mitogenic response of the KAS-6/1 cell line to IFN-α may provide an important tool to further dissect the general mechanisms of IFN-α mediated growth inhibition. Second, simultaneous analysis of myeloma cells that are growth-stimulated or growth-arrested by IFN-α should ultimately permit elucidation of the crucial, underlying differences between these cell lines. Finally, identification of the mechanisms of IFN-α-mediated growth inhibition of myeloma cells may allow development of agents that are more universally effective than IFN-α.

This work was supported by National Institutes of Health Grants CA62242 and CA62228 (awarded to D.F.J.).

References

1. Kyle RA (1995) Monoclonal gammopathy of undetermined significance (MGUS). Baillier's Clin Haematol 8:761-781
2. Kyle RA (1993) "Benign" monoclonal gammopathy - after 20 to 35 years of follow-up. Mayo Clinic Proc 68:26-36
3. Kyle RA, Lust JA (1989) Monoclonal gammopathies of undetermined significance. Semin Hematol 26:176-200
4. Greipp PR, Lust JA, O'Fallon WM, Katzmann JA, Witzig TE, Kyle RA (1993) Plasma cell labeling index and β_2-microglobulin predict survival independent of thymidine kinase and C-reactive protein in multiple myeloma. Blood 81:3382-3387
5. Greipp PR, Katzmann JA, O'Fallon WM, Kyle RA (1988) Value of β_2-microglobulin level and plasma cell labeling indices as prognostic factors in patients with newly diagnosed myeloma. Blood 72:219-223
6. Mellstedt HA, Ahre A, Bjorkholm M, Holm G, Johansson B, Strander H (1979) Interferon therapy in myelomatosis. Lancet 1:245-247
7. Oken MM (1994) Standard treatment of multiple myeloma. Mayo Clin Proc 69:781-786
8. Browman GP, Bergsagel D, Sicheri D, O'Reilly S, Wilson KS, Rubin S, Belch A, Shustik C, Barr R, Walker I, James K, Zee B, Johnston D (1995) Randomized trial of interferon maintenance in multiple myeloma: A study of the National Cancer Institute of Canada clinical trials group. J Clin Oncol 13:2354-2360
9. Ludwig H, Cohen AM, Polliack A, Huber H, Nachbaur D, Senn H-J, Morant R, Eckhardt S, Günczler P, Seewann HL, Schüller J, Rhyner K, Cavalli F, Fritz E (1995) Interferon-alpha for induction and maintenance in multiple myeloma: Results of two multicenter randomized trials and summary of other studies. Annals of Oncol 6:467-476
10. Brenning G (1985) The in vitro effect of leucocyte α-interferon on human myeloma cells in a semisolid agar culture system. Scand J Haematol 35:178-185
11. Brenning G, Ahre A, Nilsson K (1985) Correlation between in vitro and in vivo sensitivity to human leucocyte interferon in patients with multiple myeloma. Scand J Haematol 35:543-549
12. Brenning G, Jernberg H, Gidlund M, Sjöberg and Nilsson K (1986) The effect of α and γ-interferon on proliferation and production of IgE and β_2-microglobulin in the human myeloma cell line U-266 and in an α-interferon resistant U-266 subline. Scand J Haematol 37:280-288

13. Portier M, Zhang X-G, Caron E, Lu Z-Y, Bataille R, Klein B (1993) γ-interferon in multiple myeloma: Inhibition of interleukin-6 (IL-6)-dependent myeloma cell growth and downregulation of IL-6-receptor expression in vitro. Blood 81:3076-3082
14. Jelinek DF, Ahmann GJ, Greipp PR, Jalal SM, Westendorf JJ, Katzmann JA, Kyle RA, Lust JA (1993) Coexistence of aneuploid subclones within a myeloma cell line that exhibits clonal immunoglobulin gene rearrangement: Clinical implications. Can Res 53:5320-5327
15. Westendorf JJ, Ahmann GJ, Greipp PR, Witzig TE, Kyle RA, Lust JA, Jelinek DF (1996) Establishment and characterization of three myeloma cell lines that demonstrate variable cytokine responses and abilities to produce autocrine interleukin-6. Leukemia 10:866-876
16. Jelinek DF, Aagaard-Tillery KM, Arendt BK, Arora T, Tschumper RC, Westendorf JJ (1997) Differential human multiple myeloma cell line responsiveness to interferon-α: Analysis of transcription factor activation and interleukin 6 receptor expression. J Clin Invest, in press
17. Ihle JN (1995) The Janus protein tyrosine kinase family and its role in cytokine signaling. Adv Immunol 60:1-35
18. Schindler C, Darnell Jr JE (1995) Transcriptional responses to polypeptide ligands: The JAK/STAT pathway. Annu Rev Biochem 64:621-651
19. Sadowski HB, Shuai K, Darnell Jr JE, Gilman MZ (1993) A common nuclear signal transduction pathway activated by growth factor and cytokine receptors. Science 261:1739-1744
20. Einat M, Resnitzky D, Kimchi A (1985) Close link between reduction of c-myc expression by interferon and G_0/G_1 arrest. Nature 313:597-600
21. Bladé J, López-Guillermo A, Tassies D, Montserrat E, Rozman C (1991) Development of aggressive plasma cell leukaemia under interferon-alpha therapy. Br J Haematol 79:523-525
22. Sawamura M, Murayama K, Ui G, Matsushima T, Tamura J, Murakami H, Naurse T, Tsuchiya J (1992) Plasma cell leukaemia with alpha-interferon therapy in myeloma. Br J Haematol 82:631

Investigation of Aberrant Translational Control of c-*myc* in Cell Lines Derived from Patients with Multiple Myeloma

A. E. WILLIS, F. E. M. PAULIN, M. J. WEST and R. L. WHITNEY
Department of Biochemistry, University of Leicester, University Road, Leicester LE1 7RH, United Kingdom

Abstract

In cell lines derived from patients with multiple myeloma (MM) we have found an elevation in the amount of the c-*myc* protein which is not accompanied by an increase in the level of mRNA or a change in the half-life of the protein. There is a 3.4 fold enhancement in the degree of association of the c-*myc* message with polysomes. This is not accompanied by an alteration in polysome size or a change in the transit time of the c-*myc* mRNA on the polysomes thus suggesting that there is an increase in the degree of mobilisation of the c-*myc* message. Sequencing of the c-*myc* 5'UTR has revealed the presence of a mutation in all the MM cell lines studied and we demonstrate that this mutation causes altered binding of cellular proteins to this RNA species.

Introduction

Multiple myeloma (MM) is a B-cell neoplasia which is characterised by the expansion of a plasma cell type in the bone marrow (Barker et. al. 1992). These plasma cells, by the production of a range of cytokines, including IL1, IL3 and IL6 (Carter et. al. 1990; Hitzler et. al.. 1991; Caligaris-Cappio et. al. 1991) stimulate the growth of certain cell types, including osteoclasts, in the bone marrow microenvironment which results in bone destruction (Neivizky et. al. 1993). Death usually occurs three to five years from the initial presentation of the disease by haemorrhage and/or infection (Niesvizky et. al. 1993). The plasma cell types that are thought to be important in MM have been extensively studied for the aberrant expression of proto-oncogenes however, no uniform oncogene deregulation has been reported to be involved with MM. Changes have been found in the p53 and *ras* genes, but these seem to be associated with the terminal stage of the disease and moreover there are discrepancies between the altered expression of these oncogenes in cell lines when compared to fresh patient material (Portier et. al. 1992, Corradini et. al. 1993; Neri et. al. 1989). In addition, no consistent changes in the expression in c-*myc* have been reported which is perhaps rather surprising given that overproduction of c-*myc* protein is often associated with B-cell neoplasias. In studies of a total of 58

MM patients only seven examples of increased mRNA stability have been observed and two examples of c-*myc* associated chromosomal translocations have been reported (Selvanyagam et. al. 1988; Lewis and McKenzie 1984; Hollis et. al. 1988).

Results

The amount of protein present in four MM cell lines and three control cell lines was determined by a quantitative ELISA (Sullivan et. al. 1989). The MM cell lines contain between 100 and 250 pg of c-*myc* per µg of cell lysate which is on average 15 fold more than the control cell lines. In the case of GM2132 more protein is produced than in the colon adenocarcinoma cell line COLO320 which contains a 40 fold amplification of the c-*myc* gene (Fig. 1A). This is in direct contrast to the amount of RNA produced and it can be seen that the RNA expression in the MM cell lines is similar to that observed in the control B-cell lines (Fig. 1B). This discrepancy could be accounted for by a stabilisation of the c-*myc* protein, as this protein, in common with other proto-oncogenes has a short half life of approximately 20 minutes (Hann and Eisenman 1984). However no change in the half life of the protein of the c-*myc* protein was detected (Fig. 1C). This suggested that the up-regulation of c-*myc* was occurring by another mechanism.

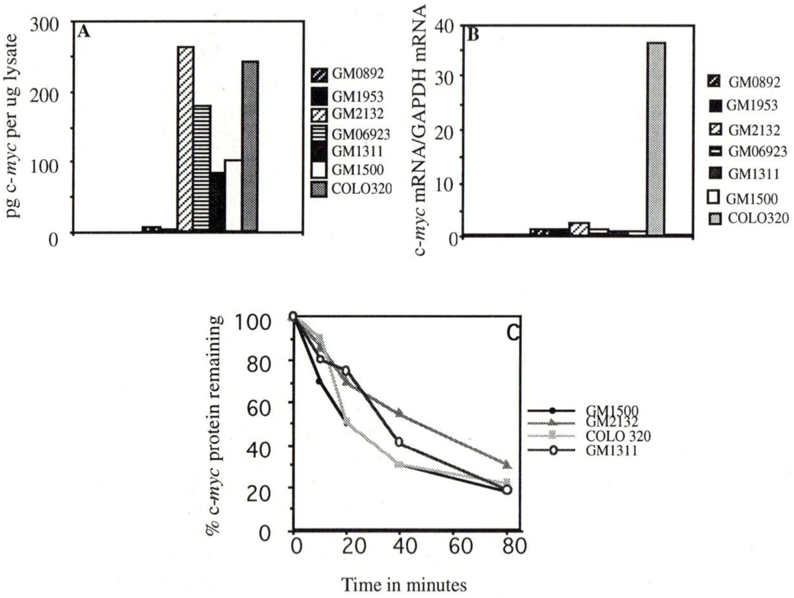

Fig 1. There is a 10-20 fold increase in the amount of c-*myc* protein (panel A) but no alteration in the level of the c-*myc* mRNA (panel B) or in the half life of the protein (panel C). MM cell lines are GM2132, GM1311, GM1500 and GM0692.3 Control B- cell lines are GM0892 and GM1953.

The data described above indicate that the aberrant regulation of c-*myc* could reside at the level of control of protein synthesis. Therefore to distinguish at which stage of the process this could be occurring, either at mobilisation, initiation, elongation or termination, sucrose gradient density centrifugation was performed (Theodorakis et. al. 1988). This technique allows the separation of the polyribosomes (polysomes), which are actively translating the mRNA, from the mRNPs which are inactive in translation. An increase in the polysome size would suggest that there was an alteration in the re-initiation rate, whilst a increase in the association of the c-*myc* mRNA with the polysomes, without a corresponding change in polysome size, would suggest that there was enhanced mobilisation of the c-*myc* message from the inactive mRNPs to the polysomes (Hershey 1991).

This analysis was performed for the MM and control cell lines and the association of the *myc* message with the polysomes relative to that of the control message glyceraldehyde 3 phosphate dehydrogenase (GAPDH) was calculated. In the control cell lines the average *myc*/GAPDH monosome/polysome ratio was found to range from 0.69-0.9 whilst in the MM cell lines the average *myc*/GAPDH ratio was higher and varied from 2.2-3.4 (Fig. 2). This shows an average increase in the degree of association of the c-*myc* message of 3.4 fold. However, no alteration in polysome size was detected (data not shown) thus suggesting that the increase in the c-*myc* protein is due to an increased mobilisation of the c-*myc* message from inactive mRNPs into actively translating polyribosomes.

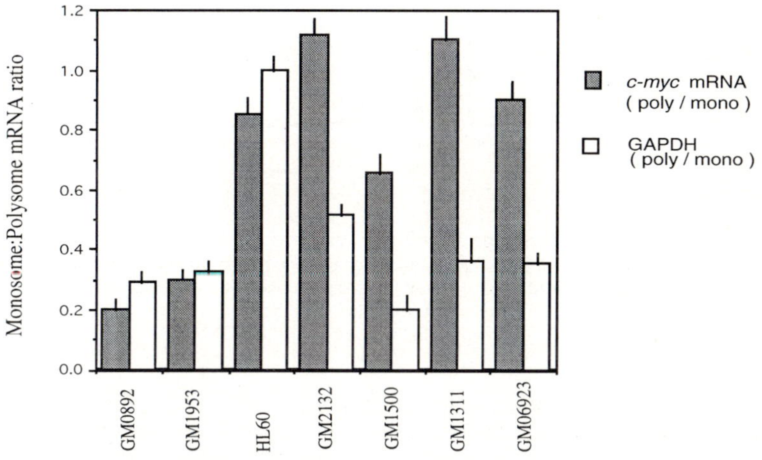

c-myc / GAPDH	0.69	0.90	0.85	2.20	3.25	3.00	2.57

Fig 2. Showing the increased association of the c-*myc* message with the polysomes in MM cell lines. (MM cell lines are GM2132, GM06923, GM1311, GM1500; control cell lines are the B-cell lines GM0892 and GM1953 and the leukaemic cell line HL60.)

To test whether the elongation rate of the c-*myc* message was also altered the transit time of the polysomes on the mRNA was determined. The MM and control cell lines were incubated with the initiation inhibitor aurintricarboxylic acid and sucrose gradient density centrifugation was carried out, thus allowing the rate at which pre-initiated polysomes could progress along the message to be determined.

No change in the transit time of the c-*myc* message on the polysomes was observed in the MM cell lines (Fig. 3, panels A[GM2132] and E [GM06923] when compared to the control cell line (Fig. 3, panel C [GM1953]) and the half life of the polysomes on the c-*myc* message was found range from 10-12 minutes. The transit time of the polysomes on the GAPDH messages was also unchanged and in all cases the half life of the polysomes on this message was found to be 7.5 minutes (Fig. 3, panels B, D, and F).

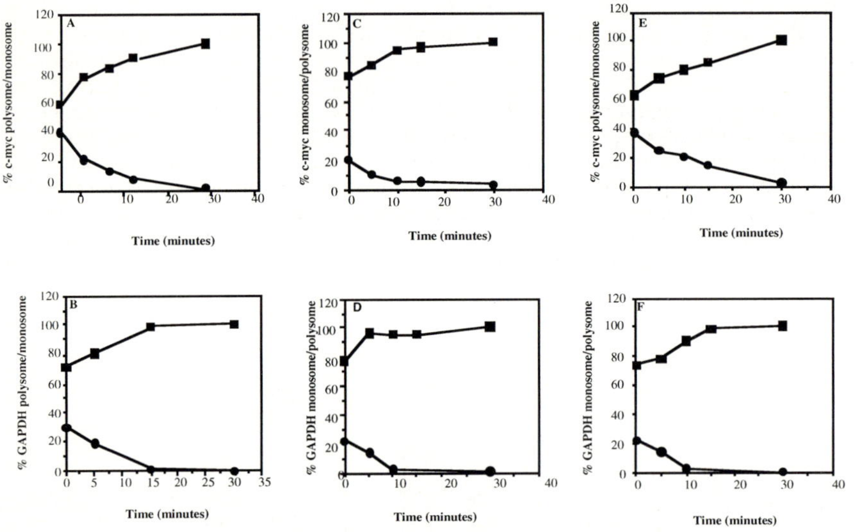

Fig. 3 Showing the transit time of the c-*myc* (panels A, C and E) or GAPDH mRNAs (panels B. D and F) on the polysomes. The closed squares denote the increased association of the message with the monosomes and the closed circles denote the disappearance of the message from the polysomes. Panels A and D, and C and F are results obtained with the MM cell lines GM2132, and GMO6923. Panels B and E are results obtained with the control cell line GM1953.

An increase in the degree of mobilisation of the c-*myc* message in MM could be brought about by either altered binding of protein factors and/or a mutation in the c-*myc* message. The 5' untranslated region of c-*myc* is mostly non-coding and has been shown previously to affect the translation of both c-*myc* and heterologous genes (Darveau et. al. 1985; Parkin et. al. 1988). This region is, therefore, a putative site for mutations which could affect translation. Thus, to determine whether mutations were present, the 5'UTR of c-*myc* was amplified by PCR and RT-PCR from genomic DNA and mRNA samples derived from MM and control cell lines. The resulting DNA products were then inserted into M13 based vectors and sequenced. A consistent change in all MM cell lines was found in the 5' UTR of c-*myc*; a C-T transition at position 2756 (Table 1).

Cell line	Sequence
Wild type	
GM3201, GM1953, GM0892	2750 2760 2770 ACT CTC CCG ACG CGG GGA GGC
MM	
GM1311, GM2132, GM0692,GM1500	2750 2760 2770 ACT CTC TCG ACG CGG GGA GGC

Table 1. Sequencing of c-*myc* exon 1 shows a mutation in all MM cell lines (numbering as in Gazin *et. al..*, 1984).

To test whether the mutation in the c-*myc* 5' UTR caused an alteration in the affinity of cellular proteins for this region of RNA, electrophoretic mobility shift assays (EMSAs) were performed. Cell extracts made from MM and control cell lines were incubated with radiolabelled RNA synthesised from the c-*myc* 5 ' UTR +/- the mutation and the reaction products separated on an agarose gel. The cellular proteins were found to bind more tightly to the RNA transcripts which harbour the mutation (Fig. 4). At a concentration of 75μg the ratio of bound transcript/bound plus free transcript is approximately 40% for the wild type sequence and between 65-70 % for the mutant sequence.

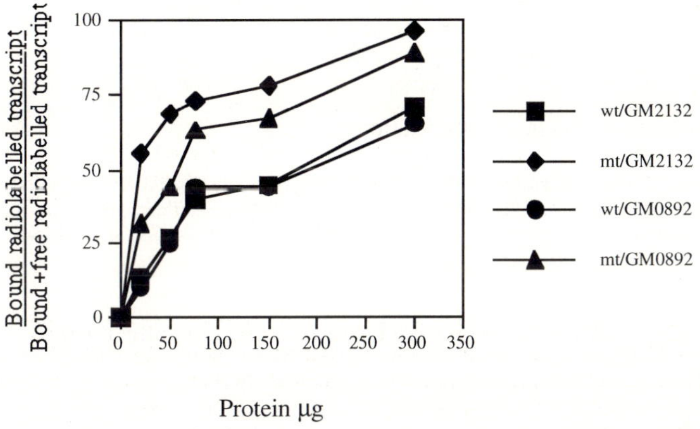

Fig. 4. Showing the enhanced binding of protein factors to the mutant sequence.
An electrophoretic mobility shift assay was performed by incubating either the radiolabelled wild type (closed squares and closed circles) or mutant (closed diamonds and closed triangles) RNA s with increasing concentrations of cell extracts from MM (GM2132) or control B-cell (GM0892) lines. The reaction products were separated by gel electrophoresis and exposed to x-ray film. The film was was sanned using a laser densitometer to quantitate the amount of radiolabel in each band and the data was plotted as shown.

Competition assays were performed using an excess of unlabelled RNA with either the wild type or the mutant RNAs that had been radiolabelled. The cellular proteins that interact with the c-*myc* RNA bind the sequence which harbours the mutation at least ten times more efficiently than the wild type sequence (Fig. 5). Hence, at a 3 fold molar excess of unlabelled transcript, the wild type sequence causes a 55% reduction in the amount of radiolabelled wild type bound, whilst the mutant sequence causes a 95% reduction. Moreover, in the converse experiment, the wild type sequence does not compete with the cellular proteins for the mutant sequence and even at a 300 molar excess of unlabelled transcript there is only a 90% reduction in the amount of radiolabelled mutant transcript bound.

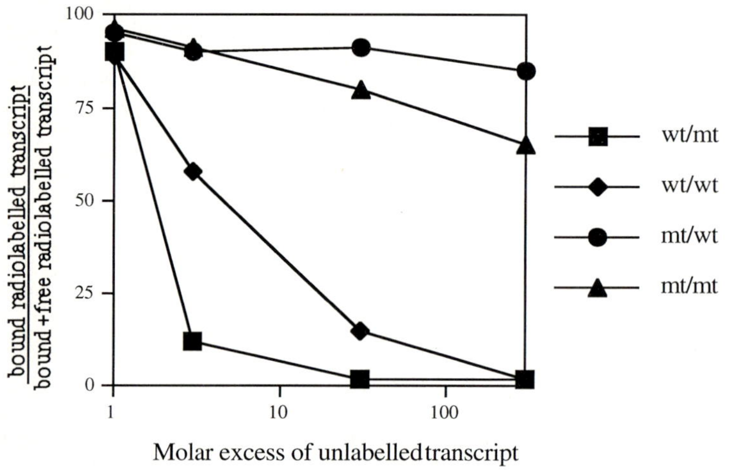

Fig 5. The effect of the addition of an excess (molar) of unlabelled wild type (closed diamonds and closed circles) or mutant (closed squares and closed trianges)c-*myc* 5' UTR to reactions containing cell extracts and wild type or mutant radiolabelled transcripts. Experiments were performed and results calculated as in Fig. 4.

In order to investigate further those protein factors which bind to the c-*myc* mRNA a number of techniques were employed including NorthWestern blotting, UV-cross linking the mRNA to the proteins and direct analysis of the RNA protein complexes formed on agarose gels. Using these disparate techniques we found that in each case a very similar group of proteins bind to the c-*myc* 5' UTR. Hence there appears to be a complex which contains four proteins with molecular weights of 98, 86, 61 and 38 KDa (Fig. 6). The wild type and the mutant transcripts appear to bind the same proteins although the binding affinity of these proteins to the mutant sequence is much higher (data not shown). Using this technique some differences in RNA binding factors between MM and control cell lines were also observed, which could either reflect the different differentiated states of the cells or the malignant phenotype of the MM cells (Paulin and Willis unpublished data).

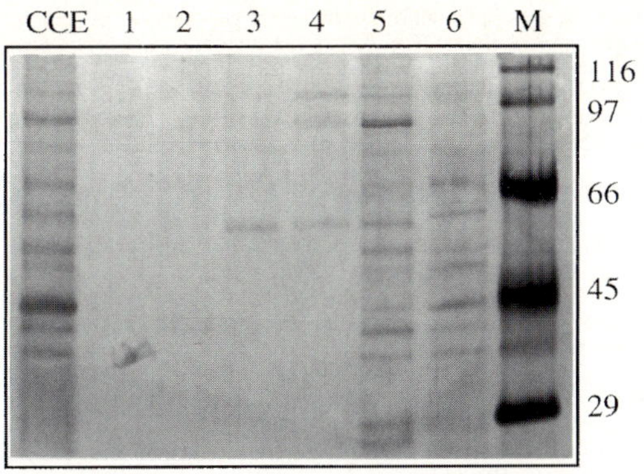

Fig. 6 An SDS polyacrylamide gel showing the proteins which associate with the *c-myc* 5' UTR. An EMSA was performed with radiolabelled mutant transcripts and MM cell extracts, the gel was cut in to six pieces and the proteins were electroelulted and separated by SDS PAGE. Numbers 1-6 represent the gel slices from which the proteins were obtained with 1 starting from the bottom of the gel.

Discussion

The mechanisms which regulate the translation of individual or specific mRNAs are, in general, poorly understood although the presence of secondary structure in untranslated regions appears to be important. Many cellular mRNAs encoding proto-oncogenes, growth factors and transcription factors contain long highly structured UTRs e.g. fibroblast growth factor, platelet derived growth factor and ornithine decarboxylase and these are often associated with a negative control of translation (Gray and Hentze 1994). The 5'UTR of c-*myc* has also been shown to cause repression of translation in certain cellular systems (Darveau et. al. 1985; Parkin et. al. 1988) and our data suggest that the altered c-*myc* expression in MM is due to a specific mutation in the c-*myc* 5' UTR which relieves this repression. This causes an enhancement in the degree of mobilisation of the c-*myc* message from inactive mRNPs to actively translating polysomes; a process that may be aided by protein factors which are specific to the MM derived cell lines. The consequence of these changes is the overproduction of the c-*myc* protein. Therefore in MM, in common with other B-cell neoplasias the expression of c-*myc* is de-regulated however, this occurs by aberrant control of translation.

References

Barker HF, Hamilton MS, Ball J, Drew M and Franklin IM. (1992). Mutiple myeloma: The biology of the malignant plasma cell. British Journal Of Haematology., 81: 331-335.

Caligaris-Cappio M, Gaidano M, Gaboli M, Schena AS, and Marchisio C. (1991) The role of bone marrow stromal cells in the growth of human mutiple myeloma. Blood:77 2688-2693

Carter A, Merchav I, Silvian-Draxler I and Tatarsky I. (1990) The role of inerleukin-1 and tumour necrosis factor alpha in human multiple myeloma. Blood 74:424-431.

Corradini P., Ladetto M, Voena C, Paulumbo A, Inghirami G, Knowles DM, Boccadoro M and Pilleri A., (1993) Mutational Activation of N- and K-ras Oncogenes in Plasma Cell Dyscrasias. Blood 81: 2708-2713.

Darveau A, Pelletier J and Sonenberg N. (1985) Differenital efficiences of in vitro translation of mouse c-myc transcripts differing in the 5' untranslated region. Proc.Natl.Acad. Sci..USA., 82:2315-2319

Gazin C, Dupont de Dinechin S, Hampe A, Masson J-M, Martin P, Stehelin D and Galibert F. (1984). Nucleotide sequence of the human c-myc locis:provocative open reading frame within the first exon. EMBO. J., 3:383-387.

Gray N and Hentze M. (1994). Regulation of protein synthesis by mRNA structure. Molecular Biology Reports, 19: 195-200.

Hann SR and Eisenman RN. (1984). Proteins expressed by the c-myc oncogene in lymphomas of human and avian origin. Mol.Cell Biol., 4: 11. 2486-2497.

Hiltzer J, Martinez-Valdez D, Berghasel M, Minden M and Messener H., (1991) Role of Interleukin-6 in the proliferation of human multiple myeloma cell lines oci-my 1 to 7 established from patients with advanced Stage of the disease. Blood 8:1996-2004.

Hollis GF, Gazdar AF, Bertness V and Kirsch IR. (1988). Complex translocational disrupts c-myc regulation in a human plasma cell myeloma. Mol. Cell. Biol., 8: 124-129.

Hershey JWB (1991). Translational control in mammalian cells. Annu. Rev. Biochem., 60:717-755.

Lewis J and MacKenzie M (1984). Non-random chromosomal aberrations associated with multiple myeloma. Haematology Oncol., 2 :307-317.

Neivizky R, Siegel D and Michaeli J. (1993). Biology and treatment of multiple myeloma. Blood, 7: 24-33

Neri A, Murphy JP, Gro L, Ferrero D, Tarella C, Baldini L and Dalla-Favera R. (1989). RAS Oncogene mutations in multiple myeloma J. Exp. Med., 170: 1715-1722.

Neri A, Baldini L, Trecca D, Gro L, Polli E and Maiolo AT. (1993). p53 Gene mutations in multiple myeloma are associated with advanced forms of malignancy. Blood, 81: 128-135.

Portier M, Moles JP, Mazars G, Jeanteur P, Bataille R and Theillet C. (1992). p53 and RAS gene mutations in multiple myeloma. Oncogene , 7: 2539-2543.

Parkin N, Darveau A, Nicholson R and Sonenberg N. (1988). cis-acting translational affects of the 5' non-coding region of the c-myc mRNA Mol.Cell.Biol., 8: 2875-2883.

Selvanayagam PM, Blick F, Narni P, van Tuinen DH, Ledbetter R, Alexanian GF, Saunders G and Barlogie B. (1988). Alteration and abnormal expression of the c-myc oncogene in human multiple myeloma. Blood, 71, 30-35.

Sullivan NF, Willis AE, Moore JP and Lindahl T. (1989). High levels of the c-myc protein in cell lines of Bloom's syndrome origin. Oncogene 4: 1509-1511.

Theodorakis NG, Banerji SS and Morimoto RI. (1988). HSP70 mRNA Translation in chicken reticulocytes is regulated at the level of elongation. J. Biol. Chem., 263 :14579-14585.

Aknowledgements

This work was supported by a grant from the Cancer Resarch Campaign which is gratefully aknowledged. Fiona Paulin was supported by a studentship from the MRC.

Dysregulation of c-myc in Multiple Myeloma

W. M. Kuehl, L. A. Brents, M. Chesi, K. Huppi[1] and P. L. Bergsagel[2]
NCI-Navy Medical Oncology Branch, Bethesda, MD 20889, USA
[1] NCI, Laboratory of Genetics, and
[2] Cornell University Medical College, New York, NY 10021, USA

Abstract

Translocation of c-myc to IgH switch regions, or less frequently to one of the IgL loci, is essentially an invariant event in murine plasmacytomas. This results in dysregulation of c-myc, manifested by selective expression of the translocated allele. Human multiple myeloma (MM) has a similarly high incidence of translocations involving IgH switch regions, but c-myc is infrequently involved as a partner in these translocations. However, in screening a panel of 20 MM cell lines, we identified six lines containing two genetically distinguishable c-myc alleles. For these six informative lines (and the corresponding tumor for one line) there is selective expression of one c-myc allele despite the apparent absence of translocation, DNA rearrangement, or amplification involving c-myc. This result suggests frequent tumor specific cis-dysregulation of c-myc in MM by a presently unknown mechanism.

Introduction

Chromosomal translocations that dysregulate c-myc are essentially invariant in murine plasmacytomas and human Burkitt's lymphoma tumors, and a frequent occurrence during progression of other B cell tumors [1,2,3,4]. Generally, the c-myc chromosomal locus is translocated to the IgH locus, with variant translocations to one of the IgL loci occurring much less frequently. In most instances, the translocated c-myc allele has mutations in non-coding exon 1 and/or intron 1, but a substantial fraction of translocated c-myc alleles also have missense mutations in exon 2. The presence of mutations in the translocated c-myc gene has enabled investigators to demonstrate that the translocated c-myc allele is expressed selectively, with the non-translocated c-myc allele expressed at a much lower or nondetectable level.

Recently, we have generated evidence indicating that chromosomal translocations involving IgH switch regions may be a nearly universal event in human multiple myeloma (MM) [5,6]. Yet the c-myc locus is rarely (<5%) involved as a partner in translocations to one of the Ig loci. Similarly, genomic DNA rearrangements and amplification of c-myc have been reported in MM, but each of these events appear to occur in only a few percent of tumors [7,8]. Despite the infrequency of genetic events affecting c-myc, it has been reported that c-myc is often over-expressed in MM, leading to speculation that c-myc is dysregulated by some other mechanism [8,9]. In this report, we summarize results showing selective expression of one c-myc allele in MM.

Results and Discussion

Selective expression of one c-myc allele in six informative MM cell lines, and confirmed in the primary tumor for one cell line.

To screen for MM cells containing c-myc genes with variant sequences, we isolated genomic DNA from 20 EBV negative MM cell lines (8226, U266, JJN-3, SK-MM1, SK-MM2, KMM-1, OPM-2, H1112, ARK, TH, MM-M1, FLAM-76, KMS-11, MM.1, Delta-47, JIM-3, UTMC-2, ANBL-6, OCI-MY5, KMS-12), and performed PCR-SSCP analyses of overlapping fragments covering all three exons [5,10]. For each line containing a variant genomic DNA SSCP pattern, we did an RT.PCR-SSCP assay of the relevant regions to determine whether normal and/or variant sequences are expressed. Fragments showing variant SSCP patterns were subjected to thermal cycle sequencing. To eliminate the possibility of genomic DNA PCR products contaminating RT.PCR reactions, these results were verified by SSCP and/or sequence analysis of RT.PCR products containing portions of 2 exons. Variant c-myc sequences were identified in 6 of 20 MM cell lines, as summarized in Table 1:

Table 1. C-Myc expression by cell lines with genetically distinguishable alleles

Line[1]	Codon[2,3]	Normal	Variant	Allele(s) Expressed[4]
Myeloma				
JJN-3	5'UT (2397)	G	A	variant
KMS-11	5'UT(2510)	C	T	variant
FLAM-76	5'UT(2510)	C	T	variant
MM.1	83 (4769)	CGG(ARG)	CGC(ARG)	normal
OPM-2	231 (5213)	CCG(PRO)	CCA(PRO)	variant
MM-M1	231 (5213)	CCG(PRO)	CCA(PRO)	variant
Other				
RAM	11 (4552)	AAC(ASN)	AGC(SER)	both
BL1	231/2(5211-14)	CCGC	CCAC?	both
HUT128	231/2[5211-14]	CCGC	CCAC?	both
ARH-77	3'UT (7266)	A	G	both

1. OPM-2, JJN-3, MM.1, KMS-11, FLAM-76, and MM-M1 are EBV negative MM lines; RAM, ARH-77, and BL1 are EBV positive lymphoblastoid cell lines; HUT128 is a lung cancer cell line from the same patient as BL1.
2. Nucleotide position from c-myc human genomic DNA (GenBank ID No.34820), with exon boundaries: 1 (2328-2881); 2 (4509-5277); 3 (6654-7526).
3. *Aci* I polymorphism detected by PCR assay for BL1 and HUT128, so that possible codons/ nucleotides altered are indicated [10].
4. All lines contain at least one normal and one variant c-myc allele .
5. Results for all lines except KMS-11, FLAM-76, MM.1, and MM-M1 are shown elsewhere[10].

As shown in Table 1, the variant sequences in the MM lines have no effect on the predicted sequence of the c-myc protein. All six MM lines contain both variant and normal c-myc alleles, and for each of these informative MM lines one of the two alleles is expressed selectively as mRNA. As controls for this analysis, we identified variant c-myc sequences in three EBV positive lymphoblastoid cell lines (LCL) and in one small cell lung cancer cell line (HUT128) that was derived from the same patient as one of the LCL (i.e. BL1). In each of these four informative lines, both c-myc alleles are expressed to a similar extent.

It was reported that 4 independent MM cell lines show hypomethylation of a unique *Hpa* II site in exon 3 of c-myc [11]. In a preliminary survey of 10 MM lines, we confirmed hypomethylation of this site in 8 MM lines (JJN-3, OPM-2, MM-M1, KMS-11, ARK, 8226, KMS-12, KMM-1). In each of these cell lines, the site is approximately 50% methylated, consistent with one methylated allele and one unmethylated c-myc allele in each cell. In contrast, this site is fully methylated in all 6 LCL examined and in 2 MM lines (H1112, SK-MM1). It remains to be determined if the methylation status of this unique *Hpa* II site in exon 3 of c-myc provides a structural correlate for the selective expression of one c-myc allele in MM lines.

With the exception of the RAM EBV positive LCL, which encodes a variant c-myc protein with an ASN>SER missense mutation at codon 11, the variant c-myc alleles would not cause changes in the encoded c-myc protein. In fact, the variant allele in RAM has been reported as a germline polymorphism [12]. The variant codon 231 sequence (OPM-2, MM-M1, BL1, HUT128) also appears to be a germline polymorphism that had been identified in 4/171 additional tumors subjected to SSCP analysis by others [10]. The variant 5'UT sequences at nucleotides 2510 (KMS-11, FLAM-76) and 2397 (JJN-3) must also represent germline polymorphisms since the same SSCP patterns were identified in a placental DNA sample and several other LCL, respectively. We also note that no missense mutations of c-myc were identified in any of the 20 MM lines screened, consistent with a report that only one exon 2 missense mutation was identified in 19 primary MM tumors [3].

From conventional karyotypic analyses, none of the six informative MM cell lines that selectively express one c-myc allele has a translocation affecting the c-myc locus. In addition, we found no evidence for c myc amplification or a DNA rearrangement occurring within 5' *Eco* RI or 3' *Hind* III sites flanking c-myc. With the exception of the H929 cell line that has a mutated c-myc allele with a 3' interstitial deletion/ translocation, we are unaware of other human MM lines in which selective expression of one c-myc allele has been reported [13].

Is the selective expression of one c-myc allele in MM cell lines an artifact of cell culture? We have not yet surveyed a panel of MM tumors, but were able to obtain primary tumor cells (JJN-3T) from the patient whose tumor generated the JJN-3 MM cell line. By analysis of IgH switch rearrangements, the JJN-3 primary tumor is identical to the cell line except for an approximately 35% contamination by normal cells. By SSCP and sequence analysis, JJN-3T contains equivalent amounts of both wild type and variant c-myc alleles but, like the cell line, selectively expresses the variant c-myc allele. Thus the selective expression of one c-myc allele is not merely an artifact of cell culture.

What is the mechanism for selective expression of one c-myc allele in MM?

The selective expression (allelic exclusion) of one c-myc allele in six informative MM cell lines is reminiscent of the situation in B cell tumors that have a translocation or DNA rearrangement involving c-myc. In general, it has been accepted that translocation or DNA rearrangement of c-myc precedes and causes selective expression of the altered allele. However, given the result for the six MM lines, one must consider the possibility that selective expression of one c-myc allele precedes the translocation or rearrangement of c-myc.

Selective expression of one c-myc allele in MM tumors is consistent with either imprinting [14] or tumor specific dysregulation (activation or inactivation) of one allele. We cannot conclusively exclude the possibility of imprinting, and particularly tissue specific imprinting (e.g. in plasma cells), but we think this to be unlikely. First, a homozygous c-myc knockout mouse is lethal, whereas hemizygous progeny from a either a male or female hemizygous knockout parent are essentially normal [15]. Second, both c-myc alleles are expressed in three LCL and one lung cancer line, which would require loss of imprinting in these cell lines or their normal tissue counterparts.

As noted above there is no evidence for a translocation, DNA rearrangement, or amplification affecting the c-myc gene in any of the six informative MM lines that selectively express one c-myc allele. Another mechanism that can dysregulate c-myc from a distance is rearrangements affecting the PVT1 locus, which includes a region about 20 to 300 kb downstream (telomeric) of c-myc [16,17]. Retroviral insertion into Mlvi 4 (20 kb 3' of c-myc) or Mlvi 1 (270 kb 3' of c-myc) have been reported to activate c-myc in rat T lymphomas[18]. Similarly, variant translocations into the PVT1 locus in both murine plasmacytomas and human Burkitt's lymphomas can cis-dysregulate c-myc [1,2]. It was reported that rearrangements about 20 kb downstream of c-myc (human MLVI 4 region) are present in 7/42 (16%) of primary MM bone marrow samples [19], although this was not confirmed in 15 MM samples analyzed in another study [20]. We also found no rearrangements of the MLVI 4 region in our panel of 20 MM cell lines.

In an incomplete survey of rearrangement in the PVT1 locus in the panel of 20 MM cell line DNAs, we found one line (JJN-3) with a DNA rearrangement about 300 kb downstream of c-myc. We obtained molecular clones of this region and determined by sequence analysis that the rearrangement is due to insertion of a 308 bp Alu transposon. Using a PCR assay, we determined that insertion of the transposon at this site is not found in a panel of other normal and tumor genomic DNAs. **Is this inserted sequence present in the primary tumor?** We analyzed the JJN-3T primary tumor sample (contaminated with about 35% non-tumor cells) using the same PCR assay, and identified roughly equal amounts of the normal and variant (inserted transposon) sequence. Unfortunately, since we do not have a source of normal cells from this patient, we cannot formally prove that the variant PVT1 sequence is unique to the tumor. **Furthermore, is the inserted sequence linked to the expressed, variant c-myc allele or to the unexpressed, normal c-myc allele?** We do not yet have an answer to this critical question.

In conclusion, selective expression of one c-myc allele apparently occurs frequently in MM, but the significance and mechanism of this finding remain to be determined.

Acknowledgments

We thank the many laboratories that generously provided their MM cell lines to us for analysis. In addition, we are particularly grateful to Ian Maclennan who provided primary tumor material (JJN-3T) corresponding to the JJN-3 MM cell line.

References

1. Potter M, Wiener F (1992) Plasmacytomagenesis in mice: model of neoplastic development dependent upon chromosomal translocations. Carcinogenesis 13:1681-1697
2. Dalla-Favera R Chromosomal translocations involving the c-myc oncogene in lymphoid neoplasia. *In:* I. R. Kirsch (eds.), Chromosomal translocations involving the c-myc oncogene in lymphoid neoplasia, pp. 313-332. New York: CRC Press, 1993.
3. Bhatia K, Spangler G, Hamdy N, Neri A, Brubaker G, Levin A, Magrath I (1994) Mutations in the coding region of c-myc occur independently of mutations in the regulatory regions and are predominantly associated with myc/Ig translocation. Current Topics Micobiol Immunol 194:389-398
4. Raffeld M, Yano T, Hoang AT, Lewis B, Clark HM, Otsuki T, Dang CV (1994) Clustered mutations in the transcriptional activation domain of myc in 8q24 translocated lymphomas and their functional consequences. Current Topics Micobiol Immunol 194:265-272
5. Bergsagel PL, Chesi MC, Nardini E, Brents LA, Kirby SL, Kuehl WM (1996) Promiscuous translocations into immunoglobulin heavy chain switch regions in multiple myeloma. Proc Nat Acad Sci 93:13931-13936
6. Bergsagel PL, Nardini E, Chesi M, Kuehl WM IgH Translocations in Multiple Myeloma: a nearly universal event that rarely involves c-myc. Current Topics Microbiol Immunol In Press (this volume):
7. Bakkus MHC, Brakel-van Peer KMJ, Michiels JJ, van't Veer MB, Benner R (1990) Amplification of the c-myc and the pvt-like region in human multiple myeloma. Oncogene 5:1359-1364
8. Barlogie B, Hoover R, Epstein J (1994) Multiple myeloma - recent developments in molecular and cellular biology. Current Topics In Microbiology And Immunology 194:37-41
9. Skopelitou A, Hadjiyannakis M, Tsenga A, Theocharis S, Alexopoulou V, Kittas C, Agnantis N (1993) Expression of c-myc p62 oncoprotein in multiple myeloma: an immunohistochemical study of 180 cases. Anticancer Res 13:1091-1096
10. Kuehl WM, Brents LA, Chesi M, Bergsagel PL (1996) Selective expression of one c-myc allele in two human myeloma cell lines. Cancer Res 56:4370-4373
11. Ohtsuki T, Nishitani K, Hatamochi A, Yawata Y, Namba M (1991) Analysis of methylation in the c-myc gene in five human myeloma cell lines. British Journal Of Haematology 77:172-179
12. Rothberg PG, Otto YM (1995) A polymorphic variant of human c-Myc: Asn11>Ser. Mammalian Genome 6:209-211
13. Hollis GF, Gazdar AF, Bertness V, Kirsch IR (1988) Complex translocation disrupts c-myc regulation in a human plasma cell myeloma. Mol Cell Biol 8:124-129
14. Barlow DP (1995) Genetic imprinting in mammals. Science 270:1610-1613
15. Davis AC, Wims M, Spotts GD, Hann SR, Bradley A (1993) A null c-myc mutation causes lethality before 10.5 days of gestation in homozygotes and reduced fertility in heterozygous female mice. Genes & Develop 7:671-682
16. Huppi K, Siwarski D, Goodnight J, Skurla RMJ, Mushinski JF (1992) Alternative splicing of Pvt-1 transcripts in murine B-lymphocytic neoplasms accompanies amplification and chromosomal translocation. Int J Oncol 1:525-532

17. Henglein B, Synovzik H, Groitl P, Bornkamm G, Hartl P, Lipp M (1989) Three breakpoints of variant t(2;8) translocations in Burkitt's lymphoma cells fall within a region 140 kb distal from c-myc. Mol Cell Biol 9:2105-2113
18. Lazo PA, Lee JS, Tsichlis PN (1990) Long-distance activation of the myc protooncogene by provirus insertion in Mlvi-1 or Mlvi-4 in rat T-cell lymphomas. Proceedings National Academy Of Science 87:170-173
19. Palumbo AP, Boccadoro M, Battaglio S, Corradini P, Tsichlis PN, Huebner K, Pileri A, Croce CM (1990) Human homologue of Moloney leukemia virus integration-4 locus(Mlvi-4) located 20 kilobases 3' of the myc gene, is rearranged in multiple myelomas. Cancer Research 50:6487-6482
20. Ladanyi M, Wang S, Niesvizky R, Feiner H, Michaeli J (1992) Proto-oncogene analysis in multiple myeloma. Amer J Pathol 141:949-953

IgH Translocations in Multiple Myeloma: A Nearly Universal Event that Rarely Involves c-myc

P. L. Bergsagel, E. Nardini, L. Brents[1], M. Chesi[1] and W. M. Kuehl[1]
Cornell University Medical College, New York, NY 10021, USA, and
[1] NCI-Navy Medical Oncology Branch, Bethesda, MD 20889, USA

Abstract

Dysregulation of c-myc by translocation to the switch regions of the IgH locus occurs in most murine plasmacytomas. Translocations involving 14q32 have been reported in 20-40% of abnormal karyotypes from human multiple myeloma (MM), and involve a variety of loci. Using cytogenetics, FISH and a Southern blot assay, we analyzed 21 MM cell lines and one plasma cell leukemia and identified evidence of a 14q32 translocation in 20/22 samples. The partner loci involved are 11q13 in 6 (associated with cyclin D1 expression), 4p16 in 6 (associated with FGFR3 expression), unidentified in 3 and 1p13, 6, 8q24, 12q24, 16q23, and 21q22 once each. We conclude that conventional karyotypes underestimate the frequency of 14q32 translocations in MM, where they appear to be a nearly universal event. The translocations most frequently involve IgH switch regions, and include two recurrent partner loci (11q13 and 4p16) and a promiscuous array of other partner loci. Although c-myc appears to be cis-dysregulated frequently in MM, it is only rarely translocated to the IgH locus.

Introduction

A translocation to the IgH locus is a seminal event in the pathogenesis of many B cell malignancies. In murine plasmacytomas, dysregulation of c-myc frequently occurs by translocation into the IgH switch regions [1]. Although we have identified evidence of frequent c-myc cis-dysregulation in MM [2,3], this infrequently occurs by IgH translocation, and the mechanism responsible is undefined. In contrast, 14q32 translocations are identified in 20-40% of abnormal karyotypes in MM [4,5]. By analogy to murine plasmacytomas, and because MM is a tumor of mature, isotype switched plasma cells, we postulated that these translocations would also occur into the switch regions. We developed a comprehensive Southern blot assay to identify illegitimate switch recombination fragments (ISRFs), markers of potential translocation breakpoints involving switch regions [6]. The assay uses paired probes located on either side (5' and 3') of the

Table 1. Illegitimate switch recombinations in 21 human MM cell lines and one tumor

Line/Tumor[a]	14q32[b] abnormality	Illegitimate switch[c,d] 5' probe	3' probe	Oncogene[e]
FLAM-76	11q13	NONE	NONE	Cyclin D1
MM-M1	11q13	NONE	NONE	Cyclin D1
H1112	(11)	NONE	NONE	Cyclin D1
SK-MM2	11q13	NONE	Sγ [11q13]	Cyclin D1
KMS-12	11q13	Sμ, Sα	Sγ [11q13], Sμ [14]	Cyclin D1
U266	NONE	Sγ	Sα [11q13]	Cyclin D1
DELTA-47	14q+	NONE	σμ	
TH	14q+	Sμ	NONE	
8226	1p13	NONE	Sγ	
MM.1	12q24	Sμ	Sγ	
JJN-3 (T)	14q+	5'σμ	Sμ [16q23]	
SK-MM1	14q+	Sμ	Sμ [6], Sγ	
JIM-3 (T)	14q+	Sμ	Sγ [4p16]	? FGFR3
KMS-11	NONE	Sμ (4p16)	Sμ [4p16], Sμ, Sγ	FGFR3
H929 (T)	NONE	Sμ [4p16]	Sα (4p16)	FGFR3
TUMOR	NONE	Sμ [4p16]	Sγ (4p16)	FGFR3
UTMC-2 (T)	(4p16)	Sμ (4p16)	Sμ (4p16)	FGFR3
OPM-2	(4p16)	Sμ	Sγ	FGFR3
KMM-1	NONE	σμ [8q24]	σδ [21q22]	? C-MYC
ANBL-6	NONE	Sμ	Sμ	
ARK	NONE	NONE	NONE	
OCI-MY5	ND	NONE	NONE	

[a]The translocation breakpoint identified in the cell lines followed by (T) was also identified in the corresponding primary tumor.

[b]14q32 translocation identified by cytogenetics, those identified only by FISH are indicated in parentheses.

[c]An illegitimate switch recombination fragment hybridizes only to a single 5' or 3' probe, and to no other probes.

[d]Chromosomal partner in cloned breakpoint indicated within square brackets, and in Southern blot mapped breakpoints in round brackets.

[e]Oncogene expressed at a high level in these lines

five switch regions (σμ/σδ, Sμ, Sγ, Sα, Sε), and restriction enzymes (*Bgl*II, *Hind*III and *Sph*I) with sites that flank the probes. A legitimate switch recombination occurs between two switch regions, and generates one or two switch recombination fragments, each of which hybridizes to two switch probes. An illegitimate switch recombination occurs between a switch and a non-switch region, and generates two switch recombination fragments that each hybridize with only one switch probe. We analyzed 21 MM cell lines and one plasma cell leukemia sample using this assay, and in this report we summarize and update our results [6,7,8].

Results

We detected ISRFs in 17/22 samples (Table 1). By cloning or Southern blotting we have shown that 16/18 ISRFs are translocation breakpoints. We have confirmed by Southern blot or PCR in four of these samples (JJN-3, JIM-3, H929 and UTMC-2) that the same translocation breakpoint was present in the corresponding primary

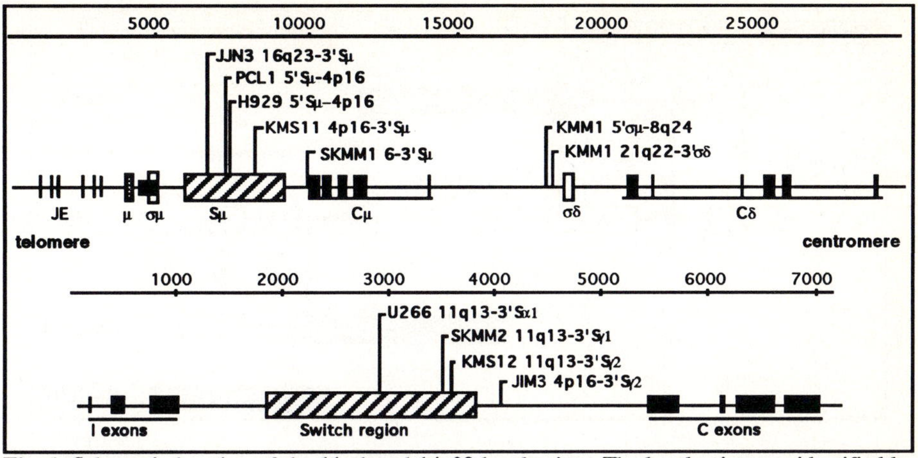

Fig. 1. Schematic location of the 11 cloned 14q32 breakpoints. The breakpoints are identified by the cell line or tumor from which they were cloned, and the source of the sequences on either side of the breakpoint. Since the alpha and gamma switch regions are all different sizes, this map simply gives an approximation of the relative location of the breakpoints.

tumor that gave rise to the cell line. In 6 of the cell lines there was a high level of expression of cyclin D1 mRNA by Northern blot. We detected and cloned ISRFs from SK-MM2, KMS-12, and U266, and in each case identified sequences from 11q13 juxtaposed to Sα or Sγ. In FLAM-76, MM-M1 and H1112 we did not detect any ISRFs, although they had cytogenetic evidence of t(11;14)(q13;q32) [6,7]. In 5 cell lines, and the plasma cell leukemia sample we identified a t(4;14)(p16;q32) by cloning the breakpoint (JIM-3, KMS-11, H929, and the tumor sample), by Southern blot mapping (UTMC-2), and by FISH (OPM-2, UTMC-2). The breakpoints occur in a 50 kb region approximately 100 kb upstream of FGFR3. With the exception of JIM-3 these samples have a variably elevated level of expression of FGFR3 detected by RT-PCR, Northern blot and Western blot [8]. In addition, we cloned 14q32 breakpoints involving 16q23 in JJN-3, chromosome 6 in SK-MM1, and 8q24 and 21q22 in KMM-1. The relative location within the IgH locus and nature of the cloned breakpoints is shown schematically in Fig. 1.

Complex reciprocal translocations involving 8q24, 14q32, and 21q22 in KMM-1

We identified one cell line, KMM-1, with a translocation involving the c-myc locus at 8q24 (Fig 2). It is a complex reciprocal translocation involving three chromosomes: 8, 14 and 21. The telomere of 14 is translocated to der(8). On this allele there is a deletion of sequences starting in σμ and ending downstream of Cμ membrane exons, followed by a translocation breakpoint upstream of σδ that is juxtaposed to sequences from 8q24 upstream (centromeric) to c-myc (Fig. 2). Approximately 300 bp (upstream of σδ) have been deleted between the reciprocal breakpoints. On der(14) the reciprocal breakpoint immediately upstream of σδ is juxtaposed to sequences from 21q22 (that map by radiation hybrids in the vicinity of AML-1). In this example, c-myc is not translocated to the IgH locus, and the cytogenetic location of the translocated c-myc and of AML-1 with respect to the 21q22 breakpoint are not known. If this is a reciprocal three-way translocation, then c-myc is translocated onto der(21). This differs from other B cell tumors where the translocated c-myc is associated with the Ig locus. In KMM-1, the

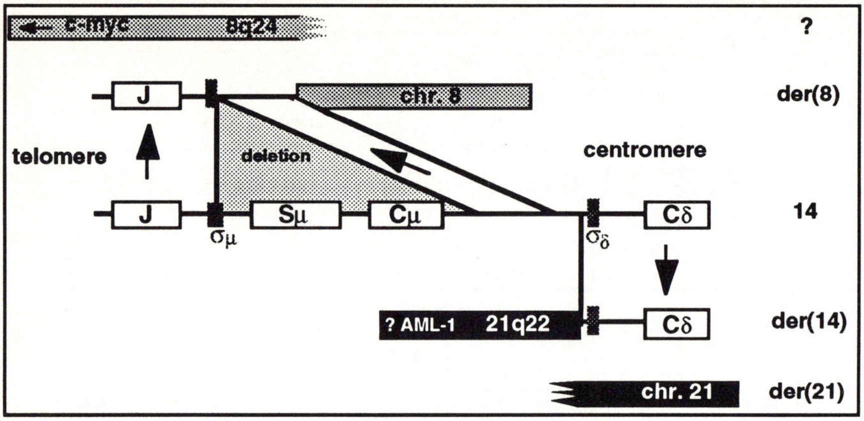

Fig. 2. Complex 8q24;14q32 and 14q32;21q22 translocations in KMM-1. C-myc is not associated with the IgH locus, although the exact cytogenetic locations of the translocated c-myc, and of AML-1 with respect to the breakpoints, are not known.

deletion on der 8 and the reciprocal translocation breakpoints are all located near or in sequences that are important for switching to delta. This suggests that the translocation may have occurred as a result of an error during switching to delta.

Discussion

It is clear from this analysis that conventional cytogenetics underestimates the frequency of 14q32 translocations in MM. We have shown that 16/18 ISRFs represent translocation breakpoints, indicating that they are a good marker of IgH translocations. We identified ISRFs in 8/9 samples lacking a karyotypically detectable 14q32 abnormality, and have so far confirmed a translocation in 7. That 5 of these involve 4p16 indicates that t(4;14) translocations are frequently missed by routine cytogenetics, which may be explained by the telomeric location of the breakpoints. By combining cytogenetics with the results of our Southern blot assay, 20/22 samples have evidence of a 14q32 translocation, most frequently into a switch region. There are two recurrent loci: 11q13, associated with cyclin D1 expression, and 4p16, associated with FGFR3 expression. In addition, there is a promiscuous array of other loci that have been identified once in the cell lines: 1p13, 6, 8q24, 12q24, 16q23, and 21q22. Other loci identified in published karyotypes include: 1q21, 3p11, 6p21, 7q11, 11q23 and 18q21 [5,9]. The translocation to 8q24 that we have cloned is a complex translocation from a region 5' of c-myc into a region 5' of σδ, that appears to be related to switching to delta. Unlike translocations involving the myc locus in other B cell tumors, in this example, c-myc is not associated with the Ig locus, and its location remains undefined.

We speculate that when the legitimate switch recombination occurs on the productive allele, an illegitimate switch recombination occurs on the non-productive allele, resulting in a chromosome translocation. Since monoclonal gammopathy, and the MM that develops from it, share the same legitimate switch on the productive allele, we postulate that they will share the same illegitimate switch on the non-productive allele. If so, a translocation to the IgH locus may be one of the first events in the development of plasma cell neoplasms. The translocations presumably act by dysregulating the expression of a gene critical for the growth, differentiation or survival of the cell. In approximately 25% the gene is cyclin D1, in another 25% it is FGFR3, and in the remaining 50% it appears to be a variety of other genes, occasionally c-myc. We hypothesize that as in the lymphomas, myelomas with the same 14q32 translocations will have similar morphology, histology, clinical course, and response to treatment and will correspond to clinically significant sub-types of the disease.

Acknowledgments

We are particularly grateful to Ian Maclennan for sending us primary tumor corresponding to the cell lines JJN-3 and JIM-3, and to Alan Solomon for sending us primary tumor corresponding to the cell line UTMC-2. In addition, we thank the many investigators who provided us with the cell lines used in this analysis.

References

1. Potter M, Wiener F (1992) Plasmacytomagenesis in mice: model of neoplastic development dependent upon chromosomal translocations. Carcinogenesis 13:1681-97
2. Kuehl WM, Brents LA, Chesi M, Huppi K, Bergsagel PL (1997) Dysregulation of c-myc in multiple myeloma. Curr Top Microbiol Immunol
3. Kuehl WM, Brents LA, Chesi M, Bergsagel PL (1996) Selective expression of one c-myc allele in two human myeloma cell lines. Cancer Res 56:4370-4373
4. Lai JL, Zandecki M, Mary JY, Bernardi F, Izydorczyk V, Flactif M, Morel P, Jouet JP, Bauters F, Facon T (1995) Improved cytogenetics in multiple-myeloma - a study of 151 patients including 117 patients at diagnosis. Blood 85:2490-2497
5. Sawyer JR, Waldron JA, Jagannath S, Barlogie B (1995) Cytogenetic findings in 200 patients with multiple-myeloma. Cancer Gen Cytogen 82:41-49
6. Bergsagel PL, Chesi M, Nardini E, Brents LA, Kirby SL, Kuehl WM (1996) Promiscuous translocations into IgH switch regions in multiple myeloma. Proc Natl Acad Sci USA 93:13931-13936
7. Chesi M, Bergsagel PL, Brents LA, Smith CA, Gerhard DS, Kuehl WM (1996) Dysregulation of cyclin D1 by translocation into an IgH gamma switch region in two multiple myeloma cell lines. Blood 88:674-681
8. Chesi M, Nardini E, Schrock E, Ried T, Brents LA, Kuehl WM, Bergsagel PL (1997) Frequent dysregulation of fibroblast growth factor receptor 3 by t(4;14)(p16.3;q32.3) translocation in multiple myeloma. submitted
9. Taniwaki M, Nishida K, Takashima T, Nakagawa H, Fujii H, Tamaki T, Shimazaki C, Horiike S, Misawa S, Abe T, et a (1994) Nonrandom chromosomal rearrangements of 14q32.3 and 19p13.3 and preferential deletion of 1p in 21 patients with multiple myeloma and plasma cell leukemia. Blood 84:2283-90

Subject Index

Current Topics in Microbiology and Immunology

Volumes published since 1989 (and still available)

Vol. 184: **Dunon, Dominique; Mackay, Charles R.; Imhof, Beat A. (Eds.):** Adhesion in Leukocyte Homing and Differentiation. 1993. 37 figs. IX, 260 pp. ISBN 3-540-56756-9

Vol. 185: **Ramig, Robert F. (Ed.):** Rotaviruses. 1994. 37 figs. X, 380 pp. ISBN 3-540-56761-5

Vol. 186: **zur Hausen, Harald (Ed.):** Human Pathogenic Papillomaviruses. 1994. 37 figs. XIII, 274 pp. ISBN 3-540-57193-0

Vol. 187: **Rupprecht, Charles E.; Dietzschold, Bernhard; Koprowski, Hilary (Eds.):** Lyssaviruses. 1994. 50 figs. IX, 352 pp. ISBN 3-540-57194-9

Vol. 188: **Letvin, Norman L.; Desrosiers, Ronald C. (Eds.):** Simian Immunodeficiency Virus. 1994. 37 figs. X, 240 pp. ISBN 3-540-57274-0

Vol. 189: **Oldstone, Michael B. A. (Ed.):** Cytotoxic T-Lymphocytes in Human Viral and Malaria Infections. 1994. 37 figs. IX, 210 pp. ISBN 3-540-57259-7

Vol. 190: **Koprowski, Hilary; Lipkin, W. Ian (Eds.):** Borna Disease. 1995. 33 figs. IX, 134 pp. ISBN 3-540-57388-7

Vol. 191: **ter Meulen, Volker; Billeter, Martin A. (Eds.):** Measles Virus. 1995. 23 figs. IX, 196 pp. ISBN 3-540-57389-5

Vol. 192: **Dangl, Jeffrey L. (Ed.):** Bacterial Pathogenesis of Plants and Animals. 1994. 41 figs. IX, 343 pp. ISBN 3-540-57391-7

Vol. 193: **Chen, Irvin S. Y.; Koprowski, Hilary; Srinivasan, Alagarsamy; Vogt, Peter K. (Eds.):** Transacting Functions of Human Retroviruses. 1995. 49 figs. IX, 240 pp. ISBN 3-540-57901-X

Vol. 194: **Potter, Michael; Melchers, Fritz (Eds.):** Mechanisms in B-cell Neoplasia. 1995. 152 figs. XXV, 458 pp. ISBN 3-540-58447-1

Vol. 195: **Montecucco, Cesare (Ed.):** Clostridial Neurotoxins. 1995. 28 figs. XI., 278 pp. ISBN 3-540-58452-8

Vol. 196: **Koprowski, Hilary; Maeda, Hiroshi (Eds.):** The Role of Nitric Oxide in Physiology and Pathophysiology. 1995. 21 figs. IX, 90 pp. ISBN 3-540-58214-2

Vol. 197: **Meyer, Peter (Ed.):** Gene Silencing in Higher Plants and Related Phenomena in Other Eukaryotes. 1995. 17 figs. IX, 232 pp. ISBN 3-540-58236-3

Vol. 198: **Griffiths, Gillian M.; Tschopp, Jürg (Eds.):** Pathways for Cytolysis. 1995. 45 figs. IX, 224 pp. ISBN 3-540-58725-X

Vol. 199/I: **Doerfler, Walter; Böhm, Petra (Eds.):** The Molecular Repertoire of Adenoviruses I. 1995. 51 figs. XIII, 280 pp. ISBN 3-540-58828-0

Vol. 199/II: **Doerfler, Walter; Böhm, Petra (Eds.):** The Molecular Repertoire of Adenoviruses II. 1995. 36 figs. XIII, 278 pp. ISBN 3-540-58829-9

Vol. 199/III: **Doerfler, Walter; Böhm, Petra (Eds.):** The Molecular Repertoire of Adenoviruses III. 1995. 51 figs. XIII, 310 pp. ISBN 3-540-58987-2

Vol. 200: **Kroemer, Guido; Martinez-A., Carlos (Eds.):** Apoptosis in Immunology. 1995. 14 figs. XI, 242 pp. ISBN 3-540-58756-X

Vol. 201: **Kosco-Vilbois, Marie H. (Ed.):** An Antigen Depository of the Immune System: Follicular Dendritic Cells. 1995. 39 figs. IX, 209 pp. ISBN 3-540-59013-7

Vol. 202: **Oldstone, Michael B. A.; Vitković, Ljubiša (Eds.):** HIV and Dementia. 1995. 40 figs. XIII, 279 pp. ISBN 3-540-59117-6

Vol. 203: **Sarnow, Peter (Ed.):** Cap-Independent Translation. 1995. 31 figs. XI, 183 pp. ISBN 3-540-59121-4

Vol. 204: **Saedler, Heinz; Gierl, Alfons (Eds.):** Transposable Elements. 1995. 42 figs. IX, 234 pp. ISBN 3-540-59342-X

Vol. 205: **Littman, Dan R. (Ed.):** The CD4 Molecule. 1995. 29 figs. XIII, 182 pp. ISBN 3-540-59344-6

Vol. 206: **Chisari, Francis V.; Oldstone, Michael B. A. (Eds.):** Transgenic Models of Human Viral and Immunological Disease. 1995. 53 figs. XI, 345 pp. ISBN 3-540-59341-1

Vol. 207: **Prusiner, Stanley B. (Ed.):** Prions Prions Prions. 1995. 42 figs. VII, 163 pp. ISBN 3-540-59343-8

Vol. 208: **Farnham, Peggy J. (Ed.):** Transcriptional Control of Cell Growth. 1995. 17 figs. IX, 141 pp. ISBN 3-540-60113-9

Vol. 209: **Miller, Virginia L. (Ed.):** Bacterial Invasiveness. 1996. 16 figs. IX, 115 pp. ISBN 3-540-60065-5

Vol. 210: **Potter, Michael; Rose, Noel R. (Eds.):** Immunology of Silicones. 1996. 136 figs. XX, 430 pp. ISBN 3-540-60272-0

Vol. 211: **Wolff, Linda; Perkins, Archibald S. (Eds.):** Molecular Aspects of Myeloid Stem Cell Development. 1996. 98 figs. XIV, 298 pp. ISBN 3-540-60414-6

Vol. 212: **Vainio, Olli; Imhof, Beat A. (Eds.):** Immunology and Developmental Biology of the Chicken. 1996. 43 figs. IX, 281 pp. ISBN 3-540-60585-1

Vol. 213/I: **Günthert, Ursula; Birchmeier, Walter (Eds.):** Attempts to Understand Metastasis Formation I. 1996. 35 figs. XV, 293 pp. ISBN 3-540-60680-7

Vol. 213/II: **Günthert, Ursula; Birchmeier, Walter (Eds.):** Attempts to Understand Metastasis Formation II. 1996. 33 figs. XV, 288 pp. ISBN 3-540-60681-5

Vol. 213/III: **Günthert, Ursula; Schlag, Peter M.; Birchmeier, Walter (Eds.):** Attempts to Understand Metastasis Formation III. 1996. 14 figs. XV, 262 pp. ISBN 3-540-60682-3

Vol. 214: **Kräusslich, Hans-Georg (Ed.):** Morphogenesis and Maturation of Retroviruses. 1996. 34 figs. XI, 344 pp. ISBN 3-540-60928-8

Vol. 215: **Shinnick, Thomas M. (Ed.):** Tuberculosis. 1996. 46 figs. XI, 307 pp. ISBN 3-540-60985-7

Vol. 216: **Rietschel, Ernst Th.; Wagner, Hermann (Eds.):** Pathology of Septic Shock. 1996. 34 figs. X, 321 pp. ISBN 3-540-61026-X

Vol. 217: **Jessberger, Rolf; Lieber, Michael R. (Eds.):** Molecular Analysis of DNA Rearrangements in the Immune System. 1996. 43 figs. IX, 224 pp. ISBN 3-540-61037-5

Vol. 218: **Berns, Kenneth I.; Giraud, Catherine (Eds.):** Adeno-Associated Virus (AAV) Vectors in Gene Therapy. 1996. 38 figs. IX,173 pp. ISBN 3-540-61076-6

Vol. 219: **Gross, Uwe (Ed.):** Toxoplasma gondii. 1996. 31 figs. XI, 274 pp. ISBN 3-540-61300-5

Vol. 220: **Rauscher, Frank J. III; Vogt, Peter K. (Eds.):** Chromosomal Translocations and Oncogenic Transcription Factors. 1997. 28 figs. XI, 166 pp. ISBN 3-540-61402-8

Vol. 221: **Kastan, Michael B. (Ed.):** Genetic Instability and Tumorigenesis. 1997. 12 figs.VII, 180 pp. ISBN 3-540-61518-0

Vol. 222: **Olding, Lars B. (Ed.):** Reproductive Immunology. 1997. 17 figs. XII, 219 pp. ISBN 3-540-61888-0

Vol. 223: **Tracy, S.; Chapman, N. M.; Mahy, B. W. J. (Eds.):** The Coxsackie B Viruses. 1997. 37 figs. VIII, 336 pp. ISBN 3-540-62390-6

Printing: Saladruck, Berlin
Binding: Buchbinderei Lüderitz & Bauer, Berlin